Disorders of Sleep and Circadian Rhythms in Parkinson's Disease

Aleksandar Videnovic • Birgit Högl

Editors

Disorders of Sleep and Circadian Rhythms in Parkinson's Disease

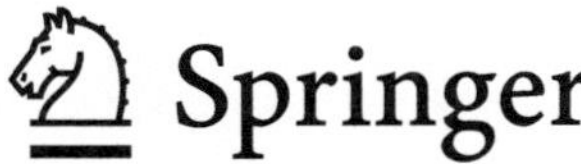 Springer

Editors
Aleksandar Videnovic, MD, MSc
Department of Neurology
Massachusetts General Hospital
Harvard Medical School
Boston, MA
USA

Birgit Högl, MD
Department of Neurology
Medical University of Innsbruck
Innsbruck
Austria

ISBN 978-3-7091-1973-0   ISBN 978-3-7091-1631-9   (eBook)
DOI 10.1007/978-3-7091-1631-9

Springer Wien Heidelberg New York Dordrecht London
© Springer-Verlag Wien 2015
Softcover reprint of the hardcover 1st edition 2015

Printed on acid-free paper

Springer-Verlag GmbH Wien is part of Springer Science+Business Media (www.springer.com)

*We dedicate this book
To our families, for their love and support,
To our patients, for their grace
and inspiration,
To our colleagues and mentors, for their
friendship and vision.*

Birgit and Aleks

Foreword

Parkinson's disease holds a firm and prominent place in the Movement Disorder section of all textbooks of Neurology. These discussions, however, usually focus on the motor components of the disease with incomplete discussions of the plethora of nonmotor disturbances. Nonmotor features of Parkinson's disease, however, have a crucial impact on quality of life, and several of them may antedate the onset of classical motor signs. As such, nonmotor aspects of Parkinson's disease are emerging as the earliest manifestations of the illness and ones that continue to provoke challenges throughout the course of the disease. Disorders of sleep and wakefulness are a prominent example for these nonmotor elements of Parkinson's disease and rank among the most prevalent and most problematic in overall burden across all stages of the disease. Their multifaceted causes include Parkinson's disease itself but also medications and comorbidities such as depression and agitation. Proper management and comprehensive patient care require accurate identification, careful evaluation, and precise treatment of sleep disruption and correction of circadian rhythms. Because of this complexity, understanding, diagnosing, and treating sleep–wake disorders in Parkinson's disease require considerable expertise and attention to detail. To this end, a key unmet need has been a comprehensive volume edited and authored by internationally renowned movement disorder experts and sleep neurologists to provide a thorough and up-to-date focus on sleep disorders and Parkinson's disease.

In *Disorders of Sleep and Circadian Rhythms in Parkinson's Disease*, Aleksandar Videnovic and Birgit Högl have expertly accomplished this goal and have assembled an outstanding group of international leaders to contribute state-of–the-art reviews on the pathophysiology, clinical manifestations, assessment, and treatment of all major types of Parkinson's disease–associated disturbances of sleep–wake regulation. These chapters are preceded by a series of five outstanding reviews covering the neurobiology of sleep and wakefulness and the general approaches to the evaluation of sleep–wake function in Parkinson's disease. The topics covered in this volume span the entire spectrum of sleep problems that clinicians encounter when managing Parkinson's disease subjects, and the respective chapters are carefully referenced and supplemented with informative tables and illustrations.

In filling this gap in the current landscape of available sources on both sleep disorders and nonmotor symptoms of Parkinson's disease, this new volume is a welcome source of reference for the expert clinician and health professional caring for Parkinson's disease patients and for students and residents trying to understand the mysteries of Parkinson's disease. Most importantly, with this text and the lessons learned, we hope that our Parkinson's disease patients will ultimately benefit and be unburdened by the plight so well captured by William Shakespeare:

O sleep! O gentle sleep!

Nature's soft nurse, how have I frighted thee,

That thou no more wilt weigh my eyelids down

And steep my senses in forgetfulness?

Innsbruck, Austria   Werner Poewe
Chicago, IL, USA   Christopher G. Goetz

Contents

Introduction: Sleep, Alertness, and Circadian Rhythms in Parkinson's Disease

Parkinson's disease is the second most common neurodegenerative disorder. Named after James Parkinson, an English surgeon, the disease was initially described in his famous *Essay on the Shaking Palsy*, published in 1817. In this essay, Dr. Parkinson writes about six patients with "paralysis agitans" or shaking palsy. His astute observations provided an excellent description of many aspects of this disease and testify to the power of clinical observation in human medicine. On page 7, Dr. Parkinson wrote "In this stage, the sleep becomes much disturbed. The tremulous motion of the limbs occur during sleep, and augment until they awaken the patient, and frequently with much agitation and alarm". Dr. Parkinson recognized sleep dysfunction in his patients early on, two centuries ago. It is only over the past three decades that disturbances of sleep and wake associated with Parkinson's disease (PD) have attracted the attention of medical and scientific community.

Disorders of sleep and alertness are very common in PD, and likely to affect every patient during the course of their disease. All described categories of sleep disorders have been associated with PD. These disorders encompass insomnia, sleep related breathing disorders, parasomnias, circadian rhythms disorders, and sleep related movement disorders. Each of these disorders has unique characteristics in PD, which likely reflect on interactions between neurodegenerative processes of PD with sleep-wake regulation mechanisms.

Sleep disorders are commonly underreported by patients, and underdiagnosed/ misdiagnosed by health care professionals. Studies have reported that impaired sleep and alertness affect quality of life of PD patients to a similar degree as motor symptoms of the disease. Further, they predispose patient to significant safety challenges. It is therefore important to timely and accurately address sleep dysfunction in PD patients, educate health professionals, and enhance public outreach related to sleep health in PD.

Systematic study of sleep, alertness and circadian function PD is challenged by many confounding factors that influence sleep-wake regulation in this population. Examples include co-existent primary sleep disorders, psychiatric co-morbidities, complex medication regimens, limited physical activity and light exposure. Further, individual variability related to the PD phenotype poses additional challenges to the study of sleep in PD. Specific expertise for the execution and interpretation of sleep studies in PD may be limited, and the wide range of ascertainment methods and associated costs may further limit the extent of sleep investigations in PD.

Specific sleep disorders have emerged as important early manifestations of synuclein related neurodegeneration specific for PD. The most robust support for this hypothesis arises from investigations in patients with idiopathic REM sleep behavior disorder (iRBD), as these patients confer a high risk for developing a synucleinopathy. Therefore, patients with iRBD may be an ideal study population for disease modifying therapies for PD, once these become available.

This book is dedicated to disorders of sleep, alertness, and circadian function in PD. The book is composed of two parts. Part I is focused on the biology of sleep and wake in general and in PD, as well as on the methods for the assessment of sleep-wake cycles in PD. In Part II, specific sleep and circadian disorders associated with PD are presented. Authors hope this book will serve as a valuable resource for neurologists, movement disorders and sleep medicine specialists, trainees and other allied health professionals.

Aleksandar Videnovic
Boston, USA

Birgit Högl
Innsbruck, Austria

Part I

Regulation of Sleep and Wake Homeostasis

Cathy A. Goldstein and Ronald D. Chervin

Contents

Abstract

The interaction of two opposing processes, the circadian rhythm and homeostatic sleep drive, governs sleep and wake. Circadian timing promotes alertness during the environmental day and sleep during the environmental night, while the homeostatic sleep drive grows with cumulative wakefulness independent of time. Homeostatic sleep drive is measured by its electroencephalogram correlate, slow-wave activity. Slow-wave activity increases not only in response to prolonged wakefulness, but also demonstrates spatial organization and increases in a local, use-dependent pattern based on previous physical and mental activity. These findings support the important hypothesis that sleep mediates homeostasis

C.A. Goldstein (✉) • R.D. Chervin
University of Michigan Health System Sleep Disorders Center, 1500 East Medical Center Drive, Med Inn C728, Ann Arbor, MI 48109-5845, USA
e-mail: cathygo@med.umich.edu; chervin@med.umich.edu

© Springer-Verlag Wien 2015

A. Videnovic, B. Högl (eds.), *Disorders of Sleep and Circadian Rhythms in Parkinson's Disease*, DOI 10.1007/978-3-7091-1631-9_1

of neuronal synapses. Therefore, the homeostatic control of sleep and wake has implications that extend beyond alertness.

1.1 Introduction

Sleep is orchestrated by a two-process model comprised of the homeostatic sleep drive (process S) and the circadian rhythm (process C) [1, 2]. Process S increases with wakefulness and dissipates with sleep. Process C times human sleep such that the highest propensity for sleep occurs during the environmental night, while an increased alerting signal promotes wake during the environmental day [3]. These processes interact as follows. During daytime wakefulness, process S increases sleep pressure. To counteract this, the circadian alerting signal increases to a peak in the evening [4]. The net influence of these opposing forces allows maintenance of wakefulness through bedtime [5]. At bedtime, the combination of a sharp drop in the circadian alerting signal (coinciding with the onset of melatonin secretion) with the elevated homeostatic sleep drive facilitates sleep onset [6]. Despite dissipation of process S-mediated sleep pressure after sleep onset, sleep continues due to a persistently low circadian alerting signal [7]. Together, these processes typically allow for approximately 16 h of consolidated wakefulness and 8 h of continuous sleep (see Fig. 1.1). The circadian rhythm will be discussed further in Chap. 9.

1.2 History of Sleep Recording

Homeostasis, as described by Cannon in 1932, is the need for organisms to achieve a steady state [8]. In 1980, Borbély introduced the term *sleep homeostasis*, which can be understood by its electrophysiological correlate, slow-wave activity [9]. Descriptions of brain wave activity during sleep began in the late 1930s after the advent of the electroencephalogram (EEG) in 1928 [10]. Recordings demonstrated the following EEG progression after sleep onset: drop out of alpha activity, appearance of low-voltage activity, emergence of high-voltage, low-frequency (delta) waves, followed by an increase in delta waves and the appearance of spindle activity. Thus, delta waves were thought to represent "real sleep" [11, 12]. In addition, delta activity was associated with an increased arousal threshold to auditory stimuli and, therefore, was thought to parallel the depth of sleep [11, 13, 14]. The EEG pattern described above was distinct from the activity recorded in rapid eye movement (REM) sleep described initially by Aserinsky and Kleitman in 1953 [15]. In 1957, Dement and Kleitman introduced a staging schema for EEG activity recorded during sleep. They separated nonrapid eye movement (NREM) from rapid eye movement (REM) sleep, and classified NREM sleep into stages 1, 2, 3, and 4 [16]. Stage 1 sleep was described as low-voltage EEG activity that lacked spindle activity [16]. As sleep continued, the EEG evolved with the development of slower activity, sleep spindles, and K complexes that mark stage 2 sleep [16]. Stage 3 sleep was defined by epochs containing at least two waves greater than 100 uV in amplitude with frequency less

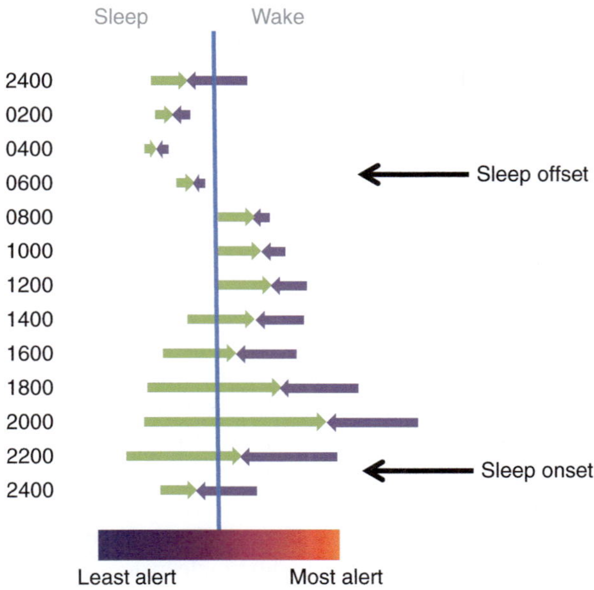

Fig. 1.1 The two-process model of sleep. *Green arrows* denote the circadian alerting signal; the longer the *arrow*, the greater the alerting signal. *Purple arrows* denote the homeostatic sleep drive. The longer the arrow, the greater the homeostatic sleep drive. The blue vertical line divides wake from sleep. The level of alertness is represented by the point at which the *arrows* meet, determined by the net effect of circadian and homeostatic forces. Propensity for sleep is high when either the magnitude of homeostatic sleep drive overcomes the circadian alerting signal, or the circadian alerting signal is sufficiently low (e.g., at 04:00–06:00). After sleep offset, homeostatic sleep drive accumulates with wakefulness. However, the circadian alerting signal increases in an opposing fashion. However, in the late afternoon the circadian alerting signal is not large enough to completely offset the effect of growing sleep pressure on alertness. Therefore, sleepiness is high at this time, referred to as the *afternoon circadian dip*. The circadian alerting signal is so high in the evening it overcomes the homeostatic sleep drive. Alertness is high at this time, which is referred to as the *forbidden zone for sleep*. The circadian alerting signal decreases about 2 h before habitual sleep onset and promotes sleep due to the already elevated homeostatic sleep drive. The initial period of the sleep bout is associated with dissipation of the homeostatic sleep need; however, sleep is maintained due to a persistently low circadian alerting signal, which reaches a nadir around 04:00. Therefore, even when the homeostatic sleep drive is less than the circadian alerting signal, if the circadian alerting signal is low, sleep will continue (as seen during the early morning hours). The above model does not take into account other factors outside of process C and process S mediating alertness

than 2 Hz [16]. During stage 4 sleep, the delta waves described above made up more than 50 % of an epoch [16]. Current sleep scoring criteria consolidates stage 3 and 4 sleep into NREM 3 (N3) sleep [17]. In addition to measuring slow-wave sleep as classically defined, the development of EEG spectral analysis allowed for the measurement of slow-wave activity [18]. Slow-wave activity is defined as the EEG power density in the 0.5–4.5 Hz range [18]. Although slow-wave sleep stages and slow-wave activity show considerable overlap, they are distinct constructs and each can generate different insight and opportunity in research and understanding of sleep homeostasis.

1.3   NREM Sleep Anatomy and Physiology

Hyperpolarization of thalamic neurons and synchronization of cortical excitatory and inhibitory postsynaptic potentials are responsible for the high-voltage, low-frequency activity seen on EEG during NREM slow-wave sleep [19, 20]. The sleep-active neurons reside in the ventrolateral preoptic nucleus (VLPO) and median preoptic nucleus (MnPN) of the preoptic area (POA) in the hypothalamus [21, 22]. When active, the VLPO and MnPN inhibit wake-promoting centers via GABAergic and galanergic projections [23–27]. As the wake-promoting centers inhibit the VLPO and MnPN, suppression of their activity releases inhibition of the VLPO and MnPN. Neurons in the VLPO and MnPN demonstrate activity that is most pronounced during NREM and REM sleep, and almost nonexistent during wake [28, 29]. Rates of neuronal discharge from the VLPO parallel the depth of NREM sleep as measured by EEG slow-wave activity [28]. Therefore, this group of neurons may play a significant role in the generation of slow-wave sleep. The inability for both the arousal and sleep-promoting centers to be activated simultaneously underlies the "sleep-switch" hypothesis [30]. This theory helps explain the stability of sleep and wake states such that under normal conditions sleep does not intrude into wakefulness and vice versa [30]. The VLPO and MnPN are regulated by direct and indirect connections from the master clock housed in the suprachiasmatic nucleus (SCN), which facilitates the circadian control of sleep (discussed further in Chap. 9). Figure 1.2 depicts the nuclei responsible for NREM sleep.

As above, the SCN is responsible for timing activity of sleep-generating neurons in the POA such that sleep demonstrates a circadian pattern. However, mechanisms that mediate the homeostatic control of sleep are less clear, but likely involve sleep-promoting neurochemicals (or *somnogens*) that act directly on the POA [31]. Prostaglandin D2 (PGD2) is a sleep-promoting hormone produced by the leptomeninges and choroid plexus [31]. PGD2 increases during sleep deprivation and acts directly on receptors near the VLPO as well as indirectly by way of other somnogens to induce sleep [31, 32]. Cytokines are also known to elicit sleep and may be most important in increasing NREM sleep during infection [31]. Growth-hormone releasing hormone promotes sleep by its direct action on the POA, and increased secretion of this hormone is seen in association with slow-wave sleep during the initial portion of the sleep period [31]. However, adenosine may be the somnogen most likely to mediate sleep homeostasis as it reflects brain energy levels. Adenosine is produced when adenosine triphosphate (ATP) is broken down in metabolically active tissues [31]. In addition, when cells are fatigued, phosphorylation of adenosine to ATP is reduced [33]; therefore, the greater the neuronal activity, the greater is the rise in adenosine. Animal experiments have demonstrated this with an increase in basal forebrain adenosine levels during wakefulness and a decrease during sleep [34]. Additionally, adenosine increases slow waves on EEG [35]. Adenosine's effects on sleep are mediated by inhibition of wake-active neurons, disinhibition of sleep-active neurons, and stimulation of sleep-active neurons primarily by action on A1 but also A2a receptors [31]. The alerting effect of caffeine occurs through adenosine receptor antagonism [36].

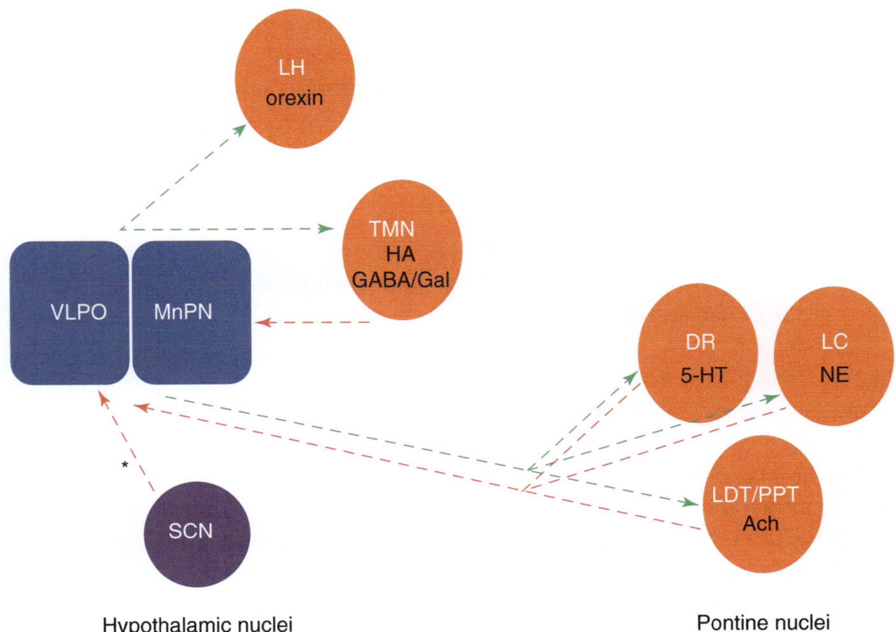

Fig. 1.2 Nuclei responsible for the generation of NREM sleep. The *orange ovals* denote nuclei that are wake promoting when active. *Blue rectangles* represent nuclei that promote sleep when active. The *purple circle* is the suprachiasmatic nucleus (SCN) of the hypothalamus, which times sleep and wake. *Projections from the SCN to the VLPO and LH are relayed via the SPZ and DMH (not shown). *Green dashed lines* illustrate the GABAergic and galanergic pathways from the VLPO/MnPN that inhibit the wake-promoting centers, allowing for sleep. The *red dashed lines* represent inhibitory efferents to the VLPO/MnPN. With inhibition of the GABA-producing neurons in the VLPO/MnPN by ACh, 5-HT, NE, Gal, and GABA (from the SPZ and DMH), wake-promoting nuclei are disinhibited, which results in alertness. The TMN inhibits the VLPO/MnPN through GABA and Gal opposed to HA, the wake-promoting transmitter of the TMN. *VLPO* ventrolateral preoptic nucleus, *MnPN* median preoptic nucleus, *LH* lateral hypothalamus, *TMN* tuberomamillary nucleus, *DR* dorsal raphe, *LC* locus coeruleus, *LDT/PPT* lateral dorsal tegmentum/pedunculopontine nucleus, *SPZ* subparaventricular zone, *DMH* dorsomedial hypothalamic nucleus, *Ach* acetylcholine, *5-HT* serotonin, *NE* norepinephrine, *Gal* galanin, *GABA* gamma-amino butyric acid [21–29]

1.4 Slow-Wave Sleep, Slow-Wave Activity, and Their Dispersion over the Course of a Normal Nocturnal Sleep Period

The early work of Dement and Kleitman demonstrated a cyclical variation of the sleep stages that occurred every 90–100 min [16]. Notably, nearly all high-voltage delta frequency activity took place during the first 3 h of sleep. After the second sleep cycle, stages 3 and 4 sleep were not seen [16]. NREM slow-wave sleep is now well known to decline over the course of subsequent sleep cycles through the night [37]. Apart from slow-wave sleep, slow-wave activity, the density of EEG activity in the 0.5–4.5 Hz range as measured by spectral analysis, demonstrates a similar pattern. Slow-wave activity displays a gradual buildup during the first NREM-REM cycle and an exponential decline from cycle 1 to cycle 3 [18]. Notably, the pattern of slow-wave sleep and slow-wave activity decay described above persists in the nonentrained state, suggesting autonomy from circadian contributions [38, 39].

1.5 Slow-Wave Sleep and Slow-Wave Activity as a Function of Prior Wakefulness

During experiments that evaluated sleep stages during naps taken in the morning, afternoon, and evening, a progressive increase was seen in the amount of slow-wave sleep recorded over the course of the day [40, 41]. This finding does not eliminate the possibility of a circadian effect. However, when healthy volunteers slept during nap opportunities at 10:00, 12:00, 14:00, 16:00, 18:00, 20:00, and 04:00, EEG power density in the delta and theta range increased in proportion to the duration of prior wakefulness [42]. Conversely, latency to sleep onset was shortest at the 16:00 and 04:00 naps, consistent with the known bimodal distribution of sleep propensity [5, 42]. In addition, when nocturnal sleep was recorded after napping, there was a significant reduction of slow-wave sleep and slow-wave activity compared to baseline nocturnal sleep that did not follow a nap [43–45].

Studies that used total sleep deprivation protocols of 40–64 h or sleep restriction to 3 h per night showed a significant increase in the amount of slow-wave sleep recorded during the recovery sleep period. In addition, shorter latency to slow-wave sleep was seen during recovery sleep [14, 19, 37, 46]. EEG spectral analysis demonstrated similar findings for slow-wave activity, with increases in delta and theta EEG power during recovery sleep [19, 39, 47–49]. The increase in lower frequency EEG activity was not confined to stages 3 and 4 sleep but also seen during stage 2 and REM sleep. The enhancement of the delta and theta band activity was maximal during the first NREM-REM cycle and the rate of build-up of slow-wave activity in this cycle was increased [19]. These findings were attenuated during subsequent cycles and on recovery day two [19]. Slow-wave activity during recovery sleep was independent of circadian timing [47]. However, slow-wave sleep did not demonstrate the same autonomy, with a reduction in the expected amounted of slow-wave sleep when the recovery period was placed at 07:00 [47]. The authors postulated that this finding was due to the higher circadian propensity for stage REM sleep at that time, such that REM sleep occurred at the expense of NREM sleep. Therefore, visually scored epochs of slow-wave sleep were not increased as expected, as opposed to slow-wave activity which was elevated in proportion to the degree of sleep deprivation [47]. As prior wakefulness does, selective deprivation of slow-wave sleep without decreasing total sleep time also increases slow-wave sleep and slow-wave activity in later portions of the sleep period and during subsequent recovery sleep periods [42, 50, 51].

In summary, slow-wave activity declines over the course of the sleep period, is dependent on prior wakefulness, rebounds when selectively suppressed, and is independent from the circadian control of alertness. Taken together, these findings strongly suggest that slow-wave activity is a useful EEG marker that reflects sleep homeostasis.

1.6   Topographic Organization of Slow-Wave Activity and Local, Use-Dependent Changes

Slow-wave activity has a topographical organization in the cerebral cortex, with an anterior-posterior gradient such that slow-wave activity is more prominent in frontal than occipital areas [52, 53]. This frontal predilection is most pronounced during the initial NREM sleep period and then declines over subsequent cycles [52, 53]. The anterior-posterior gradient is enhanced during recovery sleep following total sleep and selective slow-wave sleep deprivation [51, 53, 54]. These findings suggest a specific role for frontal brain regions in sleep homeostasis.

In addition to amount of prior wakefulness, the magnitude of activity during wake may affect the homeostatic process occurring during sleep. Physical exercise, novel mental activity, and structured social interactions all increase slow-wave sleep [55–57]. Furthermore, activation during wakefulness of specific brain regions has consequences during sleep. For example, a study by Kattler demonstrated that vibratory stimulation of the right hand during wakefulness increased delta power in the left somatosensory cortex during the first hour of sleep that followed [58]. As sensory stimulation is known to increase cerebral metabolism and blood flow in the corresponding cortical area, this finding suggests that the homeostatic process during sleep may be use dependent [58]. In contrast, among subjects subjected to arm immobilization, slow-wave activity in the contralateral sensorimotor cortex decreased during subsequent sleep [59]. The region-specific decrease in slow-wave activity was proportional to next-day deterioration of motor performance in the same limb [59]. In addition to sensorimotor manipulations, an experiment that used a cognitive task that involved specific cortical areas also resulted in locally enhanced slow-wave activity during the sleep that followed [60]. This local, use-dependent increase in slow-wave activity decayed over the course of the night. When subjects were retested, performance of the task was superior among those whose learning occurred prior to sleep; furthermore, performance correlated with the increase in slow-wave activity in the corresponding brain region [60].

Demonstration of local, use-dependent EEG changes, particularly in the setting of learning, has contributed to a synaptic homeostasis hypothesis, to explain a fundamental purpose of sleep, as advanced by Tononi and Cirelli [61, 62]. This hypothesis is based on the following premises. During wakefulness, neuronal plasticity allows the brain to strengthen and increase synapses as the individual navigates new experiences. However, synaptic potentiation comes at a high cost due to the large amount of physiological resources it requires, and therefore is not sustainable. *Synaptic pruning,* the selection of which synapses should remain, must occur to conserve energy and allow for future learning. The synaptic homeostasis hypothesis proposes that the purpose of sleep is to mediate this process, and that the footprint of this function within sleep is slow-wave activity [61, 62].

1.7 Sleep Homeostasis Across the Life Span

The homeostatic regulation of sleep may differ with age. Slow-wave sleep and slow-wave activity decline steeply during adolescence, particularly during sleep in the first NREM sleep cycle [63–70]. This pattern indicates that children, in comparison to adolescents, have a more rapid buildup of sleep pressure and need a greater amount of recovery to restore homeostasis [70]. These findings may reflect increased synaptic density in children, and provide further support for the synaptic homeostasis theory [61, 62, 70].

The changes continue throughout the life span, with decreased slow-wave sleep and slow-wave activity in older persons [71]. However, as reviewed comprehensively by Bliwise in 1993, studies that have used sleep deprivation protocols have demonstrated similar recovery sleep in elderly and younger subjects. Interestingly, changes in sleep stages after sleep deprivation are seen only in the first recovery night of older subjects, as opposed to the first and second nights in younger individuals. This suggests that aging does not necessarily impair the homeostatic process regulating sleep loss [71]. In fact, older adults in comparison to younger persons may be less affected by sleep loss, with the caveat that differences in baseline sleep among young and old subjects could in part generate these impressions [72–75]. A recent investigation demonstrated that slow-wave activity not only declines in the elderly, but that this decrement is associated with prefrontal gray matter loss and deterioration in memory consolidation [76]. These findings further support the role of slow-wave sleep and slow-wave activity in cognition.

1.8 Genetic Contributions to Sleep Homeostasis

In addition to age, genetics may affect the homeostatic regulation of sleep and wake. A polymorphism in the adenosine deaminase (ADA) gene (G>A transition at position 22 of the gene's coding region) is associated with increased amounts of slow-wave sleep and greater slow-wave activity [77–79]. The same polymorphism is associated with increased sleepiness and reduced vigilance in the setting of sleep deprivation [78]. A functional polymorphism in the brain-derived neurotrophic factor (BDNF) gene also affects slow-wave sleep and slow-wave activity in both the baseline and sleep-deprived states [80].

In addition, genes traditionally thought to modify circadian aspects of sleep are now known to participate in homeostatic mechanisms. Animal models with deletions or mutations of the circadian genes Bmal1, *Cyc*, *Clock*, *Npas2*, and *Cry* show impaired sleep homeostasis [81–85]. Additionally, the clock genes *Per1* and *Per2* have increased expression in animals undergoing sleep loss [83, 86]. In humans,

Per3 polymorphisms are involved in sleep homeostasis [87]. Subjects who are homozygous for the five repeat variable number tandem repeat (VNTR) polymorphism (*Per3 5/5*), in comparison to subjects with the four repeat VNTR polymorphism (*Per3 4/4*), show shorter sleep latencies, higher initial amounts of slow-wave activity, and more rapid slow-wave decline over the course of the night [87]. Additionally, when sleep deprived for 40 h, *Per3 5/5* subjects have increased slow rolling eye movements and greater deterioration in performance measures [87]. Interestingly, a previous study had demonstrated that the longer repeat polymorphism was associated with a morning circadian phenotype, while the shorter repeat polymorphism was more frequent in evening types and those with delayed sleep phase disorder [88].

Another gene that modifies circadian rhythms, hDEC2, has gained considerable attention [89]. A point mutation in this gene was found in a mother and daughter who both display short sleeper syndrome [89]. Individuals with this condition require shorter sleep durations, have faster buildup of slow-wave activity, and thus may function under a higher NREM sleep pressure [49]. Mice genetically modified to contain the same proline to arginine substitution found in this family also demonstrate longer active periods than mice without the mutation [89]. Therefore, hDEC2 is not only implicated in sleep timing but also modifies sleep duration requirements [89]. These findings suggest that the same molecular machinery influences both process C and process S, functions traditionally thought to oscillate autonomously.

1.9 Clinical Manifestations of Sleep Homeostasis

The homeostatic regulation of sleep has important implications in many different clinical settings. Chronic partial sleep loss is ubiquitous, as almost 40 % of American adults report sleep durations of less than 7 h on workday nights [90]. Sleep pressure builds when sleep is chronically restricted and results in reduced daytime alertness and impaired performance [91]. Shift work, as experienced by about 10 % of the US workforce, can exacerbate sleep deprivation. For example, nightshift workers average 6.1 h of sleep per 24-h period [92]. Increased homeostatic sleep pressure amplifies circadian fluctuations in performance [93, 94]. The greatest functional impairment is seen during the circadian night and is more pronounced during chronic partial sleep loss than during acute sleep deprivation [93, 94]. Repercussions can be grave among nightshift workers who undergo recurrent sleep restriction and attempt wakefulness at the circadian nadir of alertness. Naps may provide an important opportunity to mitigate the effects of increased sleep pressure on alertness and performance [95–99].

Impairment of the sleep homeostatic process may play an important role in certain sleep disorders. In idiopathic hypersomnia, excessive daytime sleepiness occurs despite adequate sleep duration and the absence of observable underlying sleep disruption. This disorder lacks the REM intrusion phenomena seen in narcolepsy. In a study that monitored 24-h EEG in 75 patients with idiopathic hypersomnia, slow-wave sleep persisted later in the night than in normal controls [100]. This observation was more prominent among patients who had idiopathic hypersomnia with long sleep time than it was among patients who had idiopathic hypersomnia without long sleep time [100]. In addition, daytime sleep episodes contained percentages of slow-wave sleep that exceed those recorded from controls [100]. Although the pathophysiology of idiopathic hypersomnia remains unknown, differences in slow-wave sleep between these patients and controls suggest involvement of the homeostatic regulation of sleep.

In patients with delayed sleep phase disorder, sleep onset and offset occurs later than desired [101]. Typical sleep onset is 2:00 AM to 6:00 AM and sleep offset is 10:00 AM to 2:00 PM [102]. The condition usually has been attributed to an abnormality in circadian timing, but a contribution from homeostatic factors also may be present. In comparison to controls, patients with delayed sleep phase disorder can demonstrate a prolonged time interval between the time of highest circadian propensity for sleep and sleep offset (abnormal *phase angle*) [103–105]. Additionally, these patients have increased amounts of slow-wave sleep in the latter portion of the sleep period, longer sleep durations, and impaired ability to recover during sleep deprivation [104, 106, 107]. Similar observations also have been made among sighted individuals with free-running circadian rhythm sleep disorder [108, 109]. Investigators hypothesize that difficulty accruing and dissipating homeostatic sleep pressure may be involved in the pathogenesis of delayed sleep phase disorder and free-running disorder in sighted individuals [106, 110]. The differences in homeostatic sleep regulation between morning and evening circadian phenotypes and the *Per3* polymorphism discussed previously may further support this hypothesis. Furthermore, morning types (individuals who prefer earlier sleep wake times) demonstrate a larger buildup of slow-wave activity in response to increased sleep pressure and show a faster decline over the course of the night compared to evening types (individuals who prefer later sleep wake times) [111–115]. However, some studies of phase angle and sleep duration have not found differences between patients with delayed sleep phase disorder and normal controls [116]. Therefore, further research is needed to delineate the role of sleep homeostasis in circadian rhythm sleep disorders.

Conclusion

In summary, sleep is regulated by a dual process model. Process S, the homeostatic sleep drive, increases with prior wakefulness and dissipates with sleep. The circadian rhythm, or process C, gates sleep pressure so that wakefulness is sustained throughout the environmental day and sleep occurs at night. The electrophysiological correlate of sleep homeostasis, slow-wave activity, is a marker of sleep need that also demonstrates local, use-dependent changes. This finding may have significant implications for the role of sleep in memory and cognition. In addition, clock genes originally found to modify circadian phase have now shown involvement in sleep and wake homeostasis. This realization, combined with data that suggest altered sleep homeostasis in different circadian phenotypes, underlines the complexity of interactions between homeostatic and circadian control of sleep and wakefulness. A better understanding of these processes and their interactions could eventually have fundamental impact on clinical care and public health.

References

1. Borbely AA. A two process model of sleep regulation. Hum Neurobiol. 1982;1(3):195–204.
2. Daan S, Beersma DG, Borbély AA. Timing of human sleep: recovery process gated by a circadian pacemaker. Am J Physiol. 1984;246(2):R161–83.
3. Wyatt JK, Ritz-De Cecco A, Czeisler CA, Dijk DJ. Circadian temperature and melatonin rhythms, sleep, and neurobehavioral function in humans living on a 20-h day. Am J Physiol. 1999;277:R1152–63.
4. Edgar DM, Dement WC, Fuller CA. Effect of SCN lesions on sleep in squirrel monkeys: evidence for opponent processes in sleep-wake regulation. J Neurosci. 1993;13(3): 1065–79.
5. Lavie P. Ultrashort sleep-waking schedule. III. 'Gates' and 'forbidden zones' for sleep. Electroencephalogr Clin Neurophysiol. 1986;63(5):414–25.
6. Lavie P. Melatonin: role in gating nocturnal rise in sleep propensity. J Biol Rhythms. 1997;12(6):657–65.
7. Dijk DJ, Czeisler CA. Paradoxical timing of the circadian rhythm of sleep propensity serves to consolidate sleep and wakefulness in humans. Neurosci Lett. 1994;166(1):63–8.
8. Cannon WB. The wisdom of the body. New York: Norton & Co., Inc.; 1932. Print.
9. Borberly AA. Sleep: circadian rhythm versus recovery process. In: Koukkou M, Lehmann D, Angst J, editors. Functional states of the brain. Their determinants. Amsterdam: Elsevier; 1980. p. 151–61.
10. Berger H. Ueber das Elektroenkephalogramm des Menschen. J Psychol Neurol. 1930;40:160–79.
11. Loomis AL, Harvey EN, Hobart G. Cerebral states during sleep, as studied by human brain potentials. J Exp Psychol. 1937;21:127–44.
12. Davis H, Davis P, Loomis A, Harvey E, Hobart G. Changes in human brain potentials during the onset of sleep. Science. 1937;86(2237):448–50.
13. Blake H, Gerard RW. Brain potentials during sleep. Am J Physiol. 1937;119:692–703.
14. Williams HL, Hammack JT, Day RL, Dement WC, Lubin A. Responses to auditory stimulation, sleep loss, and the EEG stages of sleep. Electroencephalogr Clin Neurophysiol. 1964;16:269–79.
15. Aserinsky E, Klietman N. Regularly occurring periods of eye motility, and concomitant phenomena, during sleep. Science. 1953;118(3062):273–4.
16. Dement W, Kleitman N. Cyclic variations in EEG during sleep and their relation to eye movements, body motility, and dreaming. Electroencephalogr Clin Neurophysiol. 1957;9(4):673–90.
17. Berry RB, Brooks R, Gamaldo CE, Harding SM, Marcus CL, Vaughn BV, American Academy of Sleep Medicine. The AASM manual for the scoring of sleep and associated events: rules, terminology and technical specifications, version 2.0.1. www.aasmnet.org. Darien: American Academy of Sleep Medicine; 2013.
18. Borberly AA, Baumann F, Brandeis D, et al. Sleep deprivation: effect on sleep stages and EEG power density in man. Electroencephalogr Clin Neurophysiol. 1981;51:483–93.
19. McCormick DA, Bal T. Sleep and arousal: thalamocortical mechanisms. Annu Rev Neurosci. 1997;20:185–215.
20. McCormick DA. Cortical and subcortical generators of normal and abnormal rhythmicity. Int Rev Neurobiol. 2002;49:99–114.
21. McGinty D, Szymusiak R. Brain structures and mechanisms involved in the generation of NREM sleep: focus on the preoptic hypothalamus. Sleep Med Rev. 2001;5(4):323–42.
22. Gaus SE, Strecker RE, Tate BA, Parker RA, Saper CB. Ventrolateral preoptic nucleus contains sleep-active, galaninergic neurons in multiple mammalian species. Neuroscience. 2002;115(1):285–94.
23. Sherin JE, Shiromani PJ, McCarley RW, Saper CB. Activation of ventrolateral preoptic neurons during sleep. Science. 1996;271(5246):216–9.

24. Sherin JE, Elmquist JK, Torrealba F, Saper CB. Innervation of histaminergic tuberomammillary neurons by GABAergic and galaninergic neurons in the ventrolateral preoptic nucleus of the rat. J Neurosci. 1998;18(12):4705–21.

25. Steininger TL, Gong H, McGinty D, Szymusiak R. Subregional organization of preoptic area/anterior hypothalamic projections to arousal-related monoaminergic cell groups. J Comp Neurol. 2001;429(4):638–53.

26. Gong H, McGinty D, Guzman-Marin R, Chew KT, Stewart D, Szymusiak R. Activation of c-fos in GABAergic neurones in the preoptic area during sleep and in response to sleep deprivation. J Physiol. 2004;556:935–46.

27. Uschakov A, Gong H, McGinty D, Szymusiak R. Efferent projections from the median preoptic nucleus to sleep- and arousal-regulatory nuclei in the rat brain. Neuroscience. 2007;150(1):104–20.

28. Szymusiak R, Alam N, Steininger TL, McGinty D. Sleep-waking discharge patterns of ventrolateral preoptic/anterior hypothalamic neurons in rats. Brain Res. 1998;803(1–2):178–88.

29. Takahashi K, Lin JS, Sakai K. Characterization and mapping of sleep-waking specific neurons in the basal forebrain and preoptic hypothalamus in mice. Neuroscience. 2009;161(1):269–92.

30. Saper CB, Chou TC, Scammel TE. The sleep switch: hypothalamic control of sleep and wakefulness. Trends Neurosci. 2001;12:726–31.

31. Obal Jr F, Krueger JM. Biochemical regulation of non-rapid-eye-movement sleep. Front Biosci. 2003;8:d520–50.

32. Ram A, Pandey HP, Matsumura HP, et al. CSF levels of prostaglandins, especially the level of prostaglandin D2, are correlated with increasing propensity towards sleep in rats. Brain Res. 1997;751:81–9.

33. Benington JH, Heller HC. Restoration of brain energy metabolism as a function of sleep. Prog Neurobiol. 1995;45(4):347–60.

34. Porkka-Heiskanen T, Strecker RE, Thakkar M, et al. Adenosine: a mediator of the sleep inducing effects of prior wakefulness. Science. 1997;276:1265–8.

35. Benington JH, Kodali SK, Heller HC. Stimulation of A1 adenosine receptors mimics the electroencephalographic effects of sleep deprivation. Brain Res. 1995;692:79–85.

36. Fredholm B, Battig K, Holmen J, Nehlig A, Zvartau E. Actions of caffeine in the brain with special reference to factors that contribute to its widespread use. Pharmacol Rev. 1999;51(1):83–133.

37. Webb WB, Agnew Jr HW. Stage 4 sleep: influence of time course variables. Science. 1971;174(4016):1354–6.

38. Weitzman ED, Czeisler CA, Zimmerman JC, Ronda JM. Timing of REM and stages 3+4 sleep during temporal isolation in man. Sleep. 1980;2(4):391–407.

39. Dijk DJ, Czeisler CA. Contribution of the circadian pacemaker and the sleep homeostat to sleep propensity, sleep structure, electroencephalographic slow waves, and sleep spindle activity in humans. J Neurosci. 1995;15(5 Pt 1):3526–38.

40. Karacan I, Finley W, Williams R, Hursch C. Changes in stage 1-REM and stage 4 sleep during naps. Biol Psychiatry. 1970;2:261–5.

41. Maron L, Rechtschaffen A, Wolpert E. Sleep cycle during napping. Arch Gen Psychiatry. 1964;11:503–7.

42. Dijk DJ, Beersma DG, Daan S, Bloem GM, Van den Hoofdakker RH. Quantitative analysis of the effects of slow wave sleep deprivation during the first 3 h of sleep on subsequent EEG power density. Eur Arch Psychiatry Neurol Sci. 1987;236(6):323–8.

43. Karacan I, Williams R, Finley W, Hursch C. The effects of naps on nocturnal sleep: influence on the need for stage 1-REM and stage 4 sleep. Biol Psychiatry. 1970;2:397–9.

44. Feinberg I, March J, Floyd T, et al. Homeostatic changes during post-nap sleep maintain baseline levels of delta EEG. Electroencephalogr Clin Neurophysiol. 1985;61:134–7.

45. Werth E, Dijk DJ, Achermann P, Borbély AA. Dynamics of the sleep EEG after an early evening nap: experimental data and simulations. Am J Physiol. 1996;271:501–10.

46. Webb WB, Agnew Jr HW. Sleep: effects of a restricted regime. Science. 1965;150(3704): 1745–7.
47. Dijk DJ, Brunner DP, Beersma DG, Borbély AA. Electroencephalogram power density and slow wave sleep as a function of prior waking and circadian phase. Sleep. 1990;13(5): 430–40.
48. Dijk DJ, Hayes B, Czeisler CA. Dynamics of electroencephalographic sleep spindles and slow wave activity in men: effect of sleep deprivation. Brain Res. 1993;626(1–2):190–9.
49. Aeschbach D, Cajochen C, Landolt H, Borbély AA. Homeostatic sleep regulation in habitual short sleepers and long sleepers. Am J Physiol. 1996;270(1 Pt 2):R41–53.
50. Agnew HW, Webb WB. The displacement of stages 4 and REM sleep within a full night of sleep. Psychophysiology. 1968;5:142–8.
51. Ferrara M, De Gennaro L, Curcio G, Cristiani R, Corvasce C, Bertini M. Regional differences of the human sleep electroencephalogram in response to selective slow-wave sleep deprivation. Cereb Cortex. 2002;12(7):737–48.
52. Werth E, Achermann P, Borbély AA. Fronto-occipital EEG power gradients in human sleep. J Sleep Res. 1997;6(2):102–12.
53. Finelli LA, Borbély AA, Achermann P. Functional topography of the human nonREM sleep electroencephalogram. Eur J Neurosci. 2001;13(12):2282–90.
54. Cajochen C, Foy R, Dijk DJ. Frontal predominance of a relative increase in sleep delta and theta EEG activity after sleep loss in humans. Sleep Res Online. 1999;2(3):65–9.
55. Horne JA, Moore VJ. Sleep EEG effects of exercise with and without additional body cooling. Electroencephalogr Clin Neurophysiol. 1985;60(1):33–8.
56. Horne JA, Minard A. Sleep and sleepiness following a behaviourally 'active' day. Ergonomics. 1985;28(3):567–75.
57. Naylor E, Penev PD, Orbeta L, Janssen I, Ortiz R, Colecchia EF, Keng M, Finkel S, Zee PC. Daily social and physical activity increases slow-wave sleep and daytime neuropsychological performance in the elderly. Sleep. 2000;23(1):87–95.
58. Kattler H, Dijk D, Borbely A. Effect of unilateral somatosensory stimulation prior to sleep on the sleep EEG in humans. J Sleep Res. 1994;3:159–64.
59. Huber R, Ghilardi MF, Massimini M, Ferrarelli F, Riedner BA, Peterson MJ, Tononi G. Arm immobilization causes cortical plastic changes and locally decreases sleep slow wave activity. Nat Neurosci. 2006;9(9):1169–76.
60. Huber R, Ghilardi MF, Massimini M, Tononi G. Local sleep and learning. Nature. 2004;430(6995):78–81.
61. Tononi G, Cirelli C. Sleep function and synaptic homeostasis. Sleep Med Rev. 2006;10(1): 49–62.
62. Tononi G, Cirelli C. Time to be SHY/Some comments on sleep and synaptic homeostasis. Neural Plast. 2012. Volume 2012, Article ID 415250, 12 pages.
63. Coble PA, Reynolds III CF, Kupfer DJ, Houck P. Electroencephalographic sleep of healthy children. Part II: findings using automated delta and REM sleep measurement methods. Sleep. 1987;10(6):551–62.
64. Feinberg I, Carlson VR. Sleep variables as a function of age in man. Arch Gen Psychiatry. 1968;18:239–50.
65. Feinberg I. Changes in sleep cycle patterns with age. J Psychiatr Res. 1974;10:283–306.
66. Feinberg I, March JD, Flach K, Maloney T, Chern W-J, Travis F. Maturational changes in amplitude, incidence and cyclic pattern of the 0 to 3 Hz (delta) electroencephalogram of human sleep. Brain Dysfunct. 1990;3:183–92.
67. Gaudreau H, Carrier J, Montplaisir J. Age-related modifications of NREM sleep EEG: from childhood to middle age. J Sleep Res. 2001;10:165–72.
68. Jenni OG, Carskadon MA. Spectral analysis of the sleep electroencephalogram during adolescence. Sleep. 2004;27:774–83.
69. Campbell IG, Feinberg I. Longitudinal trajectories of non-rapid eye movement delta and theta EEG as indicators of adolescent brain maturation. Proc Natl Acad Sci U S A. 2009;106: 5177–80.

70. Campbell IG, Darchia N, Higgins LM, Dykan IV, Davis NM, de Bie E, Feinberg I. Adolescent changes in homeostatic regulation of EEG activity in the delta and theta frequency bands during NREM sleep. Sleep. 2011;34(1):83–91.
71. Bliwise DL. Sleep in normal aging and dementia. Sleep. 1993;16(1):40–81.
72. Bonnet MH. Recovery of performance during sleep following sleep deprivation in older normal and insomniac adult males. Percept Mot Skills. 1985;60:323–34.
73. Bonnet MH, Rosa RR. Sleep and performance in young adults and older normals and insomniacs during acute sleep loss andrecovery. Biol Psychol. 1987;25:153–72.
74. Bonnet MH. The effect of sleep fragmentation on sleep and performance in younger and older subjects. Neurobiol Aging. 1989;10:21–5.
75. Brendel DH, Reynolds CF, Jennings JR, Hoch CC, Monk TH, Berman SR, Hall FT, Buyssee DJ, Kupfer DJ. Sleep stage physiology, mood, and vigilance responses to total sleep deprivation in healthy 80 year olds and 20 year olds. Psychophysiology. 1990;27(6):677–84.
76. Mander BA, Rao V, Lu B, Saletin JM, Lindquist JR, Ancoli-Israel S, Jagust W, Walker MP. Prefrontal atrophy, disrupted NREM slow waves and impaired hippocampal-dependent memory in aging. Nat Neurosci. 2013;16(3):357–64.
77. Rétey JV, Adam M, Honegger E, Khatami R, Luhmann UF, Jung HH, Berger W, Landolt HP. A functional genetic variation of adenosine deaminase affects the duration and intensity of deep sleep in humans. Proc Natl Acad Sci U S A. 2005;102(43):15676–81.
78. Bachmann V, Klaus F, Bodenmann S, Schäfer N, Brugger P, Huber S, Berger W, Landolt HP. Functional ADA polymorphism increases sleep depth and reduces vigilant attention in humans. Cereb Cortex. 2012;22(4):962–70.
79. Mazzotti DR, Guindalini C, de Souza AA, Sato JR, Santos-Silva R, Bittencourt LR, Tufik S. Adenosine deaminase polymorphism affects sleep EEG spectral power in a large epidemiological sample. PLoS One. 2012;7(8):e44154.
80. Bachmann V, Klein C, Bodenmann S, Schäfer N, Berger W, Brugger P, Landolt HP. The *BDNF* Val66Met polymorphism modulates sleep intensity: EEG frequency- and state-specificity. Sleep. 2012;35:335–44.
81. Laposky A, Easton A, Dugovic C, Walisser J, Bradfield C, Turek F. Deletion of the mammalian circadian clock gene BMAL/Mop3 alters baseline sleep architecture and the response to sleep deprivation. Sleep. 2005;28(4):395–409.
82. Naylor E, Bergmann BM, Krauski K, Zee PC, Takahashi JS, Vitaterna MH, Turek FW. The circadian clock mutation alters sleep homeostasis in the mouse. J Neurosci. 2000;20(21):8138–43.
83. Wisor JP, O'Hara BF, Terao A, Selby CP, Kilduff TS, Sancar A, Edgar DEM, Franken P. A role cryptochromes in sleep regulation. BMC Neurosci. 2002;3(20):1–14.
84. Franken P, Dudley CA, Estill SJ, Barakat M, Thomason R, O'Harar BF, McKnight SL. NPAS2 as a transcriptional regulator of non-rapid eye movement sleep: genotype and sex interactions. Proc Natl Acad Sci. 2006;103(18):7118–23.
85. Shaw PJ, Tononi G, Greenspan RJ, Robinson DF. Stress response genes protect against lethal effects of sleep deprivation in Drosophila. Nature. 2002;417(6886):287–91.
86. Franken P, Thomason R, Heller HC, O'Hara BF. A non-circadian role for clock-genes in sleep homeostasis: a strain comparison. BMC Neurosci. 2007;8:87.
87. Viola AU, Archer SN, James LM, Groeger JA, Lo JC, Skene DJ, von Schantz M, Dijk DJ. PER3 polymorphism predicts sleep structure and waking performance. Curr Biol. 2007;17(7):613–8.
88. Archer SN, Robilliard DL, Skene DJ, et al. A length polymorphism n the circadian clock gene Per3 is linked to delayed sleep phase syndrome and extreme diurnal preference. Sleep. 2003;26(4):413–5.
89. He Y, Jones CR, Fujiki N, Xu Y, Guo B, Holder Jr JL, Rossner MJ, Nishino S, Fu YH. The transcriptional repressor DEC2 regulates sleep length in mammals. Science. 2009;325(5942):866–70.
90. Centers for Disease Control and Prevention (CDC). Effect of short sleep duration on daily activities - United States, 2005-2008. MMWR Morb Mortal Wkly Rep. 2011;60:239–52.

91. Rupp TL, Wesensten NJ, Bliese PD, Balkin TJ. Banking sleep: realization of benefits during subsequent sleep restriction and recovery. Sleep. 2009;32(3):311–21.
92. Drake CL, Roehrs T, Richardson G, et al. Shift work sleep disorder: prevalence and consequences beyond that of symptomatic day workers. Sleep. 2004;27(8):1453–62.
93. Cohen DA, Wang W, Wyatt JK, Kronauer RE, Dijk DJ, Czeisler CA, Klerman EB. Uncovering residual effects of chronic sleep loss on human performance. Sci Transl Med. 2010;2(14):14ra3.
94. Zhou X, Ferguson SA, Mathews RW, et al. Sleep, wake, and phase dependent changes in neurobehavioral function under forced desynchrony. Sleep. 2011;34:931–41.
95. Schweitzer PK, Randazzo AC, Stone K, Erman M, Walsh JK. Laboratory and field studies of naps and caffeine as practical countermeasures for sleep-wake problems associated with night work. Sleep. 2006;29:39–50.
96. Sallinen M, Harma M, Akerstedt T, Rosa R, Lillqvist O. Promoting alertness with a short nap during a night shift. J Sleep Res. 1998;7:240–7.
97. Purnell MT, Feyer AM, Herbison GP. The impact of a nap opportunity during the night shift on the performance and alertness of 12-h shift workers. J Sleep Res. 2002;11(3):219–27.
98. Garbarino S, Mascialino B, Penco MA, et al. Professional shift-work drivers who adopt prophylactic naps can reduce the risk of car accidents during night work. Sleep. 2004;27:1295–302.
99. Bonnefond A, Muzet A, Winter-Dill AS, Bailloeuil C, Bitouze F, Bonneau A. Innovative working schedule: introducing one short nap during the night shift. Ergonomics. 2001;44:937–45.
100. Vernet C, Arnulf I. Idiopathic hypersomnia with and without long sleep time: a controlled series of 75 patients. Sleep. 2009;32(6):753–9.
101. Weitzman ED, Czeisler CA, Coleman RM, et al. Delayed sleep phase syndrome. A chronobiological disorder with sleep-onset insomnia. Arch Gen Psychiatry. 1981;38(7):737–46.
102. American Academy of Sleep Medicine. The international classification of sleep disorders: diagnostic and coding manual. 2nd ed. Westchester: American Academy of Sleep Medicine; 2005.
103. Ozaki S, Uchiyama M, Shirakawa S, et al. Prolonged interval from body temperature nadir to sleep off set in patients with delayed sleep phase syndrome. Sleep. 1996;19(1):36–40.
104. Watanabe T, Kajimura N, Kato M, et al. Sleep and circadian rhythm disturbances in patients with delayed sleep phase syndrome. Sleep. 2003;26(6):657–61.
105. Cole RJ, Smith JS, Alcala YC, et al. Bright-light mask treatment of delayed sleep phase syndrome. J Biol Rhythms. 2002;17:89–101.
106. Campbell SS, Murphy PJ. Delayed sleep phase disorder in temporal isolation. Sleep. 2007;30(9):1225–8.
107. Uchiyama M, Okawa M, Shibui K, et al. Poor compensatory function for sleep loss as a pathogenic factor in patients with delayed sleep phase syndrome. Sleep. 2000;23(4):553–8.
108. Uchiyama M, Shibui K, Hayakawa T, et al. Larger phase angle between sleep propensity and melatonin rhythms in sighted humans with non-24-hour sleep-wake syndrome. Sleep. 2002;25:83–8.
109. Hayakawa T, Uchiyama M, Kamei Y, et al. Clinical analyses of sighted patients with non-24-hour sleep-wake syndrome: a study of 57 consecutively diagnosed cases. Sleep. 2005;28(8):945–52.
110. Okawa M, Uchiyama M. Circadian rhythm sleep disorders: characteristics and entrainment pathology in delayed sleep phase and non-24-h sleep-wake syndrome. Sleep Med Rev. 2007;11(6):485–96.
111. Mongrain V, Dumont M. Increased homeostatic response to behavioral sleep fragmentation in morning types compared to evening types. Sleep. 2007;30(6):773–80.
112. Taillard J, Philip P, Coste O, Sagaspe P, Bioulac B. The circadian and homeostatic modulation of sleep pressure during wakefulness differs between morning and evening chronotypes. J Sleep Res. 2003;12:275–82.
113. Lancel M, Kerkhof GA. Sleep structure and EEG power density in morning types and evening types during a simulated day and night shift. Physiol Behav. 1991;49:1195–201.

114. Mongrain V, Carrier J, Dumont M. Difference in sleep regulation between morning and evening circadian types as indexed by antero-posterior analyses of the sleep EEG. Eur J Neurosci. 2006;23(2):497–504.

115. Schmidt C, Collette F, Leclercq Y, Sterpenich V, Vandewalle G, et al. Homeostatic sleep pressure and responses to sustained attention in the suprachiasmatic area. Science. 2009;324:516–9.

116. Chang AM, Reid KJ, Gourineni R, et al. Sleep timing and circadian phase in delayed sleep phase syndrome. J Biol Rhythms. 2009;24(4):313–21.

Neurochemistry of the Sleep-Wake Cycle in Parkinson's Disease

2

Amanda A.H. Freeman

Contents

Abstract

Many Parkinson's disease (PD) patients struggle with excessive daytime sleepiness independent of their poor nocturnal sleep quality. Unexplained by comorbid conditions, these symptoms are inherent to the underlying neuropathology of the disease. Widespread neurodegeneration in PD affects multiple neurotransmitter systems critical for regulating the sleep-wake cycle including: dopamine, acetylcholine, hypocretin/orexin, serotonin, norepinephrine, and melanin-concentrating hormone. Disruptions in these interconnected signaling pathways reduce arousal through both direct and indirect (i.e., positive and negative feedback loops)

A.A.H. Freeman, PhD
Department of Neurology, Emory University School of Medicine,
101 Woodruff Circle, WMRB, Suite 6000, Atlanta, GA 30322, USA
e-mail: aafreem@emory.edu

© Springer-Verlag Wien 2015
A. Videnovic, B. Högl (eds.), *Disorders of Sleep and Circadian Rhythms in Parkinson's Disease*, DOI 10.1007/978-3-7091-1631-9_2

mechanisms. This chapter reviews the role of each of these neurotransmitter systems in sleep-wake regulation and how degeneration of these nuclei may contribute to deficits in the sleep-wake cycle of PD patients.

2.1 Introduction

Disruptions of the sleep-wake cycle in Parkinson's disease (PD) are evident in both daytime functioning and nighttime sleep. Between 30 and 60 % of PD patients report excessive daytime sleepiness (EDS) as indicated by scores >10 on the Epworth Sleepiness Scale [1, 2], which is predictive of unintended sleep attacks [3]. Employing the multiple sleep latency test (MSLT) as an objective measure, pathological sleepiness has been observed in 20–50 % of PD patients (mean sleep latency <5 min). The presence of rapid eye movement (REM) sleep along with the short sleep latency, indicating a narcolepsy-like phenotype, has been documented in 15–39 % [4, 5].

Impairments in daytime arousal are independent of the nocturnal sleep disruptions in PD, which include sleep fragmentation, decreased slow-wave sleep, decreased REM sleep, increased REM latency, and loss of sleep spindles [4, 5]. In fact, contrary to what one might predict, poorer nocturnal sleep was associated with greater, rather than lesser, degrees of daytime alertness [5]. While daytime sleepiness correlates with disease severity [2], it cannot be explained by comorbid conditions including insomnia, periodic leg movements, or sleep apnea [4, 5]. These findings indicate that the sleep-wake disruptions are intrinsic to the neuropathology underlying the disorder rather than a secondary effect of poor sleep quality.

Progressive loss of dopaminergic neurons is the hallmark of PD, and animal models targeting dopaminergic disruption replicate some aspects of the sleepiness phenotype observed in PD patients. However, significant neuronal loss correlating with disease severity extends to additional neurotransmitter systems known to regulate arousal (e.g., acetylcholine, norepinephrine, serotonin, and hypocretin/orexin). This chapter reviews deficits in wake-promoting neurotransmitter systems, which may contribute to the disruptions in the sleep-wake cycles of Parkinson's disease patients.

2.2 Wake-Promoting Circuits

2.2.1 Dopamine

Multiple lines of converging evidence, from pharmacological interventions to genetic manipulations to targeted lesions, demonstrate that dopamine plays an essential role in the sleep-wake cycle. Drugs that increase the synaptic availability of dopamine, through stimulating release or inhibiting reuptake (e.g., amphetamine or cocaine), have long been appreciated to increase arousal. Mice [6] and flies [7] that lack functional dopamine transporters, thereby leading to increased synaptic dopamine by preventing synaptic reuptake of dopamine, demonstrate a 20 % increase in wakefulness and a >50 % decrease in rest, respectively. Administration of a selective dopamine D1 receptor agonist (SKF 38393 or A68930) increases wakefulness and decreases REM sleep and simultaneous blockade of the D1 receptor (SCH 23390) prevents the increase in arousal [8]. During their subjective day, rats spend less time awake and exhibit inappropriate REM sleep intrusions following destruction of ascending dopamine pathways from the ventral tegmental area (VTA) [9]. Lesions targeting presumptive wake-active, dopaminergic neurons in the ventral periaqueductal gray of rats increase sleep by ~20 % [10]. Sleepiness and REM intrusion into daytime naps, recapitulating the narcolepsy-like phenotype of some PD patients, is observed in a methyl,4-phenyl-1,2,3,6-tetrahydropyridine (MPTP)-induced model of parkinsonism in nonhuman primates [11]. Administration of the dopamine precursor L-DOPA or the dopamine reuptake blocker bupropion reverses these effects [11] presumably through activation of intact mesocorticolimbic circuits that are less vulnerable to MPTP. The specificity of dopamine's role in the regulation of the sleep-wake cycle, as opposed to maintenance of circadian rhythm, is emphasized by the general preservation of circadian body temperature in parkinsonian MPTP nonhuman primates [12].

Despite the evidence that dopamine promotes arousal, it has not traditionally been considered a member of the ascending reticular activating system (ARAS) because the firing rate of dopaminergic neurons does not vary across behavioral state [13]. The average firing rate, however, does not take into account that these neurons have either tonic or burst firing patterns. Extracellular dopamine concentrations increase following burst firing compared to tonic firing even when the average firing rate of the two conditions is kept constant [14]. The firing pattern of substantia nigra pars compacta (SNpc) neurons can be modulated by gluatmatergic inputs via an NMDA-receptor-dependent mechanism [15] or cholinergic inputs [16]. In the context of the sleep-wake cycle, this latter mechanism is particularly relevant considering the projections from the wake-promoting pedunculopontine tegmental nucleus to the SNpc [17].

The number of dopaminergic neurons of the SNpc decreases 50–86 % prior to clinical manifestation of symptoms [18–21], resulting in a 70–80 % decrease in dopamine concentrations at striatal nerve terminals [18]. In addition, 42–48 % of the dopaminergic neurons in the VTA degenerate, while the ventral periaqueductal gray is relatively spared (3 % loss) [19, 20]. Both, a direct and an indirect mechanism may contribute to the sleepiness observed in PD following this loss of midbrain dopaminergic neurons. The SNpc neurons project directly to thalamocortical circuits critical for promoting wakefulness including the midline, intralaminar, and reticular nuclei of the thalamus [22]. These nigrothalamic projections are, in fact, collaterals of the more well-known nigrostriatal pathway, therefore both degenerate simultaneously in PD [22]. In a manner similar to that seen elsewhere throughout the ARAS, the dopamine neurons within the SNpc, VTA, and ventral periaqueductal gray are known to feedback to the ARAS nuclei including the cortex, basal forebrain, dorsal and median raphe, locus coeruleus, pedunculopontine tegmentum,

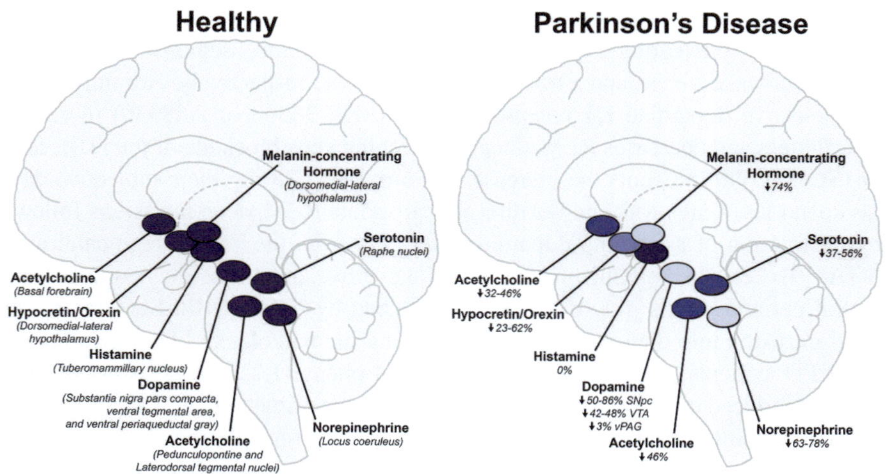

Fig. 2.1 Degree of Parkinson's disease related degeneration in sleep-wake regulating nuclei as measured by cell counts. The healthy brain depicts the nuclei, and corresponding neurotransmitter or neuropeptide, known to regulate the sleep-wake cycle. The degree of neurodegeneration is depicted by increasingly lighter shading in the Parkinson's disease brain. The percentage indicates the decreased number of neurons in Parkinson's disease compared to controls

and laterodorsal tegmentum [10, 23, 24]. Loss of an excitatory dopaminergic input to these wake-promoting nuclei may be an indirect route through which sleepiness arises from dopamine loss.

Degeneration in PD, however, is not restricted to dopaminergic neurons and the lack of strong correlation between sleepiness and the motor manifestations of the disease or the decreased nocturnal sleep efficiency suggests that deficits within other nuclei are likely to contribute to impairments in thalamocortical arousal states. Extensive neuronal cell loss occurs in multiple nondopaminergic sleep-wake-related neurotransmitter systems including acetylcholine, hypocretin/orexin, serotonin, norepinephrine, histamine, and melanin-concentrating hormone, which may contribute to these arousal deficits. Like the loss of dopamine, alterations in these signaling pathways likely have direct effects on arousal and indirect effects mediated by feedback loops to other sleep-wake regulatory nuclei (Fig. 2.1).

2.2.2 Acetylcholine

There are two primary cholinergic projection systems recognized to contribute to sleep-wake regulation: the basal forebrain and the pedunculopontine tegmental nucleus-lateral dorsal tegmental nucleus complex (PPN/LDT) in the brainstem. The primary cholinergic input to the cortex arises from the basal forebrain which includes three subpopulations: the medial septal nucleus, the diagonal band of Broca, and, in particular, the nucleus basalis of Meynert (NbM). In the brainstem, the PPN/LDT provide the major cholinergic input to the thalamus and the basal ganglia (including the SNpc) and send descending projections to the pontine reticular formation including the subcoeruleus, and the gigantocellular nucleus of the medulla [17, 25, 26].

The PPN/LDT neurons have either an equally high firing rate during both wake and REM sleep (Wake-ON) or they have significantly higher activity during REM than wake or non-REM sleep (REM-ON) [27]. Increases in activity occur 20–60 s in advance of state change [27]. This shift in firing rate prior to arousal demonstrates PPN/LDT's critical role in driving the cortical desynchronization associated with wakefulness and REM sleep.

Dysfunction within the cholinergic system occurs early in the progression of PD and can be extensive. According to the Braak PD staging criteria, Lewy neurites begin to appear simultaneously in the basal forebrain and SNpc in stage 3, prior to dramatic cell loss in the SNpc [28]. Eventually, 32–46 % of the NbM neurons degenerate in PD [29, 30]. Degree of NbM loss does not correlate with disease duration [30], but in PD with dementia the magnitude can rival that observed in Alzheimer's disease [29]. Mapping acetylcholinesterase activity in vivo with positron emission tomography indicates that the resultant decrease in cortical innervation is only 15 %; however, this can be more extensive than the deficit observed in Alzheimer's patients (9.1 %) [31]. Postmortem examinations of parkinsonian brains indicate that 46 % of PPN neurons degenerate, particularly in the pars compacta component located in the caudal portion of the nucleus [32]. This degree of neuronal loss correlates with disease severity [32]. While positron emission tomography measures of AChE indicate that Alzheimer's disease patients have no deficits in cholinergic thalamic innervation, there is a 12.8 % decrease in PD and a 19.8 % reduction in PD with dementia [33] indicative of PPN degeneration.

Deep brain stimulation (DBS) therapies reinforce the role that cholinergic brainstem nuclei play in sleep-wake regulation, and the impact that their degeneration plays in PD. Originally, the PPN was selected as a DBS target to address the postural instability and gait disturbances in PD [34]. Patients also report improvements in daytime sleepiness equivalent to a >50 % improvement on the Epworth Sleepiness Scale following bilateral PPN stimulation in comparison to STN alone [35]. Objective polysomnographic measures indicate increased sleep efficiency, a 70 % decrease in number of awakenings, and an almost twofold increase in time spent in REM sleep [35, 36]. The wake-promoting effects of PPN stimulation occur at lower stimulating frequencies (10–25 Hz), whereas high-frequency stimulation (80 Hz) can trigger sleep episodes [37]. Presumably, the higher frequency inhibits the wake-promoting thalamic projections from the PPN.

REM sleep behavioral disorder (RBD) diagnosis often precedes the clinical manifestation of PD and is considered an early manifestation of α-synucleinopathies including PD, dementia with Lewy bodies, and multiple system atrophy. Longitudinal studies of patients diagnosed with idiopathic RBD report that approximately 80 % of patients will subsequently be diagnosed with a parkinsonian disorder or dementia 12–14 years after the original onset of RBD [38, 39]. RBD is characterized by a loss of muscle atonia during REM sleep, which is traditionally maintained by a complex brainstem circuit including: PPN/LDT, locus coeruleus, subcoeruleus, medullary magnocellular reticular formation, and the ventrolateral reticulospinal tract (reviewed in [40]). Despite the strong comorbidity of RBD and PD, the severity of RBD symptoms is not correlated with impaired dopamine transporter binding as measured by positron emission tomography [41]. This suggests that the genuine pathology underlying RBD in the setting of parkinsonism involves degeneration of *nondopaminergic* circuits. Acetylcholine is an obvious candidate considering the early pathology in cholinergic circuits along with the prominent role of the PPN/LDT in the brainstem circuitry regulating atonia in rapid eye movement sleep. In PD patients, positron emission tomography reveals a significant correlation between the presence of RBD symptoms and decreased acetylcholinesterase in cortex and thalamus, but no significant relationship with either dopamine or serotonin measures [42]. Since these regions of cholinergic innervation have two different origins, the basal forebrain and the PPN/LDT, these results indicate concurrent degeneration of both pathways. PPN DBS does not reduce the increased muscle tone during REM observed in RBD patients [36]. Therefore, the decreased cholinergic innervation from the PPN is only part of the disrupted pathophysiology that underlies RBD in PD.

2.2.3 Hypocretin/Orexin

Owing to their axonal projection patterns [43] and their generally excitatory effects upon wake promoting neurons [44], the role of hypocretin/orexin (Hcrt/OX) neurons in regulating the sleep-wake cycle has long been appreciated [45, 46]. The Hcrt/OX-producing cell bodies are localized within the dorsomedial and lateral hypothalamus, including the perifornical area, and innervate histaminergic neurons in the nearby tuberomamillary nucleus and additional widespread ascending and descending projections to disparate brain regions [43]. Targets include the cortex, basal forebrain, amygdala, thalamus, SNpc, locus coeruleus, dorsal raphe, PPN/LDT, pontine reticular formation, gigantocellular nucleus of the medulla, and the spinal cord, in particular the intermediolateral cell column [43, 47]. Reciprocal innervation from these targets to the dorsomedial hypothalamus positions Hcrt/OX neurons to influence, and to be influenced by, circadian rhythms [48]. Regardless of which receptor they are binding (i.e., Hcrt1/OX1 or Hcrt2/Ox2), both Hcrt/OX peptides have excitatory downstream effects [45]. Additionally, many Hcrt/OX neurons have been found to corelease glutamate that may contribute to some of their effects on downstream targets [49].

In vivo electrophysiological investigations reveal that activation of the Hcrt/OX system is critical to orchestrating the transition between non-REM or REM sleep and wakefulness. Hcrt/OX neurons are most active during wake, particularly active waking, whereas their firing rate decreases during non-REM sleep and ceases during tonic REM sleep with a slight increase in activity during phasic REM [50, 51]. When applied experimentally, Hcrt/OX increases the firing rate of wake-promoting nuclei including: cholinergic neurons in the basal forebrain [52] and brainstem (LDT) [53], locus coeruleus [44], dorsal raphe [54], tuberomammillary nucleus [55], and the VTA [56]. Local application of Hcrt/OX into the basal forebrain [57], the locus coeruleus [58], or the LDT [59] increase wakefulness and decrease REM sleep. Optogenetic activation of the Hcrt/OX neurons triggers a transition from sleep to wakefulness, albeit with a delay between stimulation and arousal [60]. The interconnection of the multiple wake-promoting nuclei is emphasized by activation in downstream histaminergic neurons of the tuberomammillary nucleus and noradrenergic neurons of the locus coeruleus following optogenetic stimulation of the Hcrt/OX neurons [61]. Following sleep deprivation, sleep pressure overrides the effects of Hcrt/OX activation and the probability of arousal decreases and the downstream nuclei are not activated [61]. The increased firing rate of Hcrt/OX neurons throughout waking supports their hypothesized role in stabilizing the wake state, but occurrence of the highest firing rate during active wake may indicate additional roles in wake-related behaviors.

The number of Hcrt/OX neurons decreases by 23–62 % progressively over the course of PD [62]. Since the number of Hcrt/OX cells is dramatically reduced in narcolepsy [63], one might expect that the narcoleptic-like sleepiness observed in some PD patients (i.e., excessive daytime sleepiness and REM intrusions into daytime naps) would be explained by the loss of Hcrt/OX, along with the decreased dopaminergic signaling. Despite the dramatic degeneration of Hcrt/OX neurons, the level of hypocretin-1 in the CSF is not significantly reduced and does not correlate with sleep disruptions [64]. Experimental lesions in rats demonstrate that a 73 % decrease in the number of Hcrt/OX neurons is required for a concomitant 50 % reduction of Hcrt-1 in the CSF and increase in REM sleep [65]. Therefore, it seems that the remaining, viable Hcrt/OX neurons are able to compensate sufficiently to prevent significant decreases in CSF concentrations. However, the loss of excitatory drive on downstream wake-promoting nuclei still seems like a parsimonious explanation for some of the sleep-wake disturbances in PD patients. That being said, because of neuropathological heterogeneity and multiple additional factors (e.g., medications or comorbid disease) that influence sleep-wake state, it is difficult to pinpoint with certainty which parkinsonian-related sleep disturbance is attributable to the Hcrt/OX system degeneration.

2.2.4 Serotonin

Serotonin is produced in cell groups along the midline from the midbrain to the pons. The rostral potion of the serotonergic neurons in the pons and midbrain, including the dorsal raphe and median raphe, can be differentiated from the caudal portion based upon chemo- and cyto-architecture [66]. The neuroanatomical projections allow the dorsal and median raphe to be distinguished; although they project to similar areas, the terminal fields are distinct [67]. Targets of the dorsal raphe projections include the cortex, basal forebrain, thalamus, dorsomedial hypothalamus, SNpc, median raphe, locus coeruleus, PPN, subcoeruleus, and the sleep-promoting VLPO [24, 26, 68, 69]. Similarly, targets of the median raphe efferents include the cortex, basal forebrain, thalamus, dorsomedial hypothalamus, SCN, SNpc, VTA, locus coeruleus, dorsal raphe, PPN/LDT, and the subcoeruleus [26, 67].

Of the multiple serotonergic nuclei, the dorsal raphe primarily regulates sleep-wake cycles while the median raphe is integral to regulation of circadian rhythm [70–72]. The majority of serotonergic neurons within the dorsal raphe are type I, which demonstrate alterations in firing rate across behavioral state. Activity is highest during active waking, particularly when orienting to a stimulus, and decreases progressively across quiet waking and non-REM sleep [70, 72]. During REM sleep serotonergic neurons are silent, but resume wake-related levels of activity prior to the end of the episode [70, 72]. These findings indicate the dorsal raphe plays a key role in initiating the transition between stages.

In PD, decreased numbers of neurons are observed in both the dorsal raphe (37.2 %) [21] and the median raphe (56 %) [73]. Degeneration in each of these neurons may contribute separately to the sleep-wake disturbances observed in PD. Loss of the wake-promoting neurons in the dorsal raphe may contribute to the excessive sleepiness. Meanwhile, loss of circadian regulating median raphe neurons may contribute, in part, to the increased arousals at night and daytime sleepiness.

2.2.5 Norepinephrine

The locus coeruleus is the primary norepinephrine-producing nucleus in the brain. Targets of widespread noradrenergic efferents include the cortex, basal forebrain, thalamus, Hcrt/OX, dorsal raphe, PPN/LDT, subcoeruleus, and the sleep-promoting VLPO [26, 68, 74, 75]. Whether norepinephrine has excitatory or inhibitory influences on these downstream nuclei depends on the subtype of adrenergic receptors present. In the basal forebrain and dorsal raphe, excitatory effects are due to the presence of the $\alpha1$- or β-adrenoceptors [76]. The VLPO and Hcrt/OX neurons express $\alpha2$-adrenoceptors resulting in inhibitory responses [75]. In the PPN/LDT, the wake-ON neurons express $\alpha1$-adrenoceptors and the REM-on neurons express $\alpha2$-adrenoceptors allowing the effects of norepinephrine modulate state [77].

Activity of noradrenergic neurons is closely related to arousal. The neurons of the locus coeruleus are most active during wakefulness, decrease their activity during non-REM sleep, and are virtually silent during REM sleep [78]. Alterations in firing rate precede the EEG transitions to the corresponding arousal level [78]. Norepinephrine provides such a strong alerting signal that acute optogenetic stimulation results in immediate transition to wakefulness and long-term stimulation increases wakefulness and decreases non-REM sleep times [79]. Optogenetic inhibition of the locus coeruleus increases the number of sleep onsets and decreases the duration of wake episodes, but does not prolong the duration of sleep episodes [79]. However, arousals still occur during optogenetic inhibition of the locus coeruleus, indicating that this activity is not necessary and other components of the sleep-wake regulatory network can compensate in its absence [79].

In PD, 63–78 % of the neurons within the locus coeruleus degenerate [21, 80]. The extensive loss of this signaling pathway likely contributes to excessive daytime sleepiness in PD patients; the specific contributions, however, are difficult to disentangle from the effects of the degeneration in the other wake-promoting neurotransmitter systems.

2.2.6 Histamine

Histamine is produced in large cell bodies of the tuberomammillary nucleus located in the posterior hypothalamus. Widespread projections from histaminergic neurons innervate the cortex, thalamus, SNpc, VTA, locus coeruleus, dorsal raphe, LDT, pontine reticular formation, and the gigantocellular nucleus of the medulla [81]. The area of densest innervation is observed in the hypothalamus, including the Hcrt/OX cell bodies, and the basal forebrain [55, 81]. Afferents also target the sleep-promoting VLPO [68]. Four metabotropic histamine receptors have been identified (H1R-H4R); however, H4R is primarily expressed in the periphery. Signaling through both the H1R and H2R is excitatory, while H3R primarily functions as a presynaptic autoreceptor or heteroreceptor (reviewed in [82]).

Electrophysiological recordings of histaminergic neurons in freely moving mice across sleep-wake states reveal the highest firing rate during attentive or active wakefulness [83]. Activity decreases during quiet waking, ceases prior to the onset of sleep, and remains silent throughout non-REM and REM sleep [83]. Histaminergic neurons resume firing only when the animal is completely awakened, indicating that this signaling pathway is critical in the maintenance of wakefulness rather than initiating the transition from sleep to wake [83].

In contrast to all other wake-promoting nuclei, the histaminergic neurons of the tuberomammillary nucleus do not degenerate in PD [84]. In fact, the concentration of histamine is significantly increased in the SNpc (201 %) and other areas of the basal ganglia (159–234 %) [85]. In the SNpc, histaminergic innervation increases and the terminal fields are particularly dense surrounding remaining dopamine neurons [86]. This juxtaposition suggests that histamine may be important for promoting neuronal survival through stimulated release of interleukin-6 from astrocytes, which, in turn, triggers synthesis and secretion of nerve growth factor [86]. In the putamen, the concentration of the primary histamine metabolite tele-methylhistamine is the same in control and PD brains, indicating that the metabolism of histamine is unaltered despite the increased availability [85].

Pitolisant is an H3R antagonist/inverse agonist that is being developed to treat excessive daytime sleepiness. When administered to a parkinsonian feline MPTP model exhibiting daytime sleepiness, time spent awake is increased [87]. In clinical trials of PD patients, pitolisant reduced subjective sleepiness and resulted in a five-point decrease on the Epworth sleepiness scale [87].

It is difficult to know the role of increased histaminergic innervation of SNpc in general, let alone in the context of the disrupted sleep-wake cycle in PD considering the lack of information available regarding histaminergic innervation of other wake-promoting nuclei. However, the evidence indicating that histaminergic metabolism is preserved suggests that any loss of wake-promoting effect in histamine circuits would be due to degeneration of downstream targets.

2.3   Sleep-Promoting Circuit

2.3.1   Melanin-Concentrating Hormone

Melanin-concentrating hormone (MCH) neurons are intermixed with the Hcrt/OX neurons in the dorsomedial, lateral hypothalamus, but they are a distinct neuronal population [43]. Ascending and descending projections of the MCH neurons are extensive, but the relevant nuclei for sleep-wake regulation include: basal forebrain, thalamus, tuberomammillary nucleus, SNpc, VTA, PPN/LDT, dorsal and medial raphe, locus coeruleus, and the pontine reticular formation [88]. There are also reciprocal projections between the MCH neurons and the Hcrt/OX neurons [89]. MCH is an inhibitory neuropeptide, and >80 % of MCH neurons also corelease GABA [90] thereby increasing the potential inhibitory effects.

Evidence suggests that the primary role of the MCH neurons in sleep-wake regulation is to promote REM sleep. Electrophysiologically, the MCH neurons are maximally active during REM sleep and virtually silent during non-REM sleep and wakefulness [50]. Intracerebroventricular administration of MCH increases REM sleep amounts in a dose-dependent manner [91]. Optogenetic activation of MCH neurons during non-REM sleep increases the likelihood of transition to REM sleep, while activation during REM sleep increases the duration of the episode without altering the EEG power spectrum or muscle tone [90]. The extension of REM sleep duration is observed even in mice lacking the MCH receptor indicating that this effect may be mediated by the coreleased GABA rather than the MCH itself [90]. Due to the diffuse projections, it is conceivable that MCH promotion of REM sleep may occur through inhibitory projections to wake-promoting Hcrt/OX, histaminergic or basal forebrain cholinergic neurons, or by driving the REM-OFF neurons in the brainstem ARAS to cease firing. However, some evidence suggests that the MCH-histaminergic TMN or MCH-cholinergic basal forebrain circuits play key roles in mediating this effect [90].

In PD, the number of MCH neurons decreases by 74 % [62]. Loss of this signaling pathway may explain, at least in part, some of the nocturnal REM sleep deficits in PD patients. However, MCH is relatively unstudied in the context of PD and little is known about the specific impact of this deficit.

Conclusion

The neurodegeneration in PD extends beyond the hallmark nigrostriatal system and encompasses many other nuclei critical for the regulation of the sleep-wake cycle.

Due to the redundant projections and feedback loops, both negative and positive, throughout these nuclei, it is difficult to isolate the sleep-wake disruptions resulting from the loss of an individual neurotransmitter. This network must be considered to function as a unit and altered activity in one or more components impacts the output of the remaining members. The sleep-wake disruptions of PD patients reflect the integrated degeneration of multiple arousal related nuclei throughout the brain. While excessive daytime sleepiness and disrupted nocturnal sleep are inherent to the disorder itself, one cannot discount the secondary contributions of nocturnal movement disturbances or pharmacological therapies that may further worsen these symptoms.

References

1. Hogl B, Seppi K, Brandauer E, Glatzl S, Frauscher B, Niedermuller U, Wenning G, Poewe W. Increased daytime sleepiness in Parkinson's disease: a questionnaire survey. Mov Disord. 2003;18(3):319–23.
2. Ondo WG, Vuong KV, Khan H, Atassi F, Kwak C, Jankovic J. Daytime sleepiness and other sleep disorders in Parkinson's disease. Neurology. 2001;57:1392–6.
3. Tan EK, Lum SY, Fook-Chong SMC, Teoh ML, Yih Y, Tan L, Tan A, Wong MC. Evaluation of somnolence in Parkinson's disease: comparison with age and sex matched controls. Neurology. 2002;58(3):465–8.
4. Arnulf I, Konofal E, Merino-Andreu M, Houeto JL, Mesnage V, Welter ML, Lacomblez L, Golmard JL, Derenne JP, Agid Y. Parkinson's disease a sleepiness: an integral part of PD. Neurology. 2002;58:1019–24.
5. Rye DB, Bliwise DL, Dihenia B, Gurecki P. FAST TRACK: daytime sleepiness in Parkinson's disease. J Sleep Res. 2000;9(1):63–9.
6. Wisor JP, Nishino S, Sora I, Uhl GH, Mignot E, Edgar DM. Dopaminergic role in stimulant-induced wakefulness. J Neurosci. 2001;21(5):1787–94.
7. Kume K, Kume S, Park SK, Hirsh J, Jackson FR. Dopamine is a regulator of arousal in the fruit fly. J Neurosci. 2005;25(32):7377–84.
8. Trampus M, Ferri N, Adami M, Ongini E. The dopamine D1 receptor agonists, A68930 and SKF 38393, induce arousal and suppress REM sleep in the rat. Eur J Pharmacol. 1993;235(1):83–7.
9. Sakata M, Sei H, Toida K, Fujihara H, Urushihara R, Morita Y. Mesolimbic dopaminergic system is involved in diurnal blood pressure regulation. Brain Res. 2002;928(1–2):194–201.
10. Lu J, Jhou TC, Saper CB. Identification of wake-active dopaminergic neurons in the ventral periaqueductal gray matter. J Neurosci. 2006;26(1):193–202.
11. Daley JT, Turner RS, Bliwise DL, Rye DB. Nocturnal sleep and daytime alertness in the MPTP-treated primate. Sleep. 1999;22(Suppl):S218–9.
12. Almirall H, Pigarev I, de la Calzada MD, Pigareva M, Herrero MT, Sagales T. Nocturnal sleep structure and temperature slope in MPTP treated monkeys. J Neural Transm. 1999;106(11–12):1125–34.
13. Trulson ME, Preussler DW, Howell GA. Activity of substantia nigra units across the sleep-waking cycle in freely moving cats. Neurosci Lett. 1981;26(2):183–8.
14. Gonon FG. Nonlinear relationship between impulse flow and dopamine released by rat midbrain dopaminergic neurons as studied by in vivo electrochemistry. Neuroscience. 1988;24(1):19–28.
15. Chergui K, Akaoka H, Charlety PJ, Saunier CF, Buda M, Chouvet G. Subthalamic nucleus modulates burst firing of nigral dopamine neurones via NMDA receptors. Neuroreport. 1994;5(10):1185–8.
16. Kitai ST, Shepard PD, Callaway JC, Scroggs R. Afferent modulation of dopamine neuron firing patterns. Curr Opin Neurobiol. 1999;9(6):690–7.
17. Clarke PB, Hommer DW, Pert A, Skirboll LR. Innervation of substantia nigra neurons by cholinergic afferents from pedunculopontine nucleus in the rat: neuroanatomical and electrophysiological evidence. Neuroscience. 1987;23(3):1011–9.
18. Agid Y. Parkinson's disease: pathophysiology. Lancet. 1991;337(8753):1321–4.
19. German DC, Manaye K, Smith WK, Woodward DJ, Saper CB. Midbrain dopaminergic cell loss in Parkinson's disease: computer visualization. Ann Neurol. 1989;26(4):507–14.

20. Hirsch E, Graybiel AM, Agid YA. Melanized dopaminergic neurons are differentially suscep-
    tible to degeneration in Parkinson's disease. Nature. 1988;334(6180):345–8.
21. Paulus W, Jellinger K. The neuropathologic basis of different clinical subgroups of Parkinson's
    disease. J Neuropathol Exp Neurol. 1991;50(6):743–55.
22. Freeman A, Ciliax BJ, Bakay R, Daley J, Miller RD, Keating GL, Levey AI, Rye DB.
    Nigrostriatal collaterals to thalamus degenerate in parkinsonian animal models. Ann Neurol.
    2001;50:321–9.
23. Beckstead RM, Domesick VB, Nauta WJ. Efferent connections of the substantia nigra and
    ventral tegmental area in the rat. Brain Res. 1979;175(2):191–217.
24. Pasquier DA, Kemper TL, Forbes WB, Morgane PJ. Dorsal raphe, substantia nigra and locus
    coeruleus: interconnections with each other and the neostriatum. Brain Res Bull.
    1977;2(5):323–39.
25. Hallanger AE, Levey AI, Lee HJ, Rye DB, Wainer BH. The origins of cholinergic and other
    subcortical afferents to the thalamus in the rat. J Comp Neurol. 1987;262:105–24.
26. Semba K. Aminergic and cholinergic afferents to REM sleep induction regions of the pontine
    reticular formation in the rat. J Comp Neurol. 1993;330(4):543–56.
27. Steriade M, Datta S, Pare D, Oakson G, Curro Dossi RC. Neuronal activities in brain-stem
    cholinergic nuclei related to tonic activation processes in thalamocortical systems. J Neurosci.
    1990;10(8):2541–59.
28. Braak H, Tredici K, Rub U, de Vos R, Jansen Steur E, Braak E. Staging of brain pathology
    related to sproadic Parkinson's disease. Neurobiol Aging. 2003;24:197–211.
29. Gaspar P, Gray F. Dementia in idiopathic Parkinson's disease. A neuropathological study of 32
    cases. Acta Neuropathol. 1984;64(1):43–52.
30. Tagliavini F, Pilleri G, Bouras C, Constantinidis J. The basal nucleus of Meynert in idiopathic
    Parkinson's disease. Acta Neurol Scand. 1984;70(1):20–8.
31. Bohnen NI, Kaufer DI, Ivanco LS, Lopresti B, Koeppe RA, Davis JG, Mathis CA, Moore RY,
    DeKosky ST. Cortical cholinergic function is more severely affected in parkinsonian dementia
    than in Alzheimer disease: an in vivo positron emission tomographic study. Arch Neurol.
    2003;60(12):1745–8.
32. Zweig RM, Jankel WR, Hedreen JC, Mayeux R, Price DL. The pedunculopontine nucleus in
    Parkinson's disease. Ann Neurol. 1989;26(1):41–6.
33. Kotagal V, Muller ML, Kaufer DI, Koeppe RA, Bohnen NI. Thalamic cholinergic innervation
    is spared in Alzheimer disease compared to parkinsonian disorders. Neurosci Lett.
    2012;514(2):169–72.
34. Mazzone P, Lozano A, Stanzione P, Galati S, Scarnati E, Peppe A, Stefani A. Implantation of
    human pedunculopontine nucleus: a safe and clinically relevant target in Parkinson's disease.
    Neuroreport. 2005;16(17):1877–81.
35. Alessandro S, Ceravolo R, Brusa L, Pierantozzi M, Costa A, Galati S, Placidi F, Romigi A, Iani
    C, Marzetti F, Peppe A. Non-motor functions in parkinsonian patients implanted in the pedun-
    culopontine nucleus: focus on sleep and cognitive domains. J Neurol Sci. 2010;289:44–8.
36. Lim AS, Moro E, Lozano AM, Hamani C, Dostrovsky JO, Hutchison WD, Lang AE, Wennberg
    RA, Murray BJ. Selective enhancement of rapid eye movement sleep by deep brain stimulation
    of the human pons. Ann Neurol. 2009;66(1):110–4.
37. Arnulf I, Ferraye M, Fraix V, Benabid AL, Chabardes S, Goetz L, Pollak P, Debu B. Sleep
    induced by stimulation in the human pedunculopontine nucleus area. Ann Neurol.
    2010;67(4):546–9.
38. Iranzo A, Tolosa E, Gelpi E, Molinuevo JL, Valldeoriola F, Serradell M, Sanchez-Valle R,
    Vilaseca I, Lomena F, Vilas D, Llado A, Gaig C, Santamaria J. Neurodegenerative disease
    status and post-mortem pathology in idiopathic rapid-eye-movement sleep behaviour disorder:
    an observational cohort study. Lancet Neurol. 2013;12(5):443–53.
39. Schenck CH, Boeve BF, Mahowald MW. Delayed emergence of a parkinsonian disorder or
    dementia in 81% of older men initially diagnosed with idiopathic rapid eye movement sleep
    behavior disorder: a 16-year update on a previously reported series. Sleep Med.
    2013;14(8):744–8.

40. Boeve BF, Silber MH, Saper CB, Ferman TJ, Dickson DW, Parisi JE, Benarroch EE, Ahlskog JE, Smith GE, Caselli RC, Tippman-Peikert M, Olson EJ, Lin SC, Young T, Wszolek Z, Schenck CH, Mahowald MW, Castillo PR, Del Tredici K, Braak H. Pathophysiology of REM sleep behaviour disorder and relevance to neurodegenerative disease. Brain. 2007;130(Pt 11):2770–88.
41. Kim YK, Yoon IY, Kim JM, Jeong SH, Kim KW, Shin YK, Kim BS, Kim SE. The implication of nigrostriatal dopaminergic degeneration in the pathogenesis of REM sleep behavior disorder. Eur J Neurol. 2010;17(3):487–92.
42. Kotagal V, Albin RL, Muller ML, Koeppe RA, Chervin RD, Frey KA, Bohnen NI. Symptoms of rapid eye movement sleep behavior disorder are associated with cholinergic denervation in Parkinson disease. Ann Neurol. 2012;71(4):560–8.
43. Peyron C, Tighe DK, van den Pol AN, de Lecea L, Heller HC, Sutcliffe JG, Kilduff TS. Neurons containing hypocretin (orexin) project to multiple neuronal systems. J Neurosci. 1998;18(23):9996–10015.
44. Hagan JJ, Leslie RA, Patel S, Evans ML, Wattam TA, Holmes S, Benham CD, Taylor SG, Routledge C, Hemmati P, Munton RP, Ashmeade TE, Shah AS, Hatcher JP, Hatcher PD, Jones DN, Smith MI, Piper DC, Hunter AJ, Porter RA, Upton N. Orexin A activates locus coeruleus cell firing and increases arousal in the rat. Proc Natl Acad Sci U S A. 1999;96(19):10911–6.
45. de Lecea L, Kilduff TS, Peyron C, Gao X, Foye PE, Danielson PE, Fukuhara C, Battenberg EL, Gautvik VT, Bartlett 2nd FS, Frankel WN, van den Pol AN, Bloom FE, Gautvik KM, Sutcliffe JG. The hypocretins: hypothalamus-specific peptides with neuroexcitatory activity. Proc Natl Acad Sci U S A. 1998;95(1):322–7.
46. Sakurai T, Amemiya A, Ishii M, Matsuzaki I, Chemelli RM, Tanaka H, Williams SC, Richardson JA, Kozlowski GP, Wilson S, Arch JR, Buckingham RE, Haynes AC, Carr SA, Annan RS, McNulty DE, Liu WS, Terrett JA, Elshourbagy NA, Bergsma DJ, Yanagisawa M. Orexins and orexin receptors: a family of hypothalamic neuropeptides and G protein-coupled receptors that regulate feeding behavior. Cell. 1998;92(4):573–85.
47. van den Pol AN. Hypothalamic hypocretin (orexin): robust innervation of the spinal cord. J Neurosci. 1999;19(8):3171–82.
48. Chou TC, Scammell TE, Gooley JJ, Gaus SE, Saper CB, Lu J. Critical role of dorsomedial hypothalamic nucleus in a wide range of behavioral circadian rhythms. J Neurosci. 2003;23(33):10691–702.
49. Torrealba F, Yanagisawa M, Saper CB. Colocalization of orexin a and glutamate immunoreactivity in axon terminals in the tuberomammillary nucleus in rats. Neuroscience. 2003;119(4):1033–44.
50. Hassani OK, Lee MG, Jones BE. Melanin-concentrating hormone neurons discharge in a reciprocal manner to orexin neurons across the sleep-wake cycle. Proc Natl Acad Sci U S A. 2009;106(7):2418–22.
51. Mileykovskiy BY, Kiyashchenko LI, Siegel JM. Behavioral correlates of activity in identified hypocretin/orexin neurons. Neuron. 2005;46(5):787–98.
52. Eggermann E, Serafin M, Bayer L, Machard D, Saint-Mleux B, Jones BE, Muhlethaler M. Orexins/hypocretins excite basal forebrain cholinergic neurones. Neuroscience. 2001;108(2):177–81.
53. Burlet S, Tyler CJ, Leonard CS. Direct and indirect excitation of laterodorsal tegmental neurons by Hypocretin/Orexin peptides: implications for wakefulness and narcolepsy. J Neurosci. 2002;22(7):2862–72.
54. Brown RE, Sergeeva OA, Eriksson KS, Haas HL. Convergent excitation of dorsal raphe serotonin neurons by multiple arousal systems (orexin/hypocretin, histamine and noradrenaline). J Neurosci. 2002;22(20):8850–9.
55. Eriksson KS, Sergeeva O, Brown RE, Haas HL. Orexin/hypocretin excites the histaminergic neurons of the tuberomammillary nucleus. J Neurosci. 2001;21(23):9273–9.
56. Uramura K, Funahashi H, Muroya S, Shioda S, Takigawa M, Yada T. Orexin-a activates phospholipase C- and protein kinase C-mediated Ca2+ signaling in dopamine neurons of the ventral tegmental area. Neuroreport. 2001;12(9):1885–9.

57. Espana RA, Baldo BA, Kelley AE, Berridge CW. Wake-promoting and sleep-suppressing actions of hypocretin (orexin): basal forebrain sites of action. Neuroscience. 2001;106(4):699–715.

58. Bourgin P, Huitron-Resendiz S, Spier AD, Fabre V, Morte B, Criado JR, Sutcliffe JG, Henriksen SJ, de Lecea L. Hypocretin-1 modulates rapid eye movement sleep through activation of locus coeruleus neurons. J Neurosci. 2000;20(20):7760–5.

59. Xi MC, Morales FR, Chase MH. Effects on sleep and wakefulness of the injection of hypocretin-1 (orexin-A) into the laterodorsal tegmental nucleus of the cat. Brain Res. 2001;901(1–2):259–64.

60. Adamantidis AR, Zhang F, Aravanis AM, Deisseroth K, de Lecea L. Neural substrates of awakening probed with optogenetic control of hypocretin neurons. Nature. 2007;450(7168):420–4.

61. Carter ME, Adamantidis A, Ohtsu H, Deisseroth K, de Lecea L. Sleep homeostasis modulates hypocretin-mediated sleep-to-wake transitions. J Neurosci. 2009;29(35):10939–49.

62. Thannickal TC, Lai YY, Siegel JM. Hypocretin (orexin) cell loss in Parkinson's disease. Brain. 2007;130(Pt 6):1586–95.

63. Thannickal TC, Moore RY, Nienhuis R, Ramanathan L, Gulyani S, Aldrich M, Cornford M, Siegel JM. Reduced number of hypocretin neurons in human narcolepsy. Neuron. 2000;27(3):469–74.

64. Wienecke M, Werth E, Poryazova R, Baumann-Vogel H, Bassetti CL, Weller M, Waldvogel D, Storch A, Baumann CR. Progressive dopamine and hypocretin deficiencies in Parkinson's disease: is there an impact on sleep and wakefulness? J Sleep Res. 2012;21(6):710–7.

65. Gerashchenko D, Murillo-Rodriguez E, Lin L, Xu M, Hallett L, Nishino S, Mignot E, Shiromani PJ. Relationship between CSF hypocretin levels and hypocretin neuronal loss. Exp Neurol. 2003;184(2):1010–6.

66. Dahlstroem A, Fuxe K. Evidence for the existence of monoamine-containing neurons in the central nervous system. I. Demonstration of monoamines in the cell bodies of brain stem neurons. Acta Physiol Scand Suppl. 1964;Suppl 232:231–55.

67. Vertes RP, Fortin WJ, Crane AM. Projections of the median raphe nucleus in the rat. J Comp Neurol. 1999;407(4):555–82.

68. Chou TC, Bjorkum AA, Gaus SE, Lu J, Scammell TE, Saper CB. Afferents to the ventrolateral preoptic nucleus. J Neurosci. 2002;22(3):977–90.

69. Vertes RP. A PHA-L analysis of ascending projections of the dorsal raphe nucleus in the rat. J Comp Neurol. 1991;313(4):643–68.

70. McGinty DJ, Harper RM. Dorsal raphe neurons: depression of firing during sleep in cats. Brain Res. 1976;101(3):569–75.

71. Meyer-Bernstein EL, Morin LP. Differential serotonergic innervation of the suprachiasmatic nucleus and the intergeniculate leaflet and its role in circadian rhythm modulation. J Neurosci. 1996;16(6):2097–111.

72. Trulson ME, Jacobs BL. Raphe unit activity in freely moving cats: correlation with level of behavioral arousal. Brain Res. 1979;163(1):135–50.

73. Halliday GM, Blumbergs PC, Cotton RG, Blessing WW, Geffen LB. Loss of brainstem serotonin- and substance P-containing neurons in Parkinson's disease. Brain Res. 1990;510(1):104–7.

74. Lindvall O, Bjorklund A. The organization of the ascending catecholamine neuron systems in the rat brain as revealed by the glyoxylic acid fluorescence method. Acta Physiol Scand Suppl. 1974;412:1–48.

75. Yamanaka A, Muraki Y, Tsujino N, Goto K, Sakurai T. Regulation of orexin neurons by the monoaminergic and cholinergic systems. Biochem Biophys Res Commun. 2003;303(1):120–9.

76. Berridge CW, Isaac SO, Espana RA. Additive wake-promoting actions of medial basal forebrain noradrenergic alpha1- and beta-receptor stimulation. Behav Neurosci. 2003;117(2):350–9.

77. Hou YP, Manns ID, Jones BE. Immunostaining of cholinergic pontomesencephalic neurons for alpha 1 versus alpha 2 adrenergic receptors suggests different sleep-wake state activities and roles. Neuroscience. 2002;114(3):517–21.
78. Aston-Jones G, Bloom FE. Activity of norepinephrine-containing locus coeruleus neurons in behaving rats anticipates fluctuations in the sleep-waking cycle. J Neurosci. 1981;1(8):876–86.
79. Carter ME, Yizhar O, Chikahisa S, Nguyen H, Adamantidis A, Nishino S, Deisseroth K, de Lecea L. Tuning arousal with optogenetic modulation of locus coeruleus neurons. Nat Neurosci. 2010;13(12):1526–33.
80. Mann DM. The locus coeruleus and its possible role in ageing and degenerative disease of the human central nervous system. Mech Ageing Dev. 1983;23(1):73–94.
81. Panula P, Pirvola U, Auvinen S, Airaksinen MS. Histamine-immunoreactive nerve fibers in the rat brain. Neuroscience. 1989;28(3):585–610.
82. Haas HL, Sergeeva OA, Selbach O. Histamine in the nervous system. Physiol Rev. 2008;88(3):1183–241.
83. Takahashi K, Lin JS, Sakai K. Neuronal activity of histaminergic tuberomammillary neurons during wake-sleep states in the mouse. J Neurosci. 2006;26(40):10292–8.
84. Nakamura S, Ohnishi K, Nishimura M, Suenaga T, Akiguchi I, Kimura J, Kimura T. Large neurons in the tuberomammillary nucleus in patients with Parkinson's disease and multiple system atrophy. Neurology. 1996;46(6):1693–6.
85. Rinne JO, Anichtchik OV, Eriksson KS, Kaslin J, Tuomisto L, Kalimo H, Roytta M, Panula P. Increased brain histamine levels in Parkinson's disease but not in multiple system atrophy. J Neurochem. 2002;81(5):954–60.
86. Anichtchik OV, Rinne JO, Kalimo H, Panula P. An altered histaminergic innervation of the substantia nigra in Parkinson's disease. Exp Neurol. 2000;163(1):20–30.
87. Arnulf I. Results of clinical trials of tiprolisant in narcolepsy and Parkinson's disease. Eur Neuropsychopharmacol. 2009;19:S204.
88. Bittencourt JC, Presse F, Arias C, Peto C, Vaughan J, Nahon JL, Vale W, Sawchenko PE. The melanin-concentrating hormone system of the rat brain: an immuno- and hybridization histochemical characterization. J Comp Neurol. 1992;319(2):218–45.
89. Bayer L, Mairet-Coello G, Risold PY, Griffond B. Orexin/hypocretin neurons: chemical phenotype and possible interactions with melanin-concentrating hormone neurons. Regul Pept. 2002;104(1–3):33–9.
90. Jego S, Glasgow SD, Herrera CG, Ekstrand M, Reed SJ, Boyce R, Friedman J, Burdakov D, Adamantidis AR. Optogenetic identification of a rapid eye movement sleep modulatory circuit in the hypothalamus. Nat Neurosci. 2013;6(11):1637–43.
91. Verret L, Goutagny R, Fort P, Cagnon L, Salvert D, Leger L, Boissard R, Salin P, Peyron C, Luppi PH. A role of melanin-concentrating hormone producing neurons in the central regulation of paradoxical sleep. BMC Neurosci. 2003;4:19.

Impaired Sleep and Alertness in Parkinson's Disease: "What Did We Learn from Animal Models?"

3

Pierre-Hervé Luppi, Olivier Clément, Sara Valencia Garcia, Frédéric Brischoux, and Patrice Fort

Contents

P.-H. Luppi (✉)
"SLEEP" team, INSERM, U1028, CNRS, UMR5292, Lyon Neuroscience Research Center,
Team Physiopathologie des réseaux neuronaux du cycle veille-sommeil,
7 Rue Guillaume Paradin, F-69372 Lyon, France

University of Lyon, F-69000 Lyon, France

University Claude Bernard Lyon 1, F-69000 Lyon, France

Faculté de Médecine RTH Laennec, UMR5167 CNRS,
7 Rue Guillaume Paradin, Lyon 69372, France
e-mail: luppi@sommeil.univ-lyon1.fr

O. Clément • S. Valencia Garcia • F. Brischoux • P. Fort
"SLEEP" team, INSERM, U1028, CNRS, UMR5292, Lyon Neuroscience Research Center,
Team Physiopathologie des réseaux neuronaux du cycle veille-sommeil,
7 Rue Guillaume Paradin, F-69372 Lyon, France

University of Lyon, F-69000 Lyon, France

University Claude Bernard Lyon 1, F-69000 Lyon, France

© Springer-Verlag Wien 2015
A. Videnovic, B. Högl (eds.), *Disorders of Sleep and Circadian Rhythms in Parkinson's Disease*, DOI 10.1007/978-3-7091-1631-9_3

Abstract

The aim of this review is to try to provide a conceptual framework on the mechanisms potentially responsible for sleep alteration in Parkinson's disease (PD) based on data obtained in animals. We first provide state-of-the-art hypotheses on the mechanisms responsible for the succession of the three vigilance states, namely waking, non-rapid eye movement (non-REM) also called slow-wave sleep (SWS) and REM sleep also called paradoxical sleep (PS). We then review our knowledge on the role of dopamine in sleep-waking regulation. We pursue by discussing the results obtained on sleep in MPTP animal model of PD. We complete our review by providing hypotheses on the mechanisms responsible for REM sleep behavior disorder known to occur in half of the Parkinson's patients based on studies of RBD animal models.

3.1   Introduction

Sleep disturbances, excessive daytime sleepiness, and rapid eye movement sleep behavior disorder (RBD) are among the most frequent and disabling manifestations of PD [1–3]. They often precede the motor features of the disease by years and may serve as early biomarkers of the premotor phase of PD [3–6]. The pathophysiology of these sleep alterations is still not comprehended. In particular, it is still discussed as to whether the underlying mechanisms of sleep disturbances in PD are due to dopamine (DA) deficiency. In the following, we review our current knowledge on the neuronal networks responsible for the sleep-waking cycle and on the animal models available to provide possible mechanisms at the origin of sleep disturbances in PD.

3.2   Populations of Neurons Responsible for Waking

In most mammals, there are three vigilance states, which are characterized by clear differences in electroencephalogram (EEG), electromyogram (EMG) and electro-oculogram (EOG) recordings. The waking state is characterized by high-frequency, low-amplitude (desynchronized) activity on the EEG, sustained EMG activity and ocular movements; non-rapid eye movement (non-REM), also named slow-wave sleep (SWS) (synchronized), is characterized by low-frequency, high-amplitude delta oscillations on the EEG, low muscular activity on the EMG, and no ocular movement; and rapid eye movement (REM), also called paradoxical sleep (PS), is characterized by an activated low-amplitude EEG similar to the waking EEG, but with complete disappearance of postural muscle tone and the occurrence of rapid eye movements and muscle twitches.

The activation of the cortex during waking is induced by the activity of multiple neurochemical systems. These neurochemical systems include the serotonergic neurons, which are mainly localized in the dorsal raphe nucleus, noradrenergic neurons in the locus coeruleus, the histaminergic neurons localized in the tuberomammillary nucleus, and the orexin (hypocretin) neurons localized in the tuberal hypothalamus [7]. In addition, the cholinergic neurons in the pontine brainstem and the basal forebrain are implicated both in cortical activation during waking and paradoxical sleep. Altogether, these systems induce waking characterized by high-frequency, low-amplitude cortical activation [8] by means of their extensive projection to the thalamus and/or the neocortex.

3.3 Mechanisms Involved in Non-REM (Slow-Wave Sleep, SWS) Sleep

During sleep, it is believed that the waking-inducing systems are all inhibited by gamma-aminobutyric acid (GABA), the main inhibitory neurotransmitter in the brain [9, 10]. When the waking systems are inactivated, the thalamocortical network oscillates in the delta range (i.e., the slow-wave mode of activity typical of SWS) [7].

SWS-active neurons were localized by using expression of the immediate early gene – Fos – as a marker of neuronal activation in rats that had slept for a long period before sacrifice [11]. These neurons are distributed diffusely in the POA but are more densely packed in the median preoptic nucleus (MnPn) and the ventrolateral preoptic nucleus (VLPO). Studies showed that the number of Fos-immunoreactive neurons in the VLPO and MnPn positively correlated with sleep quantity and sleep consolidation during the last hour preceding sacrifice [11, 12]. It was later demonstrated that VLPO and the suprachiasmatic nucleus (SCN), a critical site in circadian rhythm network, have synchronized activity [13]. Considering that both areas are interconnected and receive inputs from the retinal ganglion cells, it is, thus, possible that circadian- and photic-linked information may be conveyed to modulate VLPO activity [7].

Electrophysiology experiments in behaving rats have shown that neurons recorded in the VLPO and MnPn are active during SWS, generally anticipating its onset by several seconds. Functionally, bilateral neurotoxic destruction of VLPO is followed by a profound and long-lasting insomnia in rats [14]. Retrograde and anterograde tract-tracing studies indicate that VLPO and MnPn neurons are reciprocally connected with wake-active neurons such as those containing histamine in the tuberomammillary nucleus (TMN), hypocretin in the perifornical hypothalamic area (PeF), serotonin in the dorsal raphe nuclei (DRN), noradrenaline in the locus coeruleus (LC), and acetylcholine in the pontine (LDT/PPT) and basal forebrain nuclei. In these wake-promoting areas, extracellular levels of GABA increase during SWS compared to W.

Electrophysiological recordings of VLPO neurons in rat brain slices showed that it contains a homogeneous neuronal group with specific intrinsic membrane properties, a clear-cut chemo-morphology, and an inhibitory response to the major waking neurotransmitters [15]. These neurons are inhibited by noradrenaline (NA), via postsynaptic alpha2-adrenoceptors, acetylcholine, through muscarinic postsynaptic and nicotinic presynaptic actions on noradrenergic terminals. In contrast, histamine and hypocretin do not modulate VLPO neurons [15, 16]. Finally, serotonin showed complex effects inducing either inhibition (50%, Type 1) or excitation (50%, Type 2) of the VLPO neurons [7, 17]. Further, application of an adenosine A_{2A} receptor ($A_{2A}R$) agonist evoked direct excitatory effects specifically in Type 2 VLPO neurons [7, 17]. A number of studies also showed that adenosine A_1 receptors (A_1R) promote sleep through inhibition of the wake-promoting neurons, in particular cholinergic and hypocretin neurons [18, 19]. However, transgenic mice that lack A_1R exhibit normal homeostatic regulation of sleep. In contrast, the lack of $A_{2A}R$ prevents normal sleep regulation and blocks the wake-inducing effect of caffeine, suggesting that the activation of $A_{2A}R$ is crucial in SWS [20–22].

3.4 Summary: The Neuronal Network Responsible for SWS (Non-REM) Sleep

Both the VLPO and the MnPn contain neurons responsible for sleep onset and maintenance. These neurons are inhibited by noradrenergic and cholinergic inputs during waking. The majority of them start firing at sleep onset (drowsiness) in response to excitatory, homeostatic (adenosine and serotonin), and circadian drives (suprachiasmatic input). Conversely, the slow removal of excitatory influences would result in a progressive firing decrease in VLPO neurons and, therefore, an activation of the wake-promoting systems inducing awakening [17, 23].

3.5 Mechanisms Involved in Paradoxical (REM) Sleep Genesis

3.5.1 The Localization of the Neurons Generating PS in the Pontine Reticular Formation

It was first shown that a state characterized by muscle atonia and REM persists following decortication, cerebellar ablation, or brain stem transections rostral to the pons and in the "pontine cat," a preparation in which all the structures rostral to the pons have been removed [24]. These results indicated that brainstem structures are necessary and sufficient to trigger and maintain the state of PS. Electrolytic and chemical lesions showed that the dorsal part of pontis oralis (PnO) and caudalis (PnC) nuclei, also named peri-locus coeruleus α (peri-LCα), pontine inhibitory area (PIA), and subcoeruleus nucleus (SubC) contain the neurons responsible for PS onset [24]. In addition, the PnO and PnC contain many neurons that show a tonic firing selective to PS (called "PS-on" neurons) [25, 26]. More recently, a corresponding area has been identified in rats, and named sublaterodorsal tegmental nucleus (SLD). We demonstrated that most of the Fos-labeled neurons localized in the SLD after PS recovery express the vesicular glutamate transporter 2 (vGlut2) [27] and are therefore glutamatergic.

A number of recent results further suggest that PS-on glutamatergic neurons located in the SLD generate muscle atonia via descending projections to PS-on GABA/glycinergic premotoneurons located at medullary level. First, by means of intracellular recordings during PS, it has been shown that trigeminal, hypoglossal, and spinal motoneurons are tonically hyperpolarized by large inhibitory postsynaptic potentials (IPSPs) during PS. Further, when these recordings were combined with local iontophoretic application of strychnine (a specific antagonist of the inhibitory neurotransmitter, glycine), motoneurons hyperpolarization was strongly decreased, indicating that they are tonically inhibited by glycinergic neurons during PS [28–30]. It has then been shown that the levels of glycine but also that of GABA increase within hypoglossal and spinal motor pools during PS-like atonia [31]. Further, it was recently shown that combined microdialysis of bicuculline, strychnine, and phaclophen (a GABA-B antagonist) in the trigeminal nucleus is necessary to restore jaw muscle tone during PS [32]. Finally, mice with impaired glycinergic and GABAergic transmissions display PS without atonia [33]. In addition, it has been shown that the SLD sends direct efferent projections to GABA/glycinergic neurons located in the nucleus raphe magnus (RMg) and the ventral (GiV), alpha (Gia) gigantocellular and lateral paragigantocellular (LPGi) reticular nuclei [34, 35]. Further, GABA/glycinergic neurons of the Gia, GiV, LPGi, and RMg express c-Fos after PS hypersomnia [34, 36].

It has also been shown that a subpopulation of SLD PS-on neurons project to the intralaminar thalamic nuclei, the posterior hypothalamus, and the basal forebrain. In addition to the SLD, it has also been shown that cholinergic neurons located in the pedunculopontine and laterodorsal tegmental nuclei and glutamatergic neurons located in the reticular formation active both during waking and PS and projecting rostrally contribute to cortical activation during PS [7, 34].

3.5.2 Mechanisms Responsible for SLD PS-On Neurons Activation During PS

A long-lasting PS-like hypersomnia can be pharmacologically induced with a short latency in head-restrained unanesthetized rats by iontophoretic application into the SLD of bicuculline or gabazine, two GABA-A receptor antagonists [34]. Further, application of kynurenate, a glutamate antagonist, reverses the PS-like state induced by bicuculline [34]. In the head restrained rat, we also recorded neurons within the

SLD specifically active during PS and excited following bicuculline or gabazine iontophoresis [37]. Taken together, these data indicate that the activation of SLD PS-on neurons is mainly due to the removal during PS of a tonic GABAergic tone present during W and SWS combined with the continuous presence of a glutamatergic input. Combining retrograde tracing with cholera toxin b subunit (CTb) injected in SLD and glutamate decarboxylase 67 (GAD67) immunohistochemistry or Fos immunohistochemistry with GAD67mRNA "in situ hybridization" after 72 h of PS deprivation, we recently demonstrated that the ventrolateral part of the periaqueductal gray (vlPAG) and the adjacent dorsal part of the deep mesencephalic nucleus (dDPMe) are the only ponto-medullary structures containing a large number of GABAergic neurons activated during PS deprivation projecting to the SLD [36]. Further, injection of muscimol in the vlPAG and/or the dDpMe induces strong increases in PS quantities in cats [38] and rats [36]. Finally, neurochemical lesion of these two structures induces a profound increase in PS quantities [39]. These congruent experimental data led us to propose that PS-off GABAergic neurons within the vlPAG and the dDpMe gate PS by tonically inhibiting PS-on neurons of the SLD during W and SWS.

3.5.3 Neurons Inhibiting the GABAergic and Monoaminergic PS-Off Neurons at the Onset and During PS

Bicuculline application on serotonergic and noradrenergic neurons during SWS or PS restores a tonic firing pattern [9, 10, 40]. These results strongly suggest that an increased GABA release is responsible for the PS-selective inactivation of monoaminergic neurons. This hypothesis is well supported by microdialysis experiments in cats, which measured a significant increase in GABA release in the DRN and LC during PS as compared to W and SWS [41, 42]. By combining retrograde tracing with CTb and GAD immunohistochemistry in rats, the vlPAG and the dorsal paragigantocellular nucleus (DPGi) [10, 43] contained numerous GABAergic neurons projecting both to the DRN and LC. We then demonstrated by combining c-Fos and retrograde labeling that both nuclei contain numerous LC-projecting neurons selectively activated during PS rebound following PS deprivation [44, 45]. Further, the DPGi contains numerous PS-on neurons that increase their activity specifically during PS [46]. In summary, a large body of data indicate that GABAergic PS-on neurons localized in the vlPAG and the DPGi hyperpolarize the monoaminergic neurons during PS.

We first proposed that these neurons might be also responsible for the inhibition of the dDPMe/vlPAG PS-off GABAergic neurons during PS. To test this hypothesis, we recently localized the neurons active during PS hypersomnia projecting to the dDPMe/vlPAG PS-off GABAergic neurons [47]. The lateral hypothalamic area (LH) is the only brain structure containing a very large number of neurons activated during PS hypersomnia and projecting to the VLPAG/dDpMe. Forty-four percent of these neurons express the neuropeptide melanin concentrating hormone (MCH). These results indicate that LH hypothalamic neurons might play a crucial role in PS onset and maintenance by means of descending projections to the vlPAG/dDPMe PS-off GABAergic neurons.

Supporting this claim, rats receiving intracerebroventricular (icv) administration of MCH showed a strong dose-dependent increase in PS and, to a minor extent, SWS quantities, due to an increased number of PS bouts [48]. Further, subcutaneous injection of an MCH antagonist decreases SWS and PS quantities [49] and mice with genetically inactivated MCH signaling exhibit altered vigilance state architecture and sleep homeostasis [50, 51]. Finally, it was recently shown that optogenetic stimulation of MCH neurons induces PS [52, 53].

To determine the function of the LH MCH+/GABA+ and MCH-/GABA+ neurons in PS control, we inactivated all LH neurons with muscimol (a GABA-A agonist) or only those bearing alpha-2 adrenergic receptors using clonidine. Muscimol and to a lesser degree clonidine bilateral injections in the LH induce an inhibition of PS with or without an increase in SWS quantities, respectively. Our results suggest that MCH/GABAergic PS-on neurons of the LH control PS onset and maintenance by means of a direct inhibitory projection to vlPAG/dDpMe PS-off GABAergic neurons. From our results, it can be proposed that MCH/GABAergic neurons of the LH constitute a master generator of PS, which controls a slave generator located in the brainstem.

The cessation of activity of the MCH/GABAergic PS-on neurons and more largely of all the PS-on neurons at the end of PS episodes is certainly due to a completely different mechanism than the entrance into the state. Indeed, animals are entering PS slowly from SWS, while in contrast they exit from it abruptly by a microarousal [54]. This indicates that the end of PS is induced by the activation of the W systems like the monoaminergic, hypocretin or the histaminergic neurons. The mechanisms responsible for their activation remain to be identified.

3.6   Conclusion

3.6.1   A Network Model for PS Onset and Maintenance

The onset of PS would be due to the activation by intrinsic and extrinsic factors of PS-on MCH/GABAergic neurons localized in the lateral hypothalamic area (LH). These neurons would inhibit at the onset and during PS the PS-off GABAergic neurons localized in the vlPAG and the dDpMe tonically inhibiting during W and SWS the glutamatergic PS-on neurons from the SLD. The disinhibited ascending glutamatergic SLD PS-on neurons would in turn induce cortical activation via their projections to intralaminar thalamic relay neurons in collaboration with W/PS-on cholinergic and glutamatergic neurons from the LDT and PPT, mesencephalic and pontine reticular nuclei and the basal forebrain. Descending glutamatergic PS-on SLD neurons would induce muscle atonia via their excitatory projections to GABA/glycinergic premotoneurons localized in the raphe magnus, alpha and ventral gigantocellular reticular nuclei. PS-on GABAergic neurons localized in the LH, DPGi, and vlPAG would also inactivate the PS-off orexin (hypocretin) and aminergic neurons during PS. The exit from PS would be due to the activation of waking systems since PS episodes are almost always terminated by an arousal. The waking systems would reciprocally inhibit the GABAergic PS-on neurons localized in the LH, vlPAG and DPGi. Since the duration of PS is negatively coupled with the metabolic rate, we propose that the activity of the waking systems is triggered to end PS to restore crucial physiological parameters like thermoregulation.

3.6.2 Role of Dopamine in the Sleep-Waking Cycle

Early electrophysiological studies in rats and cats showed that the firing rate of dopaminergic neurons of the substantia nigra (SNC) and the ventral tegmental area (VTA) is not influenced by the sleep-wake cycle [55, 56]. More recently, it was shown that dopamine neurons of the VTA display during paradoxical sleep (PS) a prominent bursting pattern [57]. The burst pattern observed during PS is similar to the activity measured during the consumption of palatable food known to induce large synaptic dopamine release. Besides, it has been shown that c-Fos expression is increased in a few or nearly no dopamine cells during a rebound of PS [58, 59]. Finally, a microdialysis study found out that extracellular levels of dopamine in nucleus accumbens and prefrontal cortex are higher both during W and PS compared to SWS [60].

Lesioning of the DA-containing neurons located in the SNC and the VTA of the cat induces no change in the quantities of each vigilance state. Waking state is characterized by akinesia, hypertonus, and a lack of behavioral arousal [61]. Wisor et al. [62] quantified sleep and W in dopamine transporter (DAT) knockout mice. These hyperdopaminergic mice show a significant increase of wake quantities and a reduction of SWS during the light phase compared with wild-type mice. It has also been shown that behavioral arousal is impaired in DA D1 receptor knockout mice [63]. Further, systemic administration of a selective DA D1 agonist induces desynchronization of the EEG and behavioral arousal, together with an increase of W and a reduction of SWS and PS. In contrast, injection of a DA D1 antagonist tends to produce sedation and to reduce W, whereas SWS and PS are increased [63]. Mice with inactivation of the D2 receptor show reduced levels of spontaneous locomotor activity. Systemic administration of DA D2 agonists induces biphasic effects, such that low doses reduce W and increase SWS and REMS, whereas large doses induce the opposite effects. Drugs with DA D2 receptor blocking properties increase NREMS and reduce W [63]. Altogether, these results suggest that DA neurons of the VTA and SNC play a role in behavioral arousal and a still to be identified role during PS.

3.6.3 Sleep in MPTP Models

Chronic treatment with 1-methyl-4-phenyl-1,2,3,6-tetrahydropyridine (MPTP) is known to induce a destruction of dopaminergic neurons of the SN and

VTA. The first study showing the induction of a sleep effect of MPTP reported a selective REM sleep suppression that lasted 6–9 days after the last administration of the neurotoxin in cats [64]. Conversely, it was then shown that MPTP-treated mice present changes in sleep architecture, with longer wakefulness and REM sleep episodes and an increase in the amount of REM sleep [65].

The abrupt ablation of REM sleep was also observed in a subsequent study in MPTP-treated monkeys [66]. They further showed that 2 weeks after cessation of MPTP treatment, REM sleep was still dramatically reduced and the animals also displayed progressive sleep deterioration and fragmentation with increased frequency and duration of wake after sleep onset and reduced sleep efficacy. The animals further showed increased daytime sleepiness [66] Interestingly, 90 days after the last MPTP injection, partial progressive but significance reemergence of REM sleep was observed (8% vs. 16% in control) [66]. Despite the general increase in tonic muscle activity, REM sleep muscle atonia still occurred but with intermittent bouts of REM sleep without atonia without occurrence of RBD.

From these results, it can be concluded that MPTP models only partly replicate the symptoms of PD. Indeed, REM sleep quantities are not reduced in Parkinson's patients, suggesting that the decrease in REM sleep quantities in MPTP models is not induced by the loss of dopaminergic neurons but rather by an effect on other types of neurons involved in PS inhibition like the serotoninergic or noradrenergic systems. In contrast, the increased daytime sleepiness might well be due to the disappearance of the dopaminergic neurons known to be involved in behavioral waking.

3.6.4   REM Sleep Behavior Disorder Models

Rapid eye movement sleep behavior disorder (RBD) is characterized by the occurrence of vivid, intense, and violent movements during rapid eye movement sleep (REM sleep, also named paradoxical sleep, PS). The patient can talk, yell, punch, kick, sit, jump from bed, and grab during REM sleep. When the patient is awakened or wakes up spontaneously during the acting, he can recall dreams that correspond to the physical activity. RBD is usually seen in middle-aged to elderly men [67]. The disorder occurs in association with various degenerative neurological diseases such as PD [68]. It has been reported that up to 65% of patients diagnosed with RBD subsequently developed PD within an average time of 12–13 years from the onset of RBD symptoms. The prevalence of RBD in PD is of 46–58% [68]. The neuronal dysfunction at the origin of the disease is not known. A large number of results suggest that RBD is not due to a dysfunction of the dopaminergic nigrostriatal system. The strongest arguments are that RBD does not occur in about half of the PD patients, the use of dopaminergic agents usually does not improve RBD, and RBD precedes for several years the onset of PD in many PD patients [68]. It is therefore more likely that RBD is due to a degeneration of the neuronal system generating muscle atonia during REM sleep. In the following, we consequently review results in animal models of RBD.

3.6.5 Animal Models of RBD

It has recently been shown that mice with impaired glycinergic and GABAergic transmissions display all features of RBD, that is, REM sleep without atonia, myoclonic jerks during NREM sleep, sleep fragmentation, and EEG slowing [33]. In addition, it has been shown that inactivation of GABA and glycinergic transmissions in the spinal cord induced the occurrence of small phasic movements during REM sleep [69]. Further, an increased tonus is seen during REM sleep in cats with GiV and Gia cytotoxic lesion [70, 71].

In addition, in cats and rats, electrolytic and neurochemical lesions of the SLD eliminate muscle atonia and induce phasic muscle activity during REM sleep. The phasic events include large limb twitches, locomotion, fear, attack, and defensive behaviors [39, 72–74]. Importantly, these lesions also induce a moderate to severe decrease in the total quantities of REM sleep depending on their location and size [24, 39, 75].

In neurodegenerative diseases where RBD is frequent, neuronal cell loss was observed in the brainstem structures controlling REM sleep, like the locus subcoeruleus (corresponding to the SLD), the pedunculopontine nucleus (PPTg), and the gigantocellular reticular nucleus (Gi), and also in their rostral afferents, especially the amygdala [68]. Importantly, RBD patients display normal quantities of REM sleep [76]. It seems therefore unlikely that RBD is due to a degeneration of a large proportion of the SLD REM-on glutamatergic neurons since large SLD lesions in cats and rats induce a moderate to strong decrease in REM sleep quantities [24, 39, 75]. One possibility is that in RBD patients, only the descending REM-on neurons of the SLD specifically responsible for muscle atonia degenerated. It would imply that REM-on glutamatergic neurons of the SLD are divided in at least two subpopulations, one descending responsible for muscle atonia and the other one inducing the state of REM sleep itself and EEG activation. Data obtained in cats support the existence of two populations of SLD REM-on cells (see above). However, these two populations have not yet been identified in rats.

Another possibility is that the premotor PS-on GABA/glycinergic neurons of the RMg, Gia, and GiV degenerate in RBD patients. Indeed, lesions of these structures in cats induced PS without atonia and only a moderate decrease in REM sleep quantities [70]. Further, the duration of REM sleep episodes but not the total quantities of REM sleep was decreased in RBD mice with disrupted GABA and glycinergic transmissions [33]. These results are in favor of the hypothesis that RBD is due to a degeneration of GABA/glycinergic REM-on neurons.

Finally, it should be mentioned that neurons located in the ventral mesencephalic reticular formation could also be implicated in RBD since neurochemical lesions of this area in cats increased muscle tone and phasic muscle activity during REM sleep with or without inducing a decrease in REM sleep quantities [77].

3.6.6 Mechanisms Responsible for Phasic Motor Activation in RBD Patients

It has been shown in rats and cats that, during REM sleep, in addition to a tonic GABA/glycinergic inhibition, the motoneurons receive during the muscle twitches phasic glutamate excitatory and glycine/GABA inhibitory inputs [78–80]. Is has been further shown that the phasic glutamatergic inputs are responsible for the occurrence of muscles twitches since the application of glutamate antagonists on motoneurons abolish them [79]. The localization of the neurons at the origin of these phasic glutamatergic inputs is not known. Glutamatergic neurons projecting to motoneurons are localized in the motor cortex, the red nucleus, the lateral vestibular nucleus, and the reticular formation [81]. Voluntary movements are induced by the phasic depolarization of motoneurons by direct and indirect (through the above structures) excitatory projections arising from the glutamatergic pyramidal cells of the motor cortex [82]. We propose that this pathway is also responsible for the muscle twitches occurring during REM sleep and the movements in RBD patients since pyramidal tract motor cortex neuronal activity, which mediates limb movements, is as high during REM sleep as it is during active wake [83, 84]. Further supporting this hypothesis, it has been shown that RBD patients can recall dreams that correspond to their physical activity [85]. In addition, it has been shown that, compared with wake movements, RBD movements in Parkinson's patients are faster and more often repeated, jerky, and pseudohallucinatory, not self-centered, never associated with tremor, and rarely involved the environment in an appropriate manner. From these results, it has been proposed that in RBD patients the motor cortex drives the movements during REM sleep without involving the basal ganglia [86]. In summary, although additional experiments are necessary to confirm such hypothesis, we propose that the motor cortex is at the origin of the twitches of REM sleep and the movements of RBD patients.

Acknowledgments This work was supported by CNRS, Fondation France Parkinson and University Claude Bernard of Lyon.

References

1. Arnulf I, Konofal E, Merino-Andreu M, Houeto JL, Mesnage V, Welter ML, Lacomblez L, Golmard JL, Derenne JP, Agid Y. Parkinson's disease and sleepiness: an integral part of PD. Neurology. 2002;58:1019–24.
2. Ghorayeb I, Loundou A, Auquier P, Dauvilliers Y, Bioulac B, Tison F. A nationwide survey of excessive daytime sleepiness in Parkinson's disease in France. Mov Disord. 2007;22:1567–72.
3. Schenck CH, Bundlie SR, Mahowald MW. REM sleep behaviour disorder (RBD) delayed emergence of parkinsonism and/or dementia in 65 % of older men initially diagnosed with idiopathic RBD, and an analysis of the maximum and minimum tonic and/or phasic electromyographic abnormalities found during REM sleep. Sleep. 2003;26(Suppl):A316.
4. Abbott RD, Ross GW, White LR, Tanner CM, Masaki KH, Nelson JS, Curb JD, Petrovitch H. Excessive daytime sleepiness and subsequent development of Parkinson disease. Neurology. 2005;65:1442–6.

5. Happe S, Baier PC, Helmschmied K, Meller J, Tatsch K, Paulus W. Association of daytime sleepiness with nigrostriatal dopaminergic degeneration in early Parkinson's disease. J Neurol. 2007;254:1037–43.

6. Postuma RB, Montplaisir J. Potential early markers of Parkinson's disease in idiopathic rapid-eye-movement sleep behaviour disorder. Lancet Neurol. 2006;5:552–3.

7. Fort P, Bassetti CL, Luppi PH. Alternating vigilance states: new insights regarding neuronal networks and mechanisms. Eur J Neurosci. 2009;29:1741–53.

8. Jones BE. Basic mechanisms of sleep-wake states. In: Kryger MH, Roth T, Dement WC, editors. Principles and practice of sleep medicine. Philadelphia: WB Saunders; 1994.

9. Gervasoni D, Darracq L, Fort P, Souliere F, Chouvet G, Luppi PH. Electrophysiological evidence that noradrenergic neurons of the rat locus coeruleus are tonically inhibited by GABA during sleep. Eur J Neurosci. 1998;10:964–70.

10. Gervasoni D, Peyron C, Rampon C, Barbagli B, Chouvet G, Urbain N, Fort P, Luppi PH. Role and origin of the GABAergic innervation of dorsal raphe serotonergic neurons. J Neurosci. 2000;20:4217–25.

11. Sherin JE, Shiromani PJ, McCarley RW, Saper CB. Activation of ventrolateral preoptic neurons during sleep. Science. 1996;271:216–9.

12. Gvilia I, Turner A, McGinty D, Szymusiak R. Preoptic area neurons and the homeostatic regulation of rapid eye movement sleep. J Neurosci. 2006;26:3037–44.

13. Novak CM, Nunez AA. Daily rhythms in Fos activity in the rat ventrolateral preoptic area and midline thalamic nuclei. Am J Physiol. 1998;275:R1620–6. JID – 0370511.

14. Lu J, Greco MA, Shiromani P, Saper CB. Effect of lesions of the ventrolateral preoptic nucleus on NREM and REM sleep. J Neurosci. 2000;20:3830–42.

15. Gallopin T, Fort P, Eggermann E, Cauli B, Luppi PH, Rossier J, Audinat E, Muhlethaler M, Serafin M. Identification of sleep-promoting neurons in vitro. Nature. 2000;404:992–5.

16. Eggermann E, Serafin M, Bayer L, Machard D, Saint-Mleux B, Jones BE, Muhlethaler M. Orexins/hypocretins excite basal forebrain cholinergic neurones. Neuroscience. 2001;108:177–81.

17. Gallopin T, Luppi PH, Cauli B, Urade Y, Rossier J, Hayaishi O, Lambolez B, Fort P. The endogenous somnogen adenosine excites a subset of sleep-promoting neurons via A2A receptors in the ventrolateral preoptic nucleus. Neuroscience. 2005;134:1377–90.

18. Porkka-Heiskanen T, Strecker RE, Mccarley RW. Brain site-specificity of extracellular adenosine concentration changes during sleep deprivation and spontaneous sleep: an in vivo microdialysis study. Neuroscience. 2000;99:507–17. JID – 7605074.

19. Rainnie DG, Grunze HC, McCarley RW, Greene RW. Adenosine inhibition of mesopontine cholinergic neurons: implications for EEG arousal. Science. 1994;263:689–92.

20. Huang ZL, Qu WM, Eguchi N, Chen JF, Schwarzschild MA, Fredholm BB, Urade Y, Hayaishi O. Adenosine A2A, but not A1, receptors mediate the arousal effect of caffeine. Nat Neurosci. 2005;8:858–9.

21. Stenberg D, Litonius E, Halldner L, Johansson B, Fredholm BB, Porkka-Heiskanen T. Sleep and its homeostatic regulation in mice lacking the adenosine A1 receptor. J Sleep Res. 2003;12:283–90.

22. Urade Y, Eguchi N, Qu WM, Sakata M, Huang ZL, Chen JF, Schwarzschild MA, Fink JS, Hayaishi O. Minireview: sleep regulation in adenosine A(2A) receptor-deficient mice. Neurology. 2003;61:S94–6.

23. Fort P, Luppi PH, Gallopin T. In vitro identification of the presumed sleep-promoting neurons of the ventrolateral preoptic nucleus (VLPO). In: Luppi PH, editor. Sleep: circuits and functions. CRC Press; 2005.

24. Jouvet M. Recherches sur les structures nerveuses et les mécanismes responsables des différentes phases du sommeil physiologique. Arch Ital Biol. 1962;100:125–206.

25. Sakai K. Neurons responsible for paradoxical sleep. In: Wauquier A, Janssen Research Foundation, editors. Sleep: neurotransmitters and neuromodulators. New York: Raven Press; 1985.

26. Sakai K, Koyama Y. Are there cholinergic and non-cholinergic paradoxical sleep-on neurones in the pons? Neuroreport. 1996;7:2449–53.
27. Clement O, Sapin E, Berod A, Fort P, Luppi PH. Evidence that neurons of the sublaterodorsal tegmental nucleus triggering paradoxical (REM) sleep are glutamatergic. Sleep. 2011;34:419–23.
28. Chase MH, Soja PJ, Morales FR. Evidence that glycine mediates the postsynaptic potentials that inhibit lumbar motoneurons during the atonia of active sleep. J Neurosci. 1989;9:743–51.
29. Soja PJ, Lopez-Rodriguez F, Morales FR, Chase MH. The postsynaptic inhibitory control of lumbar motoneurons during the atonia of active sleep: effect of strychnine on motoneuron properties. J Neurosci. 1991;11:2804–11.
30. Yamuy J, Fung SJ, Xi M, Morales FR, Chase MH. Hypoglossal motoneurons are postsynaptically inhibited during carbachol-induced rapid eye movement sleep. Neuroscience. 1999;94:11–5.
31. Kodama T, Lai YY, Siegel JM. Changes in inhibitory amino acid release linked to pontine-induced atonia: an in vivo microdialysis study. J Neurosci. 2003;23:1548–54.
32. Brooks PL, Peever JH. Identification of the transmitter and receptor mechanisms responsible for REM sleep paralysis. J Neurosci. 2012;32:9785–95.
33. Brooks PL, Peever JH. Impaired GABA and glycine transmission triggers cardinal features of rapid eye movement sleep behavior disorder in mice. J Neurosci. 2011;31:7111–21.
34. Boissard R, Gervasoni D, Schmidt MH, Barbagli B, Fort P, Luppi PH. The rat ponto-medullary network responsible for paradoxical sleep onset and maintenance: a combined microinjection and functional neuroanatomical study. Eur J Neurosci. 2002;16:1959–73.
35. Sirieix C, Gervasoni D, Luppi PH, Leger L. Role of the lateral paragigantocellular nucleus in the network of paradoxical (REM) sleep: an electrophysiological and anatomical study in the rat. PLoS One. 2012;7:e28724.
36. Sapin E, Lapray D, Berod A, Goutagny R, Leger L, Ravassard P, Clement O, Hanriot L, Fort P, Luppi PH. Localization of the brainstem GABAergic neurons controlling paradoxical (REM) sleep. PLoS One. 2009;4:e4272.
37. Boissard R, Gervasoni D, Fort P, Henninot V, Barbagli B, Luppi PH. Neuronal networks responsible for paradoxical sleep onset and maintenance in rats: a new hypothesis. Sleep. 2000;23(Suppl):107.
38. Sastre JP, Buda C, Kitahama K, Jouvet M. Importance of the ventrolateral region of the periaqueductal gray and adjacent tegmentum in the control of paradoxical sleep as studied by muscimol microinjections in the cat. Neuroscience. 1996;74:415–26.
39. Lu J, Sherman D, Devor M, Saper CB. A putative flip-flop switch for control of REM sleep. Nature. 2006;441:589–94.
40. Darracq L, Gervasoni D, Souliere F, Lin JS, Fort P, Chouvet G, Luppi PH. Effect of strychnine on rat locus coeruleus neurones during sleep and wakefulness. Neuroreport. 1996;8:351–5.
41. Nitz D, Siegel J. GABA release in the dorsal raphe nucleus: role in the control of REM sleep. Am J Physiol. 1997;273:R451–5.
42. Nitz D, Siegel JM. GABA release in the locus coeruleus as a function of sleep/wake state. Neuroscience. 1997;78:795–801.
43. Luppi PH, Peyron C, Rampon C, Gervasoni D, Barbagli B, Boissard R, Fort P. Inhibitory mechanisms in the dorsal raphe nucleus and locus coeruleus during sleep. In: Lydic R, Baghdoyan HA, editors. Handbook of behavioral state control. CRC Press; 1999.
44. Verret L, Fort P, Gervasoni D, Leger L, Luppi PH. Localization of the neurons active during paradoxical (REM) sleep and projecting to the locus coeruleus noradrenergic neurons in the rat. J Comp Neurol. 2006;495:573–86.
45. Verret L, Fort P, Luppi PH. Localization of the neurons responsible for the inhibition of locus coeruleus noradrenergic neurons during paradoxical sleep in the rat. Sleep. 2003;26:69.
46. Goutagny R, Luppi PH, Salvert D, Lapray D, Gervasoni D, Fort P. Role of the dorsal paragigantocellular reticular nucleus in paradoxical (rapid eye movement) sleep generation: a combined electrophysiological and anatomical study in the rat. Neuroscience. 2008;152:849–57.

47. Clement O, Sapin E, Libourel PA, Arthaud S, Brischoux F, Fort P, Luppi PH. The lateral hypothalamic area controls paradoxical (REM) sleep by means of descending projections to brainstem GABAergic neurons. J Neurosci. 2012;32:16763–74.

48. Verret L, Goutagny R, Fort P, Cagnon L, Salvert D, Leger L, Boissard R, Salin P, Peyron C, Luppi PH. A role of melanin-concentrating hormone producing neurons in the central regulation of paradoxical sleep. BMC Neurosci. 2003;4:19.

49. Ahnaou A, Drinkenburg WH, Bouwknecht JA, Alcazar J, Steckler T, Dautzenberg FM. Blocking melanin-concentrating hormone MCH1 receptor affects rat sleep-wake architecture. Eur J Pharmacol. 2008;579:177–88.

50. Adamantidis A, Salvert D, Goutagny R, Lakaye B, Gervasoni D, Grisar T, Luppi PH, Fort P. Sleep architecture of the melanin-concentrating hormone receptor 1-knockout mice. Eur J Neurosci. 2008;27:1793–800.

51. Willie JT, Sinton CM, Maratos-Flier E, Yanagisawa M. Abnormal response of melanin-concentrating hormone deficient mice to fasting: hyperactivity and rapid eye movement sleep suppression. Neuroscience. 2008;156:819–29.

52. Jego S, Glasgow SD, Herrera CG, Ekstrand M, Reed SJ, Boyce R, Friedman J, Burdakov D, Adamantidis AR. Optogenetic identification of a rapid eye movement sleep modulatory circuit in the hypothalamus. Nat Neurosci. 2013;16(11):1637–43.

53. Konadhode RR, Pelluru D, Blanco-Centurion C, Zayachkivsky A, Liu M, Uhde T, Glen Jr WB, van den Pol AN, Mulholland PJ, Shiromani PJ. Optogenetic stimulation of MCH neurons increases sleep. J Neurosci. 2013;33:10257–63.

54. Gervasoni D, Lin SC, Ribeiro S, Soares ES, Pantoja J, Nicolelis MA. Global forebrain dynamics predict rat behavioral states and their transitions. J Neurosci. 2004;24:11137–47.

55. Miller JD, Farber J, Gatz P, Roffwarg H, German DC. Activity of mesencephalic dopamine and non-dopamine neurons across stages of sleep and walking in the rat. Brain Res. 1983;273:133–41.

56. Trulson ME, Preussler DW. Dopamine-containing ventral tegmental area neurons in freely moving cats: activity during the sleep-waking cycle and effects of stress. Exp Neurol. 1984;83:367–77.

57. Dahan L, Astier B, Vautrelle N, Urbain N, Kocsis B, Chouvet G. Prominent burst firing of dopaminergic neurons in the ventral tegmental area during paradoxical sleep. Neuropsychopharmacology. 2007;32:1232–41.

58. Leger L, Sapin E, Goutagny R, Peyron C, Salvert D, Fort P, Luppi PH. Dopaminergic neurons expressing Fos during waking and paradoxical sleep in the rat. J Chem Neuroanat. 2010;39:262–71.

59. Maloney KJ, Mainville L, Jones BE. c-Fos expression in dopaminergic and GABAergic neurons of the ventral mesencephalic tegmentum after paradoxical sleep deprivation and recovery. Eur J Neurosci. 2002;15:774–8.

60. Lena I, Parrot S, Deschaux O, Muffat-Joly S, Sauvinet V, Renaud B, Suaud-Chagny MF, Gottesmann C. Variations in extracellular levels of dopamine, noradrenaline, glutamate, and aspartate across the sleep–wake cycle in the medial prefrontal cortex and nucleus accumbens of freely moving rats. J Neurosci Res. 2005;81:891–9.

61. Jones BE, Bobillier P, Pin C, Jouvet M. The effect of lesions of catecholamine-containing neurons upon monoamine content of the brain and EEG and behavioral waking in the cat. Brain Res. 1973;58:157–77.

62. Wisor JP, Nishino S, Sora I, Uhl GH, Mignot E, Edgar DM. Dopaminergic role in stimulant-induced wakefulness. J Neurosci. 2001;21(5):1787–94.

63. Monti JM, Monti D. The involvement of dopamine in the modulation of sleep and waking. Sleep Med Rev. 2007;11:113–33.

64. Pungor K, Papp M, Kekesi K, Juhasz G. A novel effect of MPTP: the selective suppression of paradoxical sleep in cats. Brain Res. 1990;525:310–4.

65. Monaca C, Laloux C, Jacquesson JM, Gele P, Marechal X, Bordet R, Destee A, Derambure P. Vigilance states in a parkinsonian model, the MPTP mouse. Eur J Neurosci. 2004;20:2474–8.

66. Barraud Q, Lambrecq V, Forni C, McGuire S, Hill M, Bioulac B, Balzamo E, Bezard E, Tison F, Ghorayeb I. Sleep disorders in Parkinson's disease: the contribution of the MPTP non-human primate model. Exp Neurol. 2009;219:574–82.

67. Schenck CH, Bundlie SR, Ettinger MG, Mahowald MW. Chronic behavioral disorders of human REM sleep: a new category of parasomnia. Sleep. 1986;9:293–308.

68. Iranzo A, Santamaria J, Tolosa E. The clinical and pathophysiological relevance of REM sleep behavior disorder in neurodegenerative diseases. Sleep Med Rev. 2009;13:385–401.

69. Krenzer M, Anaclet C, Vetrivelan R, Wang N, Vong L, Lowell BB, Fuller PM, Lu J. Brainstem and spinal cord circuitry regulating REM sleep and muscle atonia. PLoS One. 2011;6:e24998.

70. Holmes CJ, Jones BE. Importance of cholinergic, GABAergic, serotonergic and other neurons in the medial medullary reticular formation for sleep-wake states studied by cytotoxic lesions in the cat. Neuroscience. 1994;62:1179–200.

71. Schenkel E, Siegel JM. REM sleep without atonia after lesions of the medial medulla. Neurosci Lett. 1989;98:159–65.

72. Hendricks JC, Morrison AR, Mann GL. Different behaviors during paradoxical sleep without atonia depend on pontine lesion site. Brain Res. 1982;239:81–105.

73. Henley K, Morrison AR. A re-evaluation of the effects of lesions of the pontine tegmentum and locus coeruleus on phenomena of paradoxical sleep in the cat. Acta Neurobiol Exp (Warsz). 1974;34:215–32.

74. Sastre JP, Jouvet M. Le comportement onirique du chat [Oneiric behavior in cats]. Physiol Behav. 1979;22:979–89.

75. Webster HH, Jones BE. Neurotoxic lesions of the dorsolateral pontomesencephalic tegmentum-cholinergic cell area in the cat. II. Effects upon sleep-waking states. Brain Res. 1988;458:285–302.

76. Mahowald MW, Schenck CH. REM sleep behavior disorder. In: Kryger MH, Roth T, Dement WC, editors. Principles and practice of sleep medicine. Philadelphia: Saunders; 2000.

77. Lai YY, Hsieh KC, Nguyen D, Peever J, Siegel JM. Neurotoxic lesions at the ventral mesopontine junction change sleep time and muscle activity during sleep: an animal model of motor disorders in sleep. Neuroscience. 2008;154:431–43.

78. Brooks PL, Peever JH. Glycinergic and GABA(A)-mediated inhibition of somatic motoneurons does not mediate rapid eye movement sleep motor atonia. J Neurosci. 2008;28:3535–45.

79. Burgess C, Lai D, Siegel J, Peever J. An endogenous glutamatergic drive onto somatic motoneurons contributes to the stereotypical pattern of muscle tone across the sleep-wake cycle. J Neurosci. 2008;28:4649–60.

80. Chase MH, Morales FR. The atonia and myoclonia of active (REM) sleep. Annu Rev Psychol. 1990;41:557–84.

81. Du Beau A, Shakya Shrestha S, Bannatyne BA, Jalicy SM, Linnen S, Maxwell DJ. Neurotransmitter phenotypes of descending systems in the rat lumbar spinal cord. Neuroscience. 2012;227:67–79.

82. Holstege G. Descending motor pathways and the spinal motor system: limbic and non-limbic components. Prog Brain Res. 1991;87:307–421.

83. Evarts EV. Temporal patterns of discharge of pyramidal tract neurons during sleep and waking in the monkey. J Neurophysiol. 1964;27:152–71.

84. Evarts EV. Relation of cell size to effects of sleep in pyramidal tract neurons. Prog Brain Res. 1965;18:81–91.

85. Oudiette D, Leu-Semenescu S, Roze E, Vidailhet M, De Cock VC, Golmard JL, Arnulf I. A motor signature of REM sleep behavior disorder. Mov Disord. 2012;27:428–31.

86. Arnulf I. REM sleep behavior disorder: motor manifestations and pathophysiology. Mov Disord. 2012;27:677–89.

Objective Measures of the Sleep–Wake Cycle in Parkinson's Disease

4

Valérie Cochen De Cock

Contents

Abstract

Complaints about sleep–wake cycle are frequent in patients with Parkinson's disease (PD). Nocturnal sleep in PD may be impaired by several factors: motor phenomena related to the disease such as nocturnal bradykinesia/akinesia, rigidity, tremor or nocturia, and comorbid sleep disorders such as insomnia, restless legs syndrome (RLS), periodic limb movements (PLMs), circadian rhythm alteration, sleep disordered breathing, and rapid-eye-movement (REM) sleep behavior disorder (RBD). Moreover, daytime sleepiness and sleep attacks are frequently reported in patients with PD. Numerous studies evaluating sleep in PD have

V. Cochen De Cock
Service des pathologies du sommeil, Clinique Beau Soleil,
119 avenue de Lodève, 34070 Montpellier, France
e-mail: valerie.cochen@gmail.com

© Springer-Verlag Wien 2015

A. Videnovic, B. Högl (eds.), *Disorders of Sleep and Circadian Rhythms in Parkinson's Disease*, DOI 10.1007/978-3-7091-1631-9_4

pressed that not only the illness but also dopaminergic treatments may play an important role in these sleep disorders.

Questionnaires have been developed to identify sleep disorders in the context of PD, but objective measures are needed to confirm diagnoses and inform treatments to the patients.

Videopolysomnographic recording is the gold standard to explore sleep and to diagnose PLMs, sleep disordered breathing, and RBD. Suggested immobilization test is a useful measure to explore RLS especially in patients with PD. Excessive daytime sleepiness is usually explored as in central hypersomnia by multiple sleep latency test (MSLT) but actigraphy or 24-h ambulatory polysomnography could be interesting tools to evaluate sleepiness at home, in a more naturalistic way. Maintenance of wakefulness test (MWT) is interesting to evaluate vigilance and though the efficacy of the different treatments used to improve sleepiness.

4.1 Introduction

Sleep disorders are frequently reported in patients with Parkinson's disease (PD) [1–3]. Sleep questionnaires may allow the detection of most of these disorders, but objective measures are needed to explore sleep quality and to diagnose most of the sleep disorders associated with PD such as restless legs syndrome (RLS), periodic limb movements (PLMs), circadian rhythm alteration, sleep disordered breathing, REM sleep behavior disorder (RBD), and daytime sleepiness. Videopolysomnographic recordings, suggested immobilization test (SIT), multiple sleep latency test (MSLT), actigraphy, and maintenance of wakefulness test (MWT) are the most useful objective methods to explore sleep disorders, sleepiness, and the efficacy of treatments for sleep–wake disturbances in PD.

4.2 Videopolysomnographic Recordings

Videopolysomnography is the gold standard to explore sleep. It allows quantifying total sleep time, sleep efficiency, sleep latency, sleep architecture, sleep fragmentation, PLM, respiratory events, and RBD [4].

Videopolysomnography associates multiple channels electroencephalogram, electrooculogram, chin electromyogram (EMG), leg EMG, airflow parameters, respiratory effort parameters, oxygen saturation, position, sound and video recordings. Sleep stages, and microarousals, are scored through visual inspection of 30 epochs according to standard criteria [4].

Night sleep recordings in large studies with treated and untreated patients with PD have demonstrated decreased sleep efficiency, increased wake time after sleep onset, and sleep fragmentation [5]. Changes in slow wave sleep and REM sleep duration are inconsistent from one study to another. Impaired sleep continuity may be due to the neurodegenerative process itself, or may be associated with nocturnal bradykinesia and rigidity, medication, psychiatric complications, nocturia, and impaired circadian rhythm. Finally, PLMs sleep disordered breathing, or RBD may also disrupt sleep in PD.

4.2.1 Periodic Limb Movements

PLMs are disruptive leg movements or sometimes only muscles contractions without movement occurring mostly during sleep (for more details please refer Chap. 12).

Surface EMG from the left and right anterior tibialis muscles are used to quantify leg movements. PLMs are scored according to American Academy of Sleep Medicine (AASM) scoring manual [4], as all events lasting between 0.5 and 10 s, with a minimum amplitude increase of 8 μV from the resting EMG voltage, separated by intervals of 5–90 s and arising in series of at least four consecutive movements [4].

Patients with PD exhibit significantly higher PLM indices both during wakefulness and sleep compared to age and sex match controls [6]. PLMs are more frequent during sleep stage 1 and 2 in patients with PD as it has been reported in patients with idiopathic RLS and PLM disorder [7], but PLM index in PD is also high during REM sleep probably because of an abnormal disinhibition of the motor system during REM sleep in this extrapyramidal disorder [6]. Moreover, PLMs are also present in drug-free patients with PD showing that this movement disorder may not result from dopaminergic treatment [6].

4.2.2 Sleep Disordered Breathing

According to the AASM scoring manual [4], an apnea event is defined as a decrease of at least 90 % of the peak thermal sensor excursion lasting at least 10 s. An hypopnea event is defined as a ≥30 % decrease in nasal pressure signal excursions lasting at least 10 s with a ≥4 % decrease in SpO2 from the preceding baseline value, or as a ≥50 % decrease in nasal pressure signal excursions lasting at least 10 s with a ≥3 % decrease in SpO2 from the preceding baseline value. The apnea hypopnea index (AHI) is calculated as the total number of apnea and hypopnea events per hour of sleep. The presence of sleep apnea is defined as an apnea/hypopnea index greater than 5, and classified as mild (AHI greater than or equal to 5 and lower than or equal to 15), moderate (AHI greater than 15 and lower than or equal to 30), and severe (greater than 30) sleep apnea. Sleep apnea episodes are typically classified as obstructive sleep apnea, central sleep apnea, and mixed sleep apnea. The criterion differentiating these categories is the presence or absence of concomitant respiratory efforts [4].

When the cutoff for the AHI is set at 15 events per hour, the prevalence of obstructive sleep apnea (OSA) syndrome is estimated at about 20 % of the general population of the United States [8]. Different studies have shown that the prevalence of OSA in patients with PD ranges from 14.5 to 22.4 %, using the same cutoff value for AHI [9–12], suggesting that this disorder has a similar prevalence in the PD population as in the general population and indicating that the clinical significance of OSA as a contributor to daytime sleepiness in PD is probably low [9–12]. For more details please refer Chap. 7.

Sleep disordered breathing can also be explored by respiratory polygraphy, but in the context of PD where sleep fragmentation is important it may induce diagnostic errors (by excess or defect) and polysomnography should be preferred.

Strider, an inspiratory high pitched sound secondary to a laryngeal dysfunction is a harbinger for multiple systeme atrophy but it has also recently been described as a side effect of deep brain stimulation as in PD [13].

4.2.3 REM Sleep Behavior Disorder

Rapid-eye-movement (REM) sleep behavior disorder (RBD) is characterized by abnormal and often harmful motor behaviors associated with dream mentation that causes sleep disruption and/or injuries to the patient or the bed partner [14]. The behaviors during RBD include mostly jerks and minor movements of the limbs, gesturing, grabbing, slapping, punching, kicking, sitting up and leaping from bed, but rarely standing up and walking [15]. Nonviolent elaborate behaviors (eating, smoking, bicycling, kissing) may also occur during RBD [16].

RBD is accompanied by polysomnographic (PSG) abnormalities in REM sleep. Normally, muscle atonia and EEG desynchronization are present throughout the REM period and constitute tonic features of REM sleep in humans. Phasic events occur intermittently during REM sleep and include bursts of rapid eye movements, and facial and limb muscle twitches. In patients with RBD, both tonic and phasic components of REM sleep are altered. Partial or complete loss of tonic chin EMG atonia (REM sleep without atonia or RSWA) and increase of chin and limb phasic EMG activities are characteristic features in patients with RBD [17].

According to AASM manual [4], each 30-s epoch should be scored as tonic if chin EMG activity (EMG amplitude greater than the minimum amplitude than in non-REM sleep) is present for more than 50 % of the epoch duration. Phasic chin EMG density is scored from the submental EMG activity and represents the percentage of 3-s miniepochs containing EMG events lasting 0.1–5 s, with an amplitude exceeding four times the amplitude of background EMG activity. A tonic chin EMG density greater than 30 % and a phasic chin EMG density greater than 15 % allows for the correctly classification of 86 % of 80 patients with idiopathic RBD vs. 80 age- and sex-matched controls [17]. Sleep monitoring allows differentiating REM sleep behavior disorders from the complex movements sometimes observed during sleep apnea [18]. Simultaneous recording of the mentalis, flexor digitorum superficialis, and extensor digitorum brevis muscles provides the highest rates of REM sleep phasic EMG activity in subjects with RBD so that they should be explored [19]. RBD is present in more than 50% of the patients with PD [20, 21]. Suppeisingly patients with PD have an improvement of the quality of their movement during RBD [20].

4.2.3.1 Bruxism

It has recently been shown that bruxism could also be associated with RBD. Exploration of temporalis and masseter muscles tone could also be interesting in patients complaining of noisy or painful contractions of the jaw during sleep in order to evaluate if this contraction also appears during REM sleep [22].

4.2.4 Dystonia and Dyskinesia

In order to identify abnormal movements of the neck or the trunk, other muscles can be explored during sleep such as sternocleidomastoid, splenius, and thoraco-lumbar paraspinal muscles. Usually in PD, abnormal dyskinetic movements disappear during sleep but they can delay sleep onset and increase wakefulness during sleep.

4.3 Suggested Immobilization Test (SIT)

The SIT is a tool developed recently to objectively assess primary RLS. It assesses both subjective leg discomfort and objective leg movements during a 1-h period of immobility prior to bedtime [23].

The diagnosis of RLS is based on four clinical criteria: (1) an urge to move the legs, usually accompanied or caused by uncomfortable and unpleasant sensations in the legs; (2) symptoms begin or worsen during periods of rest or inactivity; (3) symptoms are partially or totally relieved by movement, such as walking or stretching; and (4) the urge to move or unpleasant sensations are worse in the evening or night than during the day [24]. Patients with PD frequently complain about leg discomfort and the clinical overlap between RLS, "wearing-off" related lower limb discomfort, cramps, and lower pain thresholds in PD is an important diagnostic confound [25]. Polysomnography recordings (PSG) reveal the presence of PLMs during sleep in 80 % of the patients with idiopathic RLS but PLMs during PSG are frequently reported in PD regardless of RLS status [6].

SIT is administered in the evening and lasts for 1 h. During the SIT, the patients remain in bed reclined at 45° angle with their legs outstretched. They are instructed to avoid moving voluntarily for the entire duration of the test. Surface EMG from the left and right anterior tibialis muscles is used to quantify periodic leg movements. The latter is scored according to the criteria defined by Michaud et al. [26] (i.e., all movements lasting between 0.5 and 10 s, separated by intervals of 4–90 s, and arising in series of at least four consecutive movements). The SIT periodic leg movements' index represents the number of periodic leg movements per hour of immobility. Patients report severity of leg discomfort on a visual analogue scale (VAS) ranging from 0 (no discomfort) to 100 (extreme discomfort) every 10 min during the SIT. The mean leg discomfort score is assessed using the average of the 7 values, as well as the discomfort severity at the end of the test (time 60 min). In patients with PD, the usual schedule of the dopaminergic treatment is not changed before the test.

We recently demonstrated that the mean leg discomfort score in SIT is increased in patients with PD and RLS compared to patients with PD without RLS [27]. Leg discomfort is significantly higher at the end of the test in patients with RLS compared to patients without RLS (Fig. 4.1). Using a mean leg discomfort cut-off of 11, we showed sensitivity of 91 % and specificity of 72 % for RLS diagnosis in PD during symptomatic time intervals. PLM index during SIT and during sleep did not differ between PD patients with and without RLS so that PLMs index cannot be used as

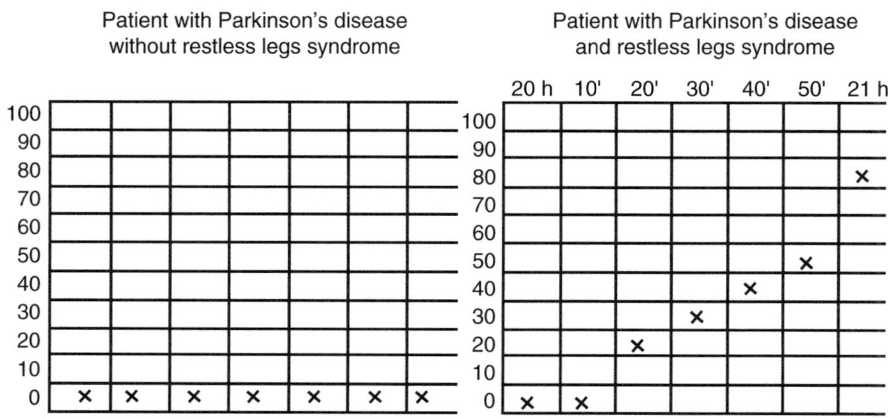

Fig. 4.1 Examples of reports of severity of leg discomfort on the visual analogue scale in a patient with PD without (*left*) and a patient with (*right*) RLS during the SIT

indirect diagnosis criteria of RLS in PD. The mean leg discomfort and the increase of leg discomfort during the 1 h of the SIT may be useful in diagnosing RLS in PD.

4.4 Multiple Sleep Latency Test (MSLT)

Since initial description of sleep attacks at the wheel in patients with PD treated with dopamine agonists [28], many reports have focused on excessive daytime sleepiness (EDS) in patients with PD but the best method to explore EDS in PD remains unclear. The subjective nature of EDS complaint, the definition used, the different populations targeted, the potential confounding factors, and the various methodological tools used to evaluate sleepiness explain most of the discrepancies between studies on EDS prevalence and risk factors in PD.

Multiple sleep latency test (MSLT) is the gold standard to objectively explore sleepiness in central hypersomnia [29]. Several studies have recorded nighttime sleep and MSLT to objectively measure hypersomnia in patients with PD [30–34]. Surprisingly, none of the controlled studies found significant differences on the mean sleep latency on MSLT between unselected patients and controls [30, 32, 33]. A narcoleptic-like phenotype was also reported in unselected patients with PD [30, 31, 33]; this propensity increased when patients were selected for sleepiness reaching 39 % [31] or hallucinations 60 % [36].

MSLT is an objective measure of daytime sleepiness. Patients receive the instruction not to fight against sleep. According to the AASM manual [4], the MSLT consists in five nap opportunities, scheduled at 2-h intervals, starting 2 h after awakening. Psychotropic drugs must be discontinued at least 2 weeks (depending on the half-life) before the recording. Each test is terminated after a 15-min sleep period or after 20 min if the patient does not fall asleep. Both sleep and REM sleep latencies are measured. Mean sleep latency below 8 min confirms the EDS. Latency below 5 min indicates severe sleepiness. Latency over 10 min is considered as normal. Between eight and ten, the interpretation depends on the clinical status of the patient. A sleep onset REM period (SOREM) defined as the occurrence of REM sleep within 15 min after sleep onset is also screened, with a narcoleptic phenotype defined as the presence of at least two SOREM on the MSLT.

As the sensitivity of MSLT to identify PD patients with disabling sleepiness remains questionable, further studies are required to validate the best methods to screen and objective hypersomnia in PD. Alternative methods to assess daytime sleepiness should be monitored in future in PD that may include the maintenance of wakefulness test or even more a prolonged 24-h continuous sleep recording in standardized conditions.

4.5 Maintenance of Wakefulness Test (MWT)

MWT is an objective measure of daytime wakefulness. It measures the ability to remain awake.

MWT consists in four 40 min tests, scheduled at 2-h intervals, starting 2 h after awakening. During the MWT the room is dimly illuminated and the subject lies in a semi-reclining position with the instruction to resist sleep [35, 36]. Subjects are not allowed to maintain wakefulness by using extraordinary measures such as slapping the face or singing. Recordings are monitored by a trained technologist. Each trial is terminated at the first onset of sleep (sleep onset) or, if sleep onset is not achieved, after a maximum in-bed duration of 40 min. Mean sleep latency below 11 min confirms the sleepiness [35, 36].

The MWT has clinical usefulness in evaluating response to treatment of sleepiness. In PD, a significant, but small, relationship between subjective (ESS) and objective (MWT) measures of daytime alertness has been observed [37]. Interestingly, using MWT, Bliwise et al. have shown that relative to unmediated patients, all classes of dopaminergic medications were associated with reduced daytime alertness, and this effect was not mediated by disease duration or disease severity. Further, the results showed that increasing dosages of dopamine agonists were associated with less daytime alertness, whereas higher levels of levodopa were associated with higher levels of alertness [37].

4.6 Ambulatory Polysomnography

PSG recording of wake and sleep activities at home or in the sleep laboratory is another way to explore sleepiness during the day in patients with PD. It allows observing sleep attacks and sleeping episodes during the day in naturalistic conditions. Only one study to our knowledge has evaluated sleep and wake cycle in PD using this method [38]. This study allowed them to show that sleep attacks are an extreme manifestation of increased daytime sleepiness.

4.7 Actigraphy

Actigraphy is a noninvasive method for monitoring human rest–activity cycles. A small accelerometer unit is worn on the wrist by the patient to measure motor activity. Absence of movement, measured by actigraphy, has proved to be a good proxy of nighttime sleep quality and correlates with PSG and subjective sleep measures [39]. It has recently been shown that actigraphy correlates to sleep measures by PSG even in patients with PD where akinesia could have been misleading [40].

Conclusion

Objective measures to explore sleep–wake cycle and sleep disorders in PD encompass videopolysomnography, suggested immobilization test, and MSLT. Other methods such as MWT, 24-h ambulatory PSG, and actigraphy have also been recently used, mainly to explore sleepiness. Even if these methods are not specific to PD, they allow good identification of most sleep disorders. However, limits such as the absence of specific criteria for sleep stages identification in a disease where EEG is frequently impaired because of neurodegeneration and the low sensibility of MSLT to objectively measure sleepiness suggest that more accurate methods should be developed for the assessment of sleep and alertness in PD.

References

1. De Cock VC, Vidailhet M, Arnulf I. Sleep disturbances in patients with parkinsonism. Nat Clin Pract Neurol. 2008;4:254–66.
2. Arnulf I, Leu S, Oudiette D. Abnormal sleep and sleepiness in Parkinson's disease. Curr Opin Neurol. 2008;21:472–7.
3. Louter M, Aarden WC, Lion J, Bloem BR, Overeem S. Recognition and diagnosis of sleep disorders in Parkinson's disease. J Neurol. 2012;259:2031–40.
4. Iber C, Ancoli-Israel S, Chesson AL, Quan SF, American Academy of Sleep Medicine. The AASM manual for the scoring of sleep and associated events: rules, terminology, and technical specifications. Westchester: American Academy of Sleep Medicine; 2007.
5. Peerally T, Yong MH, Chokroverty S, Tan EK. Sleep and Parkinson's disease: a review of case-control polysomnography studies. Mov Disord. 2012;27:1729–37.
6. Wetter TC, Collado-Seidel V, Pollmacher T, Yassouridis A, Trenkwalder C. Sleep and periodic leg movement patterns in drug-free patients with Parkinson's disease and multiple system atrophy. Sleep. 2000;23:361–7.
7. Pollmächer T, Schulz H. Periodic leg movements (PLM): their relationship to sleep stages. Sleep. 1993;16:572–7.
8. Young T, Shahar E, Nieto FJ, Redline S, Newman AB, Gottieb DJ, et al. Predictors of sleep-disordered breathing in community-dwelling adults: the Sleep Heart Health Study. Arch Intern Med. 2002;162:893–900.
9. Cochen De Cock V, Abouda M, Leu S, et al. Is obstructive sleep apnea a problem in Parkinson's disease? Sleep Med. 2010;11:247–52.
10. Diederich N, Vaillant M, Leischen M, Mancuso G, Golinval S, Nati R, et al. Sleep apnea syndrome in Parkinson's disease. A case–control study in 49 patients. Mov Disord. 2005;20:1413–8.

11. Trotti LM, Bliwise DL. No increased risk of obstructive sleep apnea in Parkinson's disease. Mov Disord. 2010;25:2246–9.

12. Takashi N, Inoue Y, Kobayashi M, Namba K, Nakashima K. Characteristics of obstructive sleep apnea in patients with Parkinson's disease. J Neurol Sci. 2013;327:22–4.

13. Fagbami OY, Donato AA. Stridor and dysphagia associated with subthalamic nucleus stimulation in Parkinson disease. J Neurosurg. 2011;115:1005–6.

14. Schenck CH, Hurwitz TD, Mahowald MW. Symposium: normal and abnormal REM sleep regulation: REM sleep behaviour disorder: an update on a series of 96 patients and a review of the world literature. J Sleep Res. 1993;2:224–31.

15. Schenck CH, Mahowald MW. REM sleep behavior disorder: clinical, developmental, and neuroscience perspectives 16 years after its formal identification in SLEEP. Sleep. 2002;25:120–38.

16. Oudiette D, De Cock VC, Lavault S, Leu S, Vidailhet M, Arnulf I. Nonviolent elaborate behaviors may also occur in REM sleep behavior disorder. Neurology. 2009;72:551–7.

17. Montplaisir J, Gagnon JF, Fantini ML, Postuma RB, Dauvilliers Y, Desautels A, et al. Polysomnographic diagnosis of idiopathic REM sleep behavior disorder. Mov Disord. 2010;25:2044–51.

18. Iranzo A, Santamaria J. Severe obstructive sleep apnea/hypopnea mimicking REM sleep behavior disorder. Sleep. 2005;28:203–6.

19. Frauscher B, Iranzo A, Högl B, Casanova-Molla J, Salamero M, Gschliesser V, Tolosa E, Poewe W, Santamaria J. Quantification of electromyographic activity during REM sleep in multiple muscles in REM sleep behavior disorder. Sleep. 2008;31:724–31.

20. De Cock VC, Vidailhet M, Leu S, et al. Restoration of normal motor control in Parkinson's disease during REM sleep. Brain. 2007;130:450–6.

21. Sixel-Doring F, Trautmann E, Mollenhauer B, Trenkwalder C. Associated factors for REM sleep behavior disorder in Parkinson disease. Neurology. 2011;77:1048–54.

22. Abe S, Gagnon JF, Montplaisir JY, Postuma RB, Rompré PH, Huynh NT, Kato T, Kawano F, Lavigne GJ. Sleep bruxism and oromandibular myoclonus in rapid eye movement sleep behavior disorder: a preliminary report. Sleep Med. 2013;14:1024–30.

23. Michaud M, Lavigne G, Desautels A, Poirier G, Montplaisir J. Effects of immobility on sensory and motor symptoms of restless legs syndrome. Mov Disord. 2002;17:112–5.

24. Allen RP, Picchietti D, Hening WA, Trenkwalder C, Walters AS, Montplaisi J. Restless legs syndrome: diagnostic criteria, special considerations, and epidemiology. A report from the restless legs syndrome diagnosis and epidemiology workshop at the National Institutes of Health. Sleep Med. 2003;4:101–19.

25. Garcia-Borreguero D, Odin P, Serrano C. Restless legs syndrome and PD: a review of the evidence for a possible association. Neurology. 2003;61:S49–55.

26. Michaud M, Poirier G, Lavigne G, Montplaisir J. Restless Legs Syndrome: scoring criteria for leg movements recorded during the suggested immobilization test. Sleep Med. 2001;2:317–21.

27. De Cock VC, Bayard S, Yu H, Grini M, Carlander B, Postuma R, Charif M, Dauvilliers Y. Suggested immobilization test for diagnosis of restless legs syndrome in Parkinson's disease. Mov Disord. 2012;27:743–9.

28. Frucht S, Rogers JD, Greene PE, Gordon MF, Fahn S. Falling asleep at the wheel: motor vehicle mishaps in persons taking pramipexole and ropinirole. Neurology. 1999;52:1908–10.

29. Littner MR, Kushida C, Wise M, Standards of Practice Committee of the American Academy of Sleep Medicine, et al. Practice parameters for clinical use of the multiple sleep latency test and the maintenance of wakefulness test. Sleep. 2005;28:113–21.

30. Rye DB, Bliwise DL, Dihenia B, Gurecki P. FAST TRACK: daytime sleepiness in Parkinson's disease. J Sleep Res. 2000;9:63–9.

31. Arnulf I, Konofal E, Merino-Andreu M, et al. Parkinson's disease and sleepiness: an integral part of PD. Neurology. 2002;58:1019–26.

32. Shpirer I, Miniovitz A, Klein C, Goldstein R, Prokhorov T, Theitler J, et al. Excessive daytime sleepiness in patients with Parkinson's disease: a polysomnography study. Mov Disord. 2006;21:1432–8.

33. Yong MH, Fook-Chong S, Pavanni R, Lim LL, Tan EK. Case control polysomnographic studies of sleep disorders in Parkinson's disease. PLoS One. 2011;6:e22511.
34. Arnulf I, Bonnet AM, Damier P, Bejjani BP, Seilhean D, Derenne JP, Agid Y. Hallucinations, REM sleep, and Parkinson's disease: a medical hypothesis. Neurology. 2000;55:281–8.
35. Doghramji K, Mitler MM, Sangal RB, et al. A normative study of the maintenance of wakefulness test (MWT). Electroencephalogr Clin Neurophysiol. 1997;103:554–62.
36. Sangal RB, Thomas L, Mitler MM. Maintenance of wakefuness test and multiple sleep latency test. Measurement of different abilities in patients with sleep disorders. Chest. 1992;101:898–902.
37. Bliwise DL, Shpirer I, Miniovitz A, Klein C, Goldstein R, Prokhorov T, Theitler J, et al. Daytime alertness in Parkinson's disease: potentially dose-dependent, divergent effects by drug class. Mov Disord. 2012;27:1118–24.
38. Manni R, Terzaghi M, Sartori I, Mancini F, Pacchetti C. Dopamine agonists and sleepiness in PD: review of the literature and personal findings. Sleep Med. 2004;5:189–93.
39. Stavitsky JL, Saurman P, McNamara A, Cronin-Golomb A. Sleep in Parkinson's disease: a comparison of actigraphy and subjective measures. Parkinsonism Relat Disord. 2010;16:280–3.
40. Kotschet K, Johnson W, McGregor S, Kettlewell J, Kyoong A, O'Driscoll DM, Turton AR, Griffiths RI, Horne MK. Daytime sleep in Parkinson's disease measured by episodes of immobility. Parkinsonism Relat Disord. 2014;20:578–83.

Subjective Assessment of Sleep and Sleepiness in Parkinson's Disease

5

Joan Santamaria

Contents

Abstract

Sleep disturbances in Parkinson's disease (PD) are common and need appropriate diagnosis and care. Sleep can be assessed in two ways: subjectively by asking patients about their symptoms and objectively with the help of electrophysiological sleep recordings. There are a number of validated scales to evaluate sleep in PD as well as electrophysiological sleep recordings. No validated scale or sleep test, however, can do the job of a thorough sleep history taken with the patient and bed partner. This needs time and a systematic approach defining the problem, schedules, behavior before sleep, during sleep, presence and timing of midnight awakenings and their cause, snoring, breathing pauses, dreaming, and abnormal movements during sleep and excessive sleepiness. Several scales can be used to screen sleep disorders, complementing – not replacing – the clinical sleep history. There is not yet an ideal scale for assessment of the whole spectrum

J. Santamaria, MD
Neurology Service and Multidisciplinary Sleep Disorders Unit, Hospital Clínic of Barcelona, University of Barcelona Medical School, Villarroel 170, 08036 Barcelona, Spain
e-mail: jsantama@clinic.cat

© Springer-Verlag Wien 2015

A. Videnovic, B. Högl (eds.), *Disorders of Sleep and Circadian Rhythms in Parkinson's Disease*, DOI 10.1007/978-3-7091-1631-9_5

of sleep problems in PD, although two have been developed specifically for use in PD, namely, the Parkinson's disease sleep scale and the SCOPA-sleep.

Sleep disturbances are frequent in Parkinson's disease (PD) and need appropriate diagnosis and care. Their evaluation is not easy, however, because the sleep complaints may be multiple, from insomnia or hypersomnia to parasomnias, and often need to be disentangled from the motor, sensory, and mood effects of the disease or its treatments. Sleep can generally be assessed in two ways: subjectively by asking patients about their symptoms and objectively with the help of electrophysiological sleep recordings. These two ways are informative and complementary with discrepancies sometimes in their results because they probably measure different aspects of the phenomenon [1, 2]. Today, there are a number of validated scales to assess sleep in PD, leaving perhaps the impression that by just using a sleep scale one can diagnose and measure the sleep problems of the patient. The same could be said about sleep recordings. As a general rule, however, no "valid" scale or sleep test can do the job of a thorough sleep history with the patient and bed partner.

In this chapter, an overview of the subjective assessment of sleep and sleepiness in PD focusing first on the clinical history and then on sleep scales is presented.

A detailed clinical sleep history is particularly necessary when a patient reports sleep complaints, either spontaneously or after questioning by the physician. One may start the interview by simply asking the *patient and bed partner* about their satisfaction with the quality of nocturnal sleep and the presence of problematic daytime sleepiness. In the absence of complaints, for routine clinical practice there is no need to ask anything else or to administer any sleep scale. One has to bear in mind, however, that sleep symptoms in patients with PD are often underreported [3] or even neglected, probably because they are considered "normal" in the context of parkinsonism, which logically attracts the attention of patients and caregivers. Therefore, when there are complaints about sleep or doubts about their presence a more detailed approach is mandatory, particularly in patients who sleep alone, or whose bed partner is unavailable.

5.1 How to Take a Sleep History

Taking a sleep history needs time and a systematic approach that can be summarized in the following seven steps.

First: *Defining the problem*. The first step is to clarify what specific problem is bothering the patient. The basic symptoms of sleep disorders are essentially three, which may appear alone or in combination: (a) inability to sleep as desired, (b) excessive daytime sleepiness, and (c) abnormal phenomena or behaviors during or around the sleep period. Each of these symptoms has many possible causes and with the clinical sleep history we have to look for the clues to identify them.

Second: *Sleep–wake schedule*. We always need to establish the characteristics of the major sleep episode, usually corresponding to nocturnal sleep, going over the sleep schedule on weekdays and weekends. A consistently shorter sleep duration during weekdays than in weekends or holidays is an indirect proof of the presence of sleep deprivation. A disorganized sleep–wake schedule will very likely be a source of problems for the patient.

Third: *Behavior before sleep*. It is useful to inquire about the routine before falling asleep. Patients may report reading, listening to an arousing radio program or watching TV, eating, etc. Important aspects are usual time to go to bed, latency to fall asleep, and presence of physically disturbing symptoms. Questions regarding restless legs syndrome are essential since RLS may produce important sleep onset difficulties . The main characteristics are an urge to move, usually accompanied by an unpleasant sensation in the legs, which appears at night or in the afternoon, particularly during rest and that improves, at least transiently, with movement [4]. Finding a comfortable body position in bed to fall asleep is an almost impossible task for those patients. The RLS symptoms usually decrease in intensity gradually during the night and disappear by early morning. In PD, however, the presentation and characteristics of RLS may be partially modified or masked by the dopaminergic agents used for the treatment of parkinsonism. Another cause of potentially troublesome sleep onset insomnia is the presence of either dyskinesia or "off" periods at the time of going to sleep. For these reasons, a detailed scrutiny of the type and schedule of antiparkinsonian agents is essential to understand the sleep problems of the patient, given that excessive amounts of dopaminergic agents or selegiline – which is converted to amphetamine [5] – may be associated with sleep-onset insomnia. The intake of caffeine, other stimulants, alcohol, or other drugs should be actively questioned. In general, patients with PD report no more difficulties in falling asleep than healthy age-matched controls, in contrast to the problems in maintaining sleep continuity which are much more often perceived [6, 7].

Fourth: *Behavior during sleep and final awakening*. A detailed interrogatory of the patient's behavior during sleep is essential and the cooperation of the bed partner here is fundamental, and should include the number, duration and time of nocturnal awakenings, type of activities during the awakenings (staying in bed, walking, going to bathroom, eating, etc.), time needed to fall asleep again after these awakenings, and time and type (spontaneous or induced) of the final awakening in the morning. One particularly frustrating symptom is awakening in the middle of the night, without any more sleepiness left. Awakening may be spontaneous or induced by snoring, arousals from sleep apnea, sudden limb jerks, pain, inability to turn in the bed, or the feeling of full bladder. Getting up at night to pass urine is one of the most common events that patients with PD report, and needs to be specifically scrutinized because it breaks sleep continuity (Table 5.2) and undermines the quality of sleep. Appearance of motor symptoms – tremor, rigidity – during the night is an indirect demonstration that sleep is broken given that the typical parkinsonian symptoms, as a rule, decrease in intensity or disappear with sleep, reappearing with arousals.

Questions about snoring or stridor, breathing pauses, and gasps during sleep should be asked to the patient and bed partner. A good imitation of the sounds by the physician may help the bed partner to identify the sounds. Also, the behavior during arousals or awakenings, presence of talking, shouting, screaming, crying or laughing, limb or other body movements such as hitting, punching, kicking involuntarily the bed partner, or falling out of bed are important points to clarify. Some of these behaviors may look to an observer as if the patients were enacting their dreams, fighting with an imaginary aggressor, and are typical of REM sleep behavior disorder (RBD). It is not always easy, however, to differentiate by clinical history the movements associated with arousals at the end of severe obstructive apneas from the dream enacting movements of RBD [9]. Also, large or brisk periodic leg movements during sleep may be confused by the bed partner with dream-enacting movements. Contusions or lacerations that are discovered at awakening by a patient that sleeps alone may give an important diagnostic clue regarding the presence of a parasomnia. Finally, the patient should be asked if after awakening in the morning he/she had enough sleep and feels refreshed or would continue sleeping more time if undisturbed and if he finds that the motor symptoms are better after sleep (sleep-effect) [10].

Fifth: *Dreaming and hallucinations*. Dream content has different patterns, depending upon the associated sleep disorder. Patients with obstructive sleep apnea may report anxious or frustrating dreams such as arriving late at an interview, missing an essential piece in a job, problems with the car engine, etc., and this usually improves after continuous positive airway pressure (CPAP) treatment [11]. Patients with NREM parasomnias (confusion arousals, somnambulism, or nocturnal terrors) may recall dreams, where they (or their loved ones) are in great danger and need to escape (flight). Patients with REM sleep behavior disorder (RBD), in contrast, typically dream that they are threatened by other people or animals and they react against the aggressor [12]. However, not every patient with dream enacting behavior recalls dreaming, even when awakened immediately after the episode, and sometimes aggressive dreams can also be reported by obstructive sleep apnea patients [9]. Abnormal dreaming in PD was reported in the old literature, before the discovery of RBD, as a side effect of levodopa [13], but it is now difficult to disentangle the possible role of this parasomnia in those cases.

Nocturnal hallucinations in PD should not be confused with dreams, but differentiation is difficult and both phenomena may occasionally occur in the same patient. A rule of thumb is that dreaming occurs with the eyes closed, even in dream enactment episodes of REM sleep behavior disorder (RBD); whereas, hallucinations occur with the patient being awake and the eyes open.

Sixth: *Daytime behavior and excessive daytime sleepiness*. It is important to ask how the sleep problems affect the daytime activities of the patient and not focus only in their nighttime symptoms. Patients with insomnia, for example, feel fatigued, unable to concentrate, with a subjective decrease in their performance, but are rarely sleepy. People with sleep onset or sleep maintenance insomnia often have stressful daytime routines that make them unable to "disconnect" easily before going to bed. The other main symptom, excessive daytime sleepiness (EDS), may cause clinically significant problems in PD, including unintended episodes of sleep [14]. From the practical standpoint, because sleepiness is a subjective feeling, the best way to measure it is asking the patient if he/she has problematic daytime sleepiness or a family member when the patient is cognitively impaired. Sleepiness is sometimes confused with tiredness or fatigue [15], another symptom that can also occur in PD. Tiredness, generally, improves with rest whereas sleepiness is worsened with relaxation. It is important to determine if sleepiness appears only in passive, relaxed situations or if it occurs even in active tasks, and to clarify if the patient feels the sleepiness before falling asleep, or, in contrast, falls asleep without feeling sleepy before. Most patients are able to feel the sleepiness and take preventive maneuvers to avoid accidents. Others, however, report that they suddenly discover they have fallen asleep without remembering any preceding sleepiness, what is called a "sleep attack." Unintended sleep episodes (or "sleep attacks") usually occur in a background of continuous sleepiness, especially in situations of minimal or moderate physical activity [16].

Seventh: *Other symptoms.* Questions about cataplexy, sleep paralysis, or hypnagogic hallucinations are sometimes very difficult to understand and may be confused with other problems. It is helpful to ask the patients to describe these symptoms using their own words rather than simply answering yes or no. Cataplexy has not been reported yet in a patient with PD, even in patients with important daytime sleepiness, although there are reports of patients with long-term narcolepsy who later in life develop PD [17]. Cataplexy is usually induced by positive emotions, rarely by negative ones, may have different intensities, is not associated with loss of consciousness (although the patient often has the eyes closed), disappears in seconds to minutes unless another triggering emotion occurs. Knee buckling, sagging of the jaw, and dropping of the head are the most common presentations but full-blown attacks can result in complete muscle paralysis with postural collapse.

Elaboration of the diagnostic hypothesis. Once all the information is available, hypothesis of what could cause the sleep problems has to be made and then decide whether any diagnostic test is needed before starting the treatment, as in any other medical situation.

5.2 Sleep Scales

To make a diagnosis of a sleep disorder problem in PD there is no better option than taking a clinical history with the patient and bed partner. However, for screening purposes, to rate specific symptoms in research studies and to complement the clinical interview, there are sleep scales. In the last 25 years, several scales designed to evaluate sleep symptoms in the general population are available, such as the Pittsburgh sleep quality index (PSQI) [18], the Epworth sleepiness scale (ESS) [19], the Stanford sleepiness scale (SSS) [20], and more focused scales for the assessment of RBD or RLS. In addition, a few scales have been specifically developed for assessment of sleep or sleepiness in PD, including the Parkinson's disease sleep scale (PDSS) version I [21] and II [8], the SCOPA-sleep [22], and the inappropriate sleep composite score [23]. Sleep scales differ in the *type of problem* evaluated (daytime sleepiness, nocturnal sleep, RBD, etc.), in the *period of time* assessed (current moment, past week, past month, recent times), and in *how are the questions answered* (the patient alone, by himself, alone but with the help of the physician or health-assistant or together with the bed partner or caregiver). The quality of the information obtained with sleep scales is entirely dependent upon the patients' ability to perceive their sleep problems, like in a traditional clinical interview. This fact becomes critical in the case of patients who sleep alone, are cognitively impaired, or are not fully aware of the severity of their problem, as it occurs in excessive daytime sleepiness or parasomnias. In PD, the information of a bed partner or caregiver, therefore, will improve the results of sleep scales particularly when the disease advances. For a variety of reasons, however, some scales were designed to be answered without the help of a bed partner.

5.2.1   Brief Description of the Scales

The Parkinson's disease sleep scale (*PDSS*) is a *self-rated scale* designed to measure *nocturnal problems*, sleep disturbance, and, in the first but not the second version, excessive daytime sleepiness in PD *over the previous week* [8, 21]. The PDSS can be used to screen daytime sleepiness and can also be used to ascertain the prevalence of general "sleep disturbance" in PD. The scale consists of *15 questions*, addressing commonly reported nocturnal symptoms occurring in patients with PD. Several of the items in the PDSS are only related with nocturnal disability. In the first version, each item was rated on a visual analogue scale from 0 (severe and always present) to 10 (not present). In the second version, each item is scored from 0 (never) to 3 (very often). The scale has been extensively used in PD population, and is credited for making an attempt to address the multidimensional nature of sleep problems in PD.

The Pittsburgh sleep quality index (*PSQI*) is a self-rating questionnaire designed to evaluate sleep quality, sleep habits, and disturbances during the previous month. It consists of 19 questions that are combined to form seven component scores (*subjective sleep quality, sleep latency, sleep duration, habitual sleep efficiency, sleep disturbances, use of sleeping medication*, and *daytime dysfunction*), scored from 0 (no difficulty) to 3 (severe difficulty). Five other questions are available to be answered by the bed partner or roommate, and provide clinical information but do not contribute to the final score.

The SCOPA-sleep [7] is a short, self-rating scale evaluating nocturnal sleep quality and daytime sleepiness specifically in patients with PD. The SCOPA includes a nighttime scale (NS), a single question about the quality of sleep with seven optional answers, not counted in the final score, and a daytime sleepiness scale (DS). In the NS, subjects indicate the extent to which their sleep was disturbed during the previous month on a scale of 0 (not at all) to 3 (very much). There are five items that include sleep initiation, sleep fragmentation, sleep efficiency, sleep duration, and early wakening. The maximum score of this scale is 15, with higher scores reflecting more severe sleep problems. The DS subscale evaluates daytime sleepiness in the past month and subjects indicate how often they fell asleep unexpectedly, fell asleep in particular everyday situations, how often they had difficulty staying awake, and whether falling asleep in the daytime was considered a problem. There are six items with four response options, ranging from 0 (never) to 3 (often) and the maximum score is 18, with higher scores reflecting more severe sleepiness. An interesting point is that a single question, not used in the sum scores of the scale, the "overall sleep quality" question is probably as good to get a clinically relevant impression as the whole scale.

The *Epworth sleepiness scale* (ESS) [19] and the *Stanford sleepiness scale* (SSS) [20] are self-administered scales designed to measure sleepiness either in recent times (ESS) or right at the moment of doing the test (SSS). In the ESS, the patient has to tell how likely has been for him in recent times to fall asleep in eight routine activities, from watching TV to talking. In the SSS, the subject must choose from descriptions of different sleepiness levels (from fully awake to fully asleep) the level that best defines his/her current state, giving an instant picture only of that particular moment, which is really not much relevant clinically during routine visits or follow-up by patients. Despite their limitations, both scales, and particularly the ESS, have been used frequently in PD [24] to identify, for example, the excessive levels of sleepiness of patients with PD compared with controls [25] or to document that unintended sleep episodes occur more often in patients with abnormally high ESS [23]. A variation of the ESS is the ICSS [23], where the patients should describe the possibility of falling asleep suddenly (sleep attacks) in the eight situations of the ESS and four additional active ones (driving, working, etc.).

The Stavanger sleepiness scale [26] assesses sleepiness in a simple way, and needs to be answered by the caregiver, who will tell how much time the patient sleeps during daytime. Three possibilities are offered: *no daytime sleepiness*, *mild sleepiness*, and *excessive daytime sleepiness* corresponding to different levels of sleeping time during the day and the number of times falling asleep. The scale has the advantage that it can be used in patients with advanced stages of the disease, that have impaired mobility and do not make several of the activities asked for in the ESS or ICSS. A multicenter study group in Europe [16] used it in the evaluation of MSA and patients with PD.

A Movement Disorder Society Task force reviewed in 2010 the available sleep scales and gave recommendations for their use in PD [27]. The Task force considered that the PDSS, the PSQI, the SCOPA-sleep and the ESS could be recommended for use in PD because they had been applied to PD populations. Other groups beyond the original developing group had published data of these scales and their clinical use and there were psychometrical studies showing that these scales are valid and reliable. They concluded that the ISCS and the SSS did not meet the criteria for recommendation, although the Task force suggested their possible use as a complement to the other scales and did not recommend the Stavanger scale because only the same group that developed the scale had used it, although this has now changed [16]. It was also mentioned that none of the reviewed scales was sufficient or appropriate to diagnose specific sleep disorders and that a scale could not replace a full sleep history with the patient and caregiver. For an overview of these scales, see Table 5.1.

Table 5.1 Summary of sleep scales for evaluation of PD

Scale	Type of disorder assessed	Bed partner/ informant	Period assessed	Population studied	Number of questions	Range of scores (*cut-off value*)	Comments
PDSS-2	Nocturnal disturbance	Not required, allowed to help	Previous week	Specific for PD	15	0–60	A previous version PDSS-1 exist with several changes
PSQI	Sleep quality, both nocturnal sleep and diurnal sleepiness	Required	Previous month	Many populations, used also in PD	19, 7 components	0–21 (5)	It gives quantitative information about number of sleep hours, sleep latencies, etc. Complex scoring system
SCOPA-sleep	Sleep quality, both nocturnal sleep and diurnal sleepiness	May or may not participate	Previous month	Designed for PD	12	0–12 (5/6)	Easy to administer, appears to have selected questions from the PSQI and ESS
ESS	Daytime sleepiness	Not required	"Recent times"	General, but used in PD several times	8	0–24 (>10)	Widely used, not designed for PD but used in many studies

ISCS	Sudden onset of sleep	Not required	Not specified	PD	6	1	Good to investigate risk of unintended sleep episodes ("sleep attacks")
SSS	Current daytime sleepiness	Not required	Current moment	General, but used in PD several times	1	–	Instantaneous measure of sleepiness, not appropriate for routine follow-up of patients
Stavanger	Daytime sleepiness	Required	Not specified	Specifically designed for PD	1	0–3 (2)	It is particularly useful in patients with advanced PD disease

Modified from Högl et al. [27]

5.2.2 Problems with Sleep Scales

Many sleep scales have been "validated," a term that people automatically equals to ready for clinical use without questioning anything else. However, the fact that a sleep scale has been validated simply says that it asks about things related to sleep problems (face validity), with more or less appropriate coverage of the sleep-related problems (content validity), more or less appropriate relationship with other aspects of the disease (construct validity), and with the items composing the scale having some internal consistency [28]. These conditions, however, are apparently not very difficult to achieve and other possible scales could be made with different questions and very likely be successfully validated. Validation does not mean that all the questions of the scale have common sense or that they are all necessary. Two examples of this – the PDSS and the SCOPA-sleep scales – are illustrative.

The PSDSS-1 and PDSS-2 have both been *validated* and yet have important differences in their scoring system (a 10-cm visual analog scale from 0 = severe and always present to 10 = not present, vs a numeric score) as well as in the items asked (items 5, 9 and 15 of PDSS-1 are no longer present in PDSS-2 and items 4, 10 and 11 have different wording). In addition, there are items whose scores were not significantly different in patients and controls (items 2, 1, 14) and a few items are overrepresented, like items 4, 5, and 10, in which a patient with RLS will very likely answer yes three times for the same problem. A lower number of items would perhaps give similar relevant information and have similar clinimetric properties than the 15-item scale (see Table 5.2). In fact, it is unclear why the authors decided to make a 15-item scale.

The SCOPA-sleep scale is another validated scale, with repetitive questions. For instance in the NS part, a positive response to item 2 (have woken too often), item 3 (lying awake too long at night), or item 4 (have woken up too early) implies very likely a positive response to item 5 (had too little sleep at night) and the same happens in the Daytime sleepiness (DS) part where a positive answer to items 1, 2, 3, 4 implies very likely a positive answer to item 5. These repetitions will artificially increase the difference between patients and controls. Finally, the construct validity of the SCOPA-sleep was proved by showing a significant correlation with the ESS and the PSQI. However, items 2, 3, and 4 in the DS-sleep part are very similar to items 1, 2, 6 and probably 3 in the ESS, whereas items 1 and 3 of the NS-sleep part are very similar to items 5a and 5b in the PSQI. It is not rare then that SCOPA-sleep correlated well with ESS and PSQI.

Two other areas for improvement can be found. One is that in most sleep scales the questions asked have not been extracted directly from the patients' own way of describing their complaints – that is from how the patients describe their own problems – rather from how their doctors (ESS, PDSS, SCOPA) interpret it. An extreme case is the SCOPA, where the questions were chosen from "the literature," and the authors in fact did not see directly any of the patients or controls that participated in the study, but only the written responses to their questionnaire.

The other is that all sleep scales have assessed their construct validity by calculating the correlation between the scores on the scale with those in other scales that

Table 5.2 Frequency of nocturnal sleep complaints

PDSS-2 (item number) ordered by frequency of positive response [8]	Score (mean ± SD) (min: 0, max: 4)	Nocturnal problems reported by patients with PD [3]	Percent (%)
Getting up at night to pass urine (item 8)	2.77 ± 1.48	Need to visit lavatory	79
Difficulties staying asleep (item 3)	2.37 ± 1.63	Inability to turn over in bed	65
"Bad sleep" quality (item 1)	1.99 ± 1.33	Painful leg cramps	55
Tired and sleepy after waking in the morning (item 14)	1.69 ± 1.62	Vivid dreams/nightmares	48
Uncomfortable/immobility at night (item 9)	1.20 ± 1.63	Cannot get out of bed unaided	35
Tremor on waking (item 13)	0.88 ± 1.38	Limb/facial dystonia	34
Difficulties falling asleep (item 2)	0.84 ± 1.41	Back pain	34
Restlessness, urge to move, pain or muscle cramps in "ARMS or LEGS" (items 4, 5, 10, 11, very similar)	(Range of means in the 4 items) 0.68– 0.84 ± 1.3	Jerks of legs	33
Distressing dreams at night (item 6)	0.58 ± 1.13	Visual hallucinations	16
Snoring or difficulties in breathing (item 15)	0.36 ± 0.86	None	4
Distressing hallucinations at night (item 7)	0.28 ± 0.94	Told their doctors	45

Modified from Trenkwalder et al. [8], and from Lees et al. [3] from a list of complaints given by patients with PD to a postal survey at the British PD association. The complaints in the PDSS and in the list obtained from the patients have similarities but it is not the same. Remarkably, the most disturbing sleep symptom in both lists is the need to visit the lavatory at night.

have addressed similar constructs, but not with objective sleep recordings. Unfortunately, the older scales – such as the ESS – had limited or controversial correlations with objective tests [1].

5.3 When to Use Sleep Scales and Which to Use?

Using scales has advantages and limitations. Advantages are the homogeneity of the questions asked, which is ideal for multicenter studies or to always record the same type of information. It may also help some patients to be aware of a sleep problem that they did not consider relevant enough to tell their doctor. Limitations are inherent to the methodology: homogeneity results in lack of flexibility in evaluating symptoms that do not perfectly fit with the questions. They may also induce an error, which is relying uniquely in a scale to diagnose or measure a sleep problem.

Given the availability of sleep scales, one logical question is when a neurologist caring for patients with PD should use a sleep scale and which ones to use. There is no formal study addressing these issues. A comparative usefulness of the PDSS-I and the SCOPA-sleep scales was performed by Martinez-Martín et al. [22], reporting a relative good correlation between the two scales. The authors suggested that the PDSS could be used to assess overall nocturnal sleep quality and to obtain a profile about potential causes of "bad sleep," but not to assess daytime sleepiness. On the other hand, SCOPA-sleep assesses nocturnal sleep disorders and daytime somnolence at a similar extent, but it does not explore the potential causes.

In addition to these dedicated sleep scales, the revised version of the Unified Parkinson's Disease Rating Scale (UPDRS) [29] and the new non-motor symptom scale for PD [6] contain a few basic questions about nocturnal sleep and daytime sleepiness, which are easier to administer and give probably similar information than the more detailed sleep scales.

5.4 Scales to Evaluate RBD

In the last decade several scales (Table 5.3) have been described to screen for the presence of RBD in the general population [30, 32, 33, 35] as well as in PD [31, 34]. All but one (Gjerstad) were elaborated taking into account the reports of RBD patients (diagnosed with PSG) and bed partners and were applied to populations with several sleep disorders, including patients with PD with and without RBD [32, 34], as well as in controls. The scales also had proper validation procedures. In general, these instruments were rather sensitive to detect the parasomnia but not specific, due to the misidentification of patients with other parasomnias, epilepsy or sleep apnea. Two scales consist of only one question [31, 33], two of 13 [30, 32] and one of 9 items [35]. In order to exclude the most common misdiagnosis (sleepwalking and sleep apnea), one questionnaire incorporates two specific questions for these disorders [35].

A summary of the different scales can be found in Table 5.3. There are no formal studies comparing the different scales. In terms of simplicity and reliability the Mayo sleep questionnaire [33] is good, relies on the informant (and not on the patient, which is often unaware of the problem) but it has not been applied specifically to a PD population. The rest of the scales have been used in PD [32, 34] and shown to be sensitive to detect parasomnia. The Stavanger scale [31] is very simple and has been used in follow up of population-based study of PD but did not have formal PSG validation.

In conclusion, although there has been a lot of work in last decades trying to elaborate scales and questionnaires to evaluate sleep disorders in the general population and in specific groups such as in Parkinson's disease, there is still room for improvement. Sleep scales are useful for screening purposes, to rate specific symptoms in research studies, and to complement the clinical interview with patient and bed partner, which will always give the final answer to the clinical problem of the patient. Scales need to be created based directly on the complaints of the patients and correlated with as many objective measurements of sleep as possible.

Table 5.3 RBD screening scales

Author, year, type of scale	Type of RBD	n	Control group	n	Bed partner/ informant	Period assessed	Number of questions	Range of scores (cut-off value)	Comments
Stiasny–Kolster [30] (screening)	Narcolepsy (61 %); idiopathic RBD (35 %), PD (4 %) PSG confirmed	54	Patients with sleep disorders other than RBD, referred to a sleep lab	160	Not required	Not specified	13	0–13 (5)	6 questions need a bed partner. All patients with PD have 1 extra point (item10). RBD patients who do not recall dreams have 4 points less
Gjerstad et al. [31] (screening)	PD No PSG recording	231	Age-matched healthy elderly individuals	100	Required	Not specified, recent times implied	1	0–3 (2)	No questions about dreams, only physical activity, asleep. No PSG confirmation. Used for follow-up in a large population-based study
Li et al. [32] (screening and rating of frequency)	Idiopathic RBD (51), symptomatic (29), "RBD-like" disorder (27)	107	Mostly patients with other sleep disorders such as OSAS and insomnia	107	May or may not participate	Lifetime and last year	13	0–100 (18/19)	Repeated questions about dreaming (aggressive (item 4) or frightening (item 5). Dreams may also be "emotional" (item 3) and "nightmares" (item 2). Also items 10 and 11 are very similar
Boeve et al. [33] (screening)	Cognitively impaired and/or parkinsonism	176	–	–	Fundamental	Not specified	5	0–5 (4)	Patients without bed partner cannot do it

(continued)

Table 5.3 (continued)

Author, year, type of scale	Type of RBD	n	Control group	n	Bed partner/ informant	Period assessed	Number of questions	Range of scores (*cut-off value*)	Comments
Nomura et al. [34] (screening)	PD–RBD (19); PD without RBD (26); idiopathic RBD (31) PSG confirmed	45 PD + 31 iRBD	–	–	Required	Not specified	13	0–13 (*6*)	Same comments as that for the RBDSQ, except that the partner is required to participate
Frauscher et al. [35] (screening and rating of frequency)	Idiopathic 30, PD and alike 28; narcolepsy 8, drug-induced 4 PSG confirmed	70	Consecutive sleep laboratory patients without RBD	140	Available in most patients	Last year	7 Ratio positive/ total responses	0–1 (*0.25*)	7 RBD questions and to exclude OSAS and sleepwalking. Frequency scores did not improve discrimination. A single question compared well with whole test

References

1. Chervin RD, Aldrich MS. The Epworth Sleepiness Scale may not reflect objective measures of sleepiness or sleep apnea. Neurology. 1999;52:125–31.
2. Olson LG, Cole MF, Ambrogetti A. Correlations among Epworth Sleepiness Scale scores, multiple sleep latency tests and psychological symptoms. J Sleep Res. 1998;7:248–53.
3. Lees AJ, Blackburn NA, Campbell VL. The nighttime problems of Parkinson's disease. Clin Neuropharmacol. 1988;11:512–9.
4. Trenkwalder C, Paulus W, Walters AS. The restless legs syndrome. Lancet Neurol. 2005;4:465–75.
5. Roselaar SE, Langdon N, Lock CB, Jenner P, Parkes JD. Selegiline in narcolepsy. Sleep. 1987;10:491–5.
6. Chaudhuri KR, Martínez-Martín P, Brown RG, et al. The metric properties of a novel non-motor symptoms scale for Parkinson's disease: results from an international pilot study. Mov Disord. 2007;22:1901–11.
7. Marinus J, Visser M, van Hilten JJ, Lammers GJ, Stiggelbout AM. Assessment of sleep and sleepiness in Parkinson disease. Sleep. 2003;26:1049–54.
8. Trenkwalder C, Kohnen R, Högl B, et al. Parkinson's disease sleep scale – validation of the revised version PDSS-2. Mov Disord. 2011;25:644–52.
9. Iranzo A, Santamaria J. Severe obstructive sleep apnea/hypopnea mimicking REM sleep behavior disorder. Sleep. 2005;28:203–6.
10. Factor SA, Mc Alarney T, Sáchez-Ramos JR, Weiner WJ. Sleep disorders and sleep effect in Parkinson's disease. Mov Disord. 1990;5:280–5.
11. Carrasco E, Santamaria J, Iranzo A, et al. Changes in dreaming induced by CPAP in severe obstructive sleep apnea syndrome patients. J Sleep Res. 2006;15:430–6.
12. Uguccioni G, Golmard JL, Noël de Fontréaux A, Leu-Semenescu S, Brion A, Arnulf I. Fight or flight? Dream content during sleepwalking/sleep terrors vs rapid eye movement sleep behavior disorder. Sleep Med. 2013;14:391–8.
13. Sharf B, Moskovitz C, Lupton MD, Klawans HL. Dream phenomena induced by chronic levodopa therapy. J Neural Transm. 1978;43:143–51.
14. Santamaria J. How to evaluate excessive daytime sleepiness in Parkinson's disease. Neurology. 2004;63 suppl 3:s21–3.
15. Dement WC, Hall J, Walsh JK. Tiredness versus sleepiness: semantics or a target for public education? Sleep. 2003;26:485–6.
16. Moreno C, Santamaria J, Salamero M, et al. Excessive daytime sleepiness in multiple system atrophy (SLEEMSA study). Arch Neurol. 2011;68:223–30.
17. Economou NT, Manconi M, Ghika J, Bassetti C. Development of Parkinson and Alzheimer diseases in two cases of narcolepsy-cataplexy. Eur Neurol. 2012;67:48–50.
18. Buysse DJ, Reynolds III CF, Monk TH, Berman SR, Kupfer DJ. The Pittsburgh Sleep Quality Index: a new instrument for psychiatric practice and research. Psychiatry Res. 1989;28(2):193–213.
19. Johns MW. A new method for measuring daytime sleepiness: the Epworth sleepiness scale. Sleep. 1991;14:540–5.
20. Hoddes E, Zarcone V, Smythe H, Phillips R, Dement WC. Quantification of sleepiness: a new approach. Psychophysiology. 1973;10:431–6.
21. Chaudhuri KR, Pal S, Di Marco A, et al. The Parkinson's disease sleep scale: a new instrument for assessing sleep and nocturnal disability in Parkinson's disease. J Neurol Neurosurg Psychiatry. 2002;73:629–35.
22. Martinez-Martin P, Visser M, Rodriguez-Blazquez C, Marinus J, Chaudhuri KR, van Hilten JJ. SCOPA-sleep and PDSS: two scales for assessment of sleep disorder in Parkinson's disease. Mov Disord. 2008;12:1681–8.
23. Hobson DE, Lang AE, Martin WR, et al. Excessive daytime sleepiness and sudden-onset sleep in Parkinson's disease. A survey by the Canadian Movement Disorders Group. JAMA. 2002;287:455–63.

24. Hagell P, Broman JE. Measurement properties and hierarchical item structure of the Epworth Sleepiness Scale in Parkinson's disease. J Sleep Res. 2007;16:102–9.
25. Brodsky MA, Godbold J, Roth T, Olanow CW. Sleepiness in Parkinson's disease: a controlled study. Mov Disord. 2003;18:668–72.
26. Tandberg E, Larsen JP, Karlsen K. Excessive daytime sleepiness and sleep benefit in Parkinson's disease: a community-based study. Mov Disord. 1999;14(6):922–7.
27. Högl B, Arnulf I, Comella C, et al. Scales to assess sleep impairment in Parkinson's disease: critique and recommendations. Mov Disord. 2010;25:204–2716.
28. Bland JM, Altman DG. Validating scales and indexes. Br Med J. 2002;324:606–7.
29. Goetz CG, Tilley BC, Shaftman SR, et al. Movement Disorder Society-sponsored revision of the Unified Parkinson's Disease Rating Scale (MDS-UPDRS): Scale presentation and clinimetric results. Mov Disord. 2008;23:2129–70.
30. Stiasny-Kolster K, Mayer G, Schäfer S, Möller JC, Heinzel-Gutenbrunner M, Oertel WH. The REM sleep behavior disorder questionnaire-a new diagnostic instrument. Mov Disord. 2007;22:2386–93.
31. Gjerstad MD, Boeve B, Wentzel-Larsen T, Aarsland D, Larsen JP. Occurrence and clinical correlates of REM sleep behaviour disorder in patients with Parkinson's disease over time. J Neurol Neurosurg Psychiatry. 2008;79:387–91.
32. Li SX, Wing YK, Lam SP, et al. Validation of a new REM sleep behavior disorder questionnaire (RBD-HK). Sleep Med. 2010;11:43–8.
33. Boeve BF, Molano JR, Ferman TJ, et al. Validation of the Mayo Sleep Questionnaire to screen for REM sleep behavior disorder in an aging and dementia cohort. Sleep Med. 2011;12:445–53.
34. Nomura T, Inoue Y, Kagimura T, Uemura Y, Nakashima K. Utility of the REM sleep behavior disorder questionnaire (RBDSQ) in Parkinson's disease patients. Sleep Med. 2011;12:711–3.
35. Frauscher B, Ehrman L, Zamarian L, et al. Validation of the Innsbruck REM sleep behavior disorder inventory. Mov Disord. 2012;27:1673–8.

Part II

Insomnia in Parkinson's Disease

6

Margaret Park and Cynthia L. Comella

Contents

Abstract

Insomnia is the most common sleep disorder in Parkinson's disease (PD). Sleep maintenance insomnia is the most common type of insomnia in this population. The pathophysiology of insomnia is complex and not fully understood. Contributing factors to insomnia in PD include complex medication regimens

M. Park, MD (✉)
Rush University Medical Center, Sleep Disorders Service and Reacher Center,
710 S Paulina Street, Chicago, IL 60612, USA
e-mail: Margaret_Park@rush.edu

C.L. Comella, MD, FAAN
Rush University Medical Center, Department of Neurological Sciences,
1725 West Harrison Street, Suite 755, Chicago, IL 60612, USA

© Springer-Verlag Wien 2015
A. Videnovic, B. Högl (eds.), *Disorders of Sleep and Circadian Rhythms
in Parkinson's Disease*, DOI 10.1007/978-3-7091-1631-9_6

and comorbidities associated with the disease. A dedicated sleep interview that includes patients' bed partners or care givers is a necessary diagnostic step in the management of insomnia. Treatment options include non-pharmacological and pharmacological approaches.

6.1 Introduction

Sleep complaints are highly prevalent in patients with Parkinson's disease (PD). Up to 88 % of PD patients report nighttime sleep fragmentation and early morning awakenings, [1] which are associated with decreased overall total sleep time, increased wake periods in the middle of the night ("wake after sleep onset periods," or WASO), poor daytime function, and excessive daytime sleepiness (EDS). Up to 60 % of PD patients specifically complain of insomnia [2], which objectively correlate with daytime fatigue and sleepiness [3], impaired attention and executive functioning [4], and caregiver burden [5, 6]. Subjectively, PD patients cite insomnia as a significant source of distress [7, 8]. Insomnia is frequently the cause of low quality of life for both the PD patient and their caregivers [6, 8]. Despite this, research investigating insomnia in PD has been relatively sparse, possibly due to the complex, multifactorial nature underlying the relationship between insomnia and PD.

This chapter is intended to provide a brief overview of insomnia, discuss the phenomenon of insomnia in PD, provide suggestions regarding evaluation of insomnia and its application in PD, and review potential treatment options for insomnia in PD.

6.2 Definition

The definition of insomnia has been a source of contention for several years. There are debates regarding how to differentiate the symptom from the disorder, whether specific time thresholds should be included (e.g., how long it takes to fall asleep, duration of WASO periods), and how to combine these sleep complaints with daytime, or "wake," complaints (e.g., fatigue or sleepiness) [9]. Generally, there is consensus that the core symptoms of insomnia should involve at least one nighttime or sleep symptom (e.g., difficulty initiating or maintaining sleep, early morning awakenings, non-restorative sleep) and at least one daytime or wake symptom (e.g., fatigue, mood issues, cognitive dysfunction, social or occupational impairment, EDS) [9, 10].

Diagnostic criteria for insomnia are included within the following three different classification systems: the Diagnostic and Statistical Manual of Mental Disorders, 4th edition (*DSM-V*) [11]; the International Classification of Diseases, 10th revision (*ICD-10*) [12]; and the International Classification of Sleep Disorders, 3rd edition (*ICSD-3*) [10]. For this discussion, the *ICSD-3* criteria for chronic insomnia disorder will be used which include difficulty initiating or maintaining sleep, early morning awakening, and patients' complaints related to poor nighttime sleep.

For PD patients, risk factors for insomnia include having PD itself (e.g., motor symptoms), treatment factors (e.g., medication side effects, wearing-off effects), psychosocial disturbances (e.g., depression, anxiety), and comorbid medical disorders. It is important to note that PD patients may have overlapping insomnia and other sleep disorders. Below is a brief summary of each of these diagnoses as it may pertain to PD.

Difficulty initiating or maintaining sleep may be considered a common symptom of an underlying existing medical condition. For PD patients, motor symptoms can be especially disruptive or disturbing at night [13]. For example, bradykinesia causes difficulty turning in bed, requiring frequent readjustment of pillows and blankets. Early morning dystonia is a common complaint, when dopamine levels are low or are not supplemented by medications, leading to severe contractures that disrupt sleep. Non-motor PD symptoms can also interfere with sleep, particularly autonomic dysfunction. Urinary and gastrointestinal dysfunction during sleep is known to significantly contribute to insomnia complaints [14–16]. When these PD-related symptoms lead to concern or distress to the point of causing loss of sleep or prolonged WASO, this insomnia diagnosis should be considered.

The bidirectional relationship between insomnia and mood disorders, specifically depression and anxiety, has been well documented. Insomnia may be a symptom of a variety of mental disorders, but patients also cite insomnia as a potential trigger or exacerbator of their mood or mental disorder. In PD, depression is highly prevalent [17, 18], possibly associated with dysfunction of dopaminergic transmission, a notion that is partially supported by improvement after dopamine agonist administration [19]. Additionally, movement issues can increase anxiety and depression symptoms, which can also affect sleep quality. Mood disorders in PD must be evaluated independently of motor symptoms, as depression can lead to maladaptive behaviors that can worsen insomnia [10, 20].

Medications used to help PD-related motor symptoms may alternately cause daytime sleepiness and nighttime hyperarousal [21]. Direct effects on the sleep and wake systems may depend on dose and timing of the medications. For example, levodopa 200 mg in the evening may improve subjective sleep quality [22], but continuous dopaminergic therapy has been shown to worsen sleep fragmentation [23]. Non-selective MAO-B-inhibitors have been reported to cause both daytime sleepiness and sleep disruption, possibly due to an amphetamine-like metabolite [24] that has not been reported with selective MAO-B-inhibitors [25].

Medications that may also help with non-motor symptoms can also exert deleterious effects on sleep and wake function. For example, antidepressants can have either an alerting or sedating effect, so correct timing of these medications is important. A thorough review of medications (including over-the-counter preparations), side effects, dosage, and timing of administration is recommended.

6.3 Pathophysiology and Sleep-Wake Systems

PD pathology involves lesions in the upper brainstem and lower midbrain [15], areas that are crucial in sleep and wake regulation. Alterations of brainstem cholinergic and noradrenergic neurons can result in altered REM sleep, while loss of serotonin is associated with reduced slow wave sleep. It is important to remember that PD pathology also affects wake systems [21]. As brainstem dopaminergic, cholinergic, and serotoninergic neurons, along with forebrain acetylcholine and histamine, are integral to the arousal system, PD-related neurodegeneration fundamentally alters the ability to sustain wakefulness. PD patients may also have relative losses of orexinergic neurons in the lateral hypothalamic region, which normally provides excitatory signals to these same arousal systems [26]. The overall result is an altered arousal threshold, leading to increased susceptibility to sleep (i.e., daytime napping), which can hinder the ability to initiate and consolidate nighttime sleep.

Early involvement of PD pathology within the brainstem regions [15] may explain the high frequency of insomnia complaints even in the mild stages of PD, suggesting that insomnia steadily worsens as PD progresses. On the contrary, insomnia in PD has been shown to fluctuate over time [27]. Similarly, various imaging techniques have failed to associate sleep disturbances with specific structural abnormalities in PD [28] suggesting that PD-related insomnia is not solely attributed to brainstem neurodegeneration.

6.4 Evaluation

As with any medical disorder, evaluation of insomnia should begin with a thorough history that includes frequency and duration of symptoms, exacerbating and relieving factors, average and range of bedtimes, perceived sleep latency, number of arousals, duration of WASO, average and range of wake times, and perceived quality of sleep. Discussion regarding behavioral habits during the 24-h day may include levels of activity during the day, daytime napping habits, use of non-sleep activities while in bed such as use of electronics, and environmental factors (e.g., temperature, noise, pets). Medical and psychiatric history should be considered in the context of the timing of symptoms, along with review of medications specifically including medications attempted for treatment of sleep and wake symptoms (including over-the-counter preparations) and a review of medications that can potentially influence sleep and wake rhythms (e.g., antidepressants, steroids, antihistamines, etc.) [29, 30].

Because of the complexity of insomnia in PD, evaluation and management of PD is necessarily multifaceted. In addition to a thorough history and examination, clinicians are encouraged to reevaluate both the timing and dose of PD pharmacotherapy, as this may help insomnia by either directly helping with nighttime sleep consolidation (e.g., by reducing nocturnal akinesia or dyskinesia that may interfere with sleep) or indirectly by reducing daytime sleepiness (i.e., increasing wake periods during the day, thereby helping with nighttime sleep latency and consolidation). Concomitantly, consultation for associated comorbid medical issues (e.g., urological issues) is recommended to reduce the potential interference of nighttime sleep consolidation. Consistent reevaluation of psychiatric and psychological symptoms is recommended to adequately address symptoms of depression, anxiety, hallucinations, and panic from interfering with sleep and wake function. Finally, consultation with a clinician who is experienced with the diagnosis and management of insomnia is often helpful.

6.4.1 Evaluation Tools

For PD, six scales have been deemed to meet criteria as per the movement disorders task force [31]: the Pittsburgh sleep quality index (PSQI), the Epworth sleepiness scale (ESS), the inappropriate sleep composite score (ISCS), the Stanford sleepiness scale (SSS), the Parkinson's disease sleep scale (PDSS) [32], and the scales for outcomes in Parkinson's disease (SCOPA-sleep) [33]. The first four scales are generic sleep tools, generally limited in their ability to evaluate PD-specific sleep symptoms, while the latter two scales have been developed to be specific to PD. The PDSS is a visual analogue scale that includes PD-related nocturnal symptoms including overall quality of nighttime sleep, sleep onset and maintenance insomnia, nocturnal restlessness, nocturnal psychosis, nocturia, nocturnal motor symptoms, sleep refreshment, and daytime dozing. A modified version, the PDSS-2, includes screening for sleep apnea, and is reported to have an excellent level of validity and reliability. The SCOPA-sleep is a short, two-part scale that assesses nighttime sleep and daytime sleepiness. Although this scale has been validated, it does not incorporate other PD-specific problems such as nocturnal hallucinations, motor symptoms, or nocturia. The PDSS and SCOPA-sleep scales have been developed specifically for PD patients, with incorporation of items to assess nocturnal sleep quality and impairment. However, while more applicable to sleep symptoms in PD, neither scale has been evaluated specifically for PD-related insomnia.

Available tools for insomnia assessment typically consist of sleep diary and actigraphy measures. Sleep diaries are subjective tools that help identify patterns of sleep [34]. Patients are typically asked to keep a prospective record of their bed times, WASO, wake times, and sleep quantity and quality over a course of a few weeks. Patients are usually instructed to record this information during the morning times, using recall of the previous night's sleep to complete this information. Using these records, parameters such as time-in-bed along with subjective ratings of sleep and wake function can be estimated. Sleep diaries do not necessarily correlate with objective measures of sleep, but this data can help identify important factors related to the insomnia complaints. Further, sleep diaries can be used to assess treatment response [35, 36]. Actigraphy is an accelerometer device that monitors motion and calculates activity counts, providing objective information regarding sleep and wake patterns over several days or weeks. It is considered a useful evaluative tool for insomnia [37, 38], particularly in assessing whether certain patterns of sleep emerge or to evaluate the implementation of behavioral methods such as sleep restriction on existing patterns.

Although sleep studies (polysomnography, or PSG) are considered the gold-standard assessment for most nocturnal sleep disorders, PSG is not recommended for routine assessment of insomnia [39]. However, as comorbid sleep disorders are highly prevalent in PD patients, PSG is often utilized to evaluate potential sleep apnea, periodic limb movement disorder, and REM behavior disorder.

6.5 Differential Diagnoses

6.5.1 Other Sleep Disorders

While discussion regarding other nocturnal sleep disorders is out of the scope of this chapter, it is important to note that PD patients often have comorbid sleep disorders including sleep apnea, restless leg syndrome (RLS), periodic limb movement disorder, and REM behavior disorder that contribute to sleep fragmentation, poor sleep quality, and daytime dysfunction. Evaluation and treatment of these disorders may improve the insomnia complaint, in which case an independent diagnosis of insomnia is excluded. However, it is also possible that insomnia is persistent and separate from these other sleep disorders. Further, the existence of these sleep disorders may potentially exacerbate insomnia symptoms and interfere with treatment of insomnia [40]. For example, patients may be unable to adhere to relaxation techniques for insomnia (CBT-I) if RLS symptoms are present. The symptoms of these sleep disorders should be considered during the initial evaluation as well as during subsequent follow-up visits.

6.5.2 Circadian Rhythm Sleep Disorders

The circadian system is suspected to be affected in PD-related pathophysiology, substantiated by reports of advanced sleep-wake schedules (i.e., early bedtimes and early wake times) in PD patients. Though the suprachiasmatic nucleus of PD patients is likely not involved, aberrant clock genes [41] and abnormalities in circadian hormonal patterns [42, 43] are reported. Clinically, circadian involvement in PD is partially supported by the beneficial effect of administering bright light in PD patients [44]. However, it is yet unclear whether the clinical observation of circadian misalignment in PD is mediated directly by alterations in the circadian system or via other indirect pathways (e.g., age, depression). Evaluation of insomnia should include a review of preferred versus habitual sleep and wake times to consider circadian rhythm disorders into the differential diagnosis.

6.6 Treatment

6.6.1 Behavioral Treatment

For movement issues, the comfort of the PD patient during the night can be improved by simple measures. For example, PD patients may find relief by using sheets that do not slip, wearing silk pajamas without buttons, and placing levodopa tablets and a bottle of water on the bedside table. In advanced stages of the disease, the patient's spouse should be encouraged to sleep in a different bed or room as needed, as inadequate rest for the caregiver can make the patient's sleep disturbance intolerable and lead to early institutionalization.

Enhancing both daytime activities and assisting with calming nighttime activities can provide insomnia relief. Increased activity during the day helps to increase "sleep pressure" so that sleep latency at bedtime is reduced. Nighttime measures may include stimulus control, proper sleep hygiene, and sleep restriction. Stimulus control is a set of instructions to reinforce the association between sleep and the bed/bedroom [45]. Examples include going to bed only when feeling sleepy, avoiding activities other than sleep in the bed/bedroom (e.g., no reading or watching TV), getting out of bed if sleep is not achieved in an acceptable amount of time, keeping a routine sleep-wake schedule (e.g., same wake time regardless of the amount of sleep perceived the night before), and avoidance of daytime napping. Proper sleep hygiene habits are also advised. For example, use of evening caffeine may cause evening alertness as well as worsen PD-related urinary processes. Restriction of daytime napping is also crucial in allowing for improved nighttime sleep onset latency and nighttime sleep consolidation. Patients may also be instructed to adjust environmental influences (e.g., light, noise, temperature) that may promote or interfere with sleep [46]. Sleep restriction involves limiting the amount of time-in-bed so as to reflect, as close as possible, the actual sleep time. Sleep efficiency, which is the amount of time sleeping divided by the amount of time in bed, is one outcome that helps guide treatment efficacy. Once acceptable sleep efficiency is achieved, the time-in-bed is gradually increased. For the PD patient, the caveat in implementing these particular behavioral techniques is potential worsening of daytime sleepiness, so caution with risky behaviors during the day such as driving (especially due to potential dopaminergic influence) need to be considered.

Cognitive behavioral therapy for insomnia (CBT-I) combines several of these behavioral techniques with a cognitive approach to help with insomnia symptoms. For example, a patient may go to bed earlier than a "natural" sleep time to "allow" for more sleep, even if sleep typically does not occur at that earlier time. This may cause excessive worry to occur during this time in bed (e.g., "if I can't sleep, I will have poor work performance and get fired"). CBT-I is used to reduce excessive worrying about sleep and to help reframe beliefs regarding the association between insomnia and daytime consequences [47, 48]. CBT-I is considered the first-line treatment for insomnia [39, 49] but frequently requires a trained clinician for effective results. CBT-I [48] is a potential promising line of insomnia treatment for PD patients. One study demonstrated possible benefit of using CBT-I in PD patients [44]. This finding remains to be replicated, warranting further investigation.

6.6.2 Pharmacological Treatment

Despite clinical evidence that insomnia is widespread in PD patients, research evidence is somewhat limited. As a result, most treatment recommendations are based on small studies or on anecdotal reports. Generally, if pharmacotherapy for insomnia is considered necessary, medications should be used in conjunction with behavioral treatments for insomnia.

Pharmacotherapy management should consider modification of dopaminergic doses to address PD motor symptoms. Timing of dopaminergic doses may help to identify gaps in dopaminergic stimulation over the 24-h period, but this needs to be considered in the context of possibly causing alerting effects in the middle of the night. While low doses of dopaminergic stimulation may result in sleepiness, higher doses may induce wakefulness [21]. As a result, lower doses given during the day may induce sleepiness but the additive effect at the end of the day may result in an alerting effect [50]. Additionally, PD-related urinary symptoms often disrupt sleep. Transitory blockade of nighttime polyuria with an evening intranasal dose of desmopressin may be effective in improving sleep consolidation [51].

Generally, medications for sleep are prescribed for acute onset insomnia rather than for chronic insomnia, as the sedating effect of these medications tends to decrease over time and/or side effects become more significant [52]. Potential side effects include morning sedation, memory deficits, impaired balance, and potentially sleep-related amnestic behaviors such as sleep walking. Contraindications of benzodiazepine medications for sleep include use of other sedative drugs which may lead to synergistic and additive side effects, substance use, sleep-disordered breathing including sleep apnea, and hepatic failure. Additional long-term concerns include rebound insomnia, withdrawal symptoms, and dependence [53]. In comparison, non-benzodiazepine hypnotics generally have shorter half-lives with less impact on muscle relaxation.

In PD, eszopiclone was found to have favorable subjective improvement in insomnia symptoms for a small group of PD patients [54] but objective data and long-term evaluation have not been evaluated. If the PD patient has comorbid sleep disorders requiring benzodiazepine medication (e.g., clonazepam for REM behavior disorder), the PD patient and caregiver will need to be appraised of the particular risks associated with these medications so as to take proper safety precautions. In summary, sedative medications in general should be considered only when necessary, as the peak effect of these medications may coincide with worsening motor symptoms and wearing-off effects in the middle of the night and in the early morning period, combining to aggravate imbalance and cognitive deficits.

While other prescription medications often have sedative and hypnotic effects, there is little evidence regarding their efficacy or safety in treatment of insomnia. Trazodone is perhaps one of the most widely prescribed medications for sleep possibly because of its short half-life. However, morning sedation is a common side effect [55] and the medication tends to lose its hypnotic effect after a short period of time. Medications such as gabapentin or pregabalin are often used for chronic pain conditions and have sedative qualities that may help with sleep latency, but have not been formally studied for insomnia. Sedating antipsychotic medications (e.g., quetiapine, risperidone) are often used for sleep purposes [30]; however, these medications are not FDA-approved for insomnia and may not be advisable for insomnia treatment due to concern regarding severe outcomes including metabolic syndrome and sudden death.

For PD patients, sedative antidepressants and antipsychotics are often considered to treat both insomnia symptoms along with comorbid psychiatric symptoms.

Clozapine and quetiapine [56] have been reported to improve subjective sleep quality but were not evaluated with objective sleep measures. Doxepin also appears to be effective for insomnia in PD patients [44]. Consideration should be given regarding the timeline of insomnia symptoms, as these medications can worsen symptoms of restless leg syndrome, periodic limb movements, and REM behavior disorder.

Melatonin (*N*-acetyl-5-methoxytryptamine) is an herbal supplement, available without a prescription in the United States. Melatonin receptor agonists (e.g., ramelteon) are available by prescription only, with properties similar to endogenous melatonin. These medications may help with sleep latency and possibly sleep duration but have the additional benefit of potentially shifting circadian rhythms [57, 58]. Melatonin and its derivatives are typically less potent but also have fewer side effects than hypnotic medications.

For PD patients, melatonin can have beneficial effects in subjective sleep quality but only mild benefit in objective sleep parameters [59]. Long-term data are not available to determine whether these sleep benefits are sustained chronically. Generally, higher doses of melatonin (e.g., 50 mg) are not considered more effective than lower doses of melatonin (e.g., melatonin dose 3–5 mg) in PD.

Sodium oxybate is a prescription medication that is FDA-approved for narcolepsy patients. It is derived as the sodium salt of gamma-hydroxybutyric acid. Although the mechanism of action is officially "unknown," it likely exerts its effect via GABAergic pathways. Its heavy sedative effects allow for sleep consolidation, improving next-day alertness.

Sodium oxybate was evaluated in an open-labeled study of PD patients and found to have significant subjective improvement in sleep quality [60]. While objective sleep measures showed increased slow wave sleep and REM sleep, overall total sleep time and sleep efficiency remained unchanged. Due to its heavy sedative effect, this medication should be used only after evaluation for sleep apnea, should not be taken with other sedative medications, or be used in patients who use alcohol. Exacerbation of depressive symptoms with suicidality has been reported in trials of sodium oxybate, requiring close monitoring of depressive symptoms when using this medication in the PD patient.

Over-the-counter preparations often exert sedative effects via antihistaminergic and anticholinergic pathways. Patients should be advised regarding the limited use of over-the-counter preparations, particularly as there is limited data on the safety and efficacy of these compounds when used routinely or chronically [53].

6.6.3 Deep Brain Stimulation (DBS)

Subthalamic nucleus stimulation may improve insomnia symptoms via increasing sleep duration and/or reducing nocturnal awakenings [61]. It is unclear whether this effect is mediated by sleep pathways or by improvement in motor symptoms. However, DBS is also associated with emergence of restless leg symptoms and periodic limb movements during the period of subthalamic stimulation. This suggests that the improvement noted with DBS is mediated by pathways outside of the basal ganglia. However, these DBS effects have only been observed in the advanced stages of PD. As a result, it is unclear whether these benefits would be observed for PD patients in the early stages of the disease and whether the effect would be long-lasting.

> **Conclusion**
>
> Insomnia in Parkinson's disease is a complex phenomenon that integrates several factors including PD pathology, age, depression, and medication effect, all of which contribute to insomnia pathophysiology. Therefore, insomnia evaluation necessitates consideration of multiple factors including adjustment of medications, behavioral adaptations to help with motor symptoms, addressing non-motor issues such as psychiatric and urinary complaints, evaluation of underlying sleep disorders such as sleep apnea and restless legs syndrome, and possibly administering a combination of pharmacotherapy and behavioral treatments for insomnia. Treatment of insomnia will likely involve a multidisciplinary team of specialists including neurology, psychiatry, urology, and a sleep clinician who is experienced with the diagnosis and management of insomnia.

References

1. Factor SA, McAlarney T, Sanchez-Ramos JR, Weiner WJ. Sleep disorders and sleep effect in parkinson's disease. Mov Disord. 1990;5(4):280–5.
2. Dauvilliers Y. Insomnia in patients with neurodegenerative conditions. Sleep Med. 2007;8 Suppl 4:S27–34.
3. Adler CH, Thorpy MJ. Sleep issues in parkinson's disease. Neurology. 2005;64(12 Suppl 3):S12–20.
4. Stavitsky K, Neargarder S, Bogdanova Y, McNamara P, Cronin-Golomb A. The impact of sleep quality on cognitive functioning in parkinson's disease. J Int Neuropsychol Soc. 2012;18(1):108–17.
5. Happe S, Berger K, FAQT Study Investigators. The association between caregiver burden and sleep disturbances in partners of patients with parkinson's disease. Age Ageing. 2002;31(5):349–54.
6. Pal PK, Thennarasu K, Fleming J, Schulzer M, Brown T, Calne SM. Nocturnal sleep disturbances and daytime dysfunction in patients with parkinson's disease and in their caregivers. Parkinsonism Relat Disord. 2004;10(3):157–68.
7. Lees AJ, Blackburn NA, Campbell VL. The nighttime problems of parkinson's disease. Clin Neuropharmacol. 1988;11(6):512–9.
8. Karlsen KH, Tandberg E, Arsland D, Larsen JP. Health related quality of life in parkinson's disease: a prospective longitudinal study. J Neurol Neurosurg Psychiatry. 2000;69(5):584–9.
9. Kryger M, Roth T, Dement W. Principles and practices of sleep medicine. Saint Louis: Elsevier; 2011.
10. American Academy of Sleep Medicine. International classification of sleep disorders. 3rd ed. Darien: American Academy of Sleep Medicine; 2014.
11. American Psychiatric Association. Diagnostic and statistical manual of mental disorders. 5th ed. Washington, DC: American Psychaitric Publishing; 2013.
12. World Health Organization (WHO). International classification of diseases, 10th revision (ICD-10). Geneva: World Health Organization; 1992.
13. Schrempf W, Brandt MD, Storch A, Reichmann H. Sleep disorders in parkinson's disease. J Parkinsons Dis. 2014;4(2):211–21.

14. Perlis ML, Giles DE, Mendelson WB, Bootzin RR, Wyatt JK. Psychophysiological insomnia: the behavioural model and a neurocognitive perspective. J Sleep Res. 1997;6(3):179–88.
15. Braak H, Del Tredici K, Rub U, de Vos RA, Jansen Steur EN, Braak E. Staging of brain pathology related to sporadic parkinson's disease. Neurobiol Aging. 2003;24(2):197–211.
16. Tijero B, Somme J, Gomez-Esteban JC, Berganzo K, Adhikari I, Lezcano E, et al. Relationship between sleep and dysautonomic symptoms assessed by self-report scales. Mov Disord. 2011;26(10):1967–8.
17. Zesiewicz TA, Gold M, Chari G, Hauser RA. Current issues in depression in parkinson's disease. Am J Geriatr Psychiatry. 1999;7(2):110–8.
18. Reijnders JS, Ehrt U, Weber WE, Aarsland D, Leentjens AF. A systematic review of prevalence studies of depression in parkinson's disease. Mov Disord. 2008;23(2):183–9; quiz 313.
19. Leentjens AF, Koester J, Fruh B, Shephard DT, Barone P, Houben JJ. The effect of pramipexole on mood and motivational symptoms in parkinson's disease: a meta-analysis of placebo-controlled studies. Clin Ther. 2009;31(1):89–98.
20. Riemann D, Spiegelhalder K, Feige B, Voderholzer U, Berger M, Perlis M, et al. The hyperarousal model of insomnia: a review of the concept and its evidence. Sleep Med Rev. 2010;14(1):19–31.
21. Trotti LM, Rye DB. Neurobiology of sleep: the role of dopamine in parkinson's disease. In: Chaudhuri KR, Tolosa E, Schapira A, Poewe W, editors. Non-motor symptoms in Parkinson's disease. Oxford: Oxford University Press; 2009. p. 165–76.
22. Leeman AL, O'Neill CJ, Nicholson PW, Deshmukh AA, Denham MJ, Royston JP, et al. Parkinson's disease in the elderly: response to and optimal spacing of night time dosing with levodopa. Br J Clin Pharmacol. 1987;24(5):637–43.
23. Comella CL, Morrissey M, Janko K. Nocturnal activity with nighttime pergolide in parkinson disease: a controlled study using actigraphy. Neurology. 2005;64(8):1450–1.
24. Remick RA, Froese C, Keller FD. Common side effects associated with monoamine oxidase inhibitors. Prog Neuropsychopharmacol Biol Psychiatry. 1989;13(3–4):497–504.
25. Elmer L, Schwid S, Eberly S, Goetz C, Fahn S, Kieburtz K, et al. Rasagiline-associated motor improvement in PD occurs without worsening of cognitive and behavioral symptoms. J Neurol Sci. 2006;248(1–2):78–83.
26. Thannickal TC, Lai YY, Siegel JM. Hypocretin (orexin) and melanin concentrating hormone loss and the symptoms of parkinson's disease. Brain. 2008;131(Pt 1):e87.
27. Gjerstad MD, Wentzel-Larsen T, Aarsland D, Larsen JP. Insomnia in parkinson's disease: frequency and progression over time. J Neurol Neurosurg Psychiatry. 2007;78(5):476–9.
28. Winkelman JW, Buxton OM, Jensen JE, Benson KL, O'Connor SP, Wang W, et al. Reduced brain GABA in primary insomnia: preliminary data from 4 T proton magnetic resonance spectroscopy (1H-MRS). Sleep. 2008;31(11):1499–506.
29. Schutte-Rodin S, Broch L, Buysse D, Dorsey C, Sateia M. Clinical guideline for the evaluation and management of chronic insomnia in adults. J Clin Sleep Med. 2008;4(5):487–504.
30. Buysse DJ. Insomnia. JAMA. 2013;309(7):706–16.
31. Hogl B, Arnulf I, Comella C, Ferreira J, Iranzo A, Tilley B, et al. Scales to assess sleep impairment in parkinson's disease: critique and recommendations. Mov Disord. 2010;25(16):2704–16.
32. Chaudhuri KR, Pal S, DiMarco A, Whately-Smith C, Bridgman K, Mathew R, et al. The parkinson's disease sleep scale: a new instrument for assessing sleep and nocturnal disability in parkinson's disease. J Neurol Neurosurg Psychiatry. 2002;73(6):629–35.
33. Marinus J, Visser M, van Hilten JJ, Lammers GJ, Stiggelbout AM. Assessment of sleep and sleepiness in parkinson disease. Sleep. 2003;26(8):1049–54.
34. Buysse DJ, Ancoli-Israel S, Edinger JD, Lichstein KL, Morin CM. Recommendations for a standard research assessment of insomnia. Sleep. 2006;29(9):1155–73.
35. Carney CE, Buysse DJ, Ancoli-Israel S, Edinger JD, Krystal AD, Lichstein KL, et al. The consensus sleep diary: standardizing prospective sleep self-monitoring. Sleep. 2012;35(2):287–302.
36. Ong JC, Suh S. Diagnostic tools for insomnia. In: Kushida C, editor. The encyclopedia of sleep. Waltham: Academic; 2013. p. 268–73.

37. Ancoli-Israel S, Cole R, Alessi C, Chambers M, Moorcroft W, Pollak CP. The role of actigraphy in the study of sleep and circadian rhythms. Sleep. 2003;26(3):342–92.

38. Morgenthaler T, Alessi C, Friedman L, Owens J, Kapur V, Boehlecke B, et al. Practice parameters for the use of actigraphy in the assessment of sleep and sleep disorders: an update for 2007. Sleep. 2007;30(4):519–29.

39. Morgenthaler T, Kramer M, Alessi C, Friedman L, Boehlecke B, Brown T, et al. Practice parameters for the psychological and behavioral treatment of insomnia: an update an american academy of sleep medicine report. Sleep. 2006;29(11):1415–9.

40. Ong JC, Crisostomo MI. The more the merrier? Working towards multidisciplinary management of obstructive sleep apnea and comorbid insomnia. J Clin Psychol. 2013;69(10):1066–77.

41. Cai Y, Liu S, Sothern RB, Xu S, Chan P. Expression of clock genes Per1 and Bmal1 in total leukocytes in health and parkinson's disease. Eur J Neurol. 2010;17(4):550–4.

42. Hartmann A, Veldhuis JD, Deuschle M, Standhardt H, Heuser I. Twenty-four hour cortisol release profiles in patients with alzheimer's and parkinson's disease compared to normal controls: ultradian secretory pulsatility and diurnal variation. Neurobiol Aging. 1997;18(3):285–9.

43. Fertl E, Auff E, Doppelbauer A, Waldhauser F. Circadian secretion pattern of melatonin in de novo parkinsonian patients: evidence for phase-shifting properties of l-dopa. J Neural Transm Park Dis Dement Sect. 1993;5(3):227–34.

44. Rios RS, Creti L, Fichten CS, Bailes S, Libman E, Pelletier A, et al. Doxepin and cognitive behavioural therapy for insomnia in patients with parkinson's disease – A randomized study. Parkinsonism Relat Disord. 2013. (http://dx.doi.org/10.1016/j.parkreldis.2013.03.003).

45. Bootzin RR, Epstein D, Wood JM. Stimulus control instructions. In: Hauri PJ, editor. Case studies in insomnia. New York: Plenum Press; 1991. p. 19–28.

46. Hauri PJ. Current concepts: the sleep disorders. Kalamazoo: The Upjohn Company; 1977.

47. Morin CM, Stone J, Trinkle D, Mercer J, Remsberg S. Dysfunctional beliefs and attitudes about sleep among older adults with and without insomnia complaints. Psychol Aging. 1993;8(3):463–7.

48. Ong JC, Cvengros JA, Wyatt JK. Cognitive behavioral treatment for insomnia. Psychatr Ann. 2008;38:590–5.

49. Stepanski EJ. Hypnotics should not be considered for the initial treatment of chronic insomnia. Con. J Clin Sleep Med. 2005;1(2):125–8.

50. Bruin VM, Bittencourt LR, Tufik S. Sleep-wake disturbances in parkinson's disease: current evidence regarding diagnostic and therapeutic decisions. Eur Neurol. 2012;67(5):257–67.

51. Suchowersky O, Furtado S, Rohs G. Beneficial effect of intranasal desmopressin for nocturnal polyuria in parkinson's disease. Mov Disord. 1995;10(3):337–40.

52. Ancoli-Israel S, Richardson GS, Mangano RM, Jenkins L, Hall P, Jones WS. Long-term use of sedative hypnotics in older patients with insomnia. Sleep Med. 2005;6(2):107–13.

53. Walsh JK, Roth T. Pharmacologic treatment of insomnia: benzodiazepine receptor agonists. In: Kryger MH, Roth T, Dement WC, editors. Principles and practices of sleep medicine. 5th ed. St Louis: Elsevier; 2011. p. 905–15.

54. Menza M, Dobkin RD, Marin H, Gara M, Bienfait K, Dicke A, et al. Treatment of insomnia in parkinson's disease: a controlled trial of eszopiclone and placebo. Mov Disord. 2010;25(11):1708–14.

55. Walsh JK, Erman M, Erwin CW, Jamieson A, Mahowald M, Regestein Q, et al. Subjective hypnotic efficacy of trazodone and zolpidem in DSM-III-R primary insomnia. Hum Psychopharmacol. 1998;13(3):191–8.

56. Juri C, Chana P, Tapia J, Kunstmann C, Parrao T. Quetiapine for insomnia in parkinson disease: results from an open-label trial. Clin Neuropharmacol. 2005;28(4):185–7.

57. Buscemi N, Vandermeer B, Hooton N, Pandya R, Tjosvold L, Hartling L, et al. The efficacy and safety of exogenous melatonin for primary sleep disorders. A meta-analysis. J Gen Intern Med. 2005;20(12):1151–8.

58. Roth T, Seiden D, Sainati S, Wang-Weigand S, Zhang J, Zee P. Effects of ramelteon on patient-reported sleep latency in older adults with chronic insomnia. Sleep Med. 2006;7(4):312–8.

59. Dowling GA, Mastick J, Colling E, Carter JH, Singer CM, Aminoff MJ. Melatonin for sleep disturbances in parkinson's disease. Sleep Med. 2005;6(5):459–66.
60. Ondo WG, Perkins T, Swick T, Hull Jr KL, Jimenez JE, Garris TS, et al. Sodium oxybate for excessive daytime sleepiness in parkinson disease: an open-label polysomnographic study. Arch Neurol. 2008;65(10):1337–40.
61. Arnulf I, Bejjani BP, Garma L, Bonnet AM, Houeto JL, Damier P, et al. Improvement of sleep architecture in PD with subthalamic nucleus stimulation. Neurology. 2000;55(11):1732–4.

Sleep Disordered Breathing in Parkinson's Disease

Michael K. Scullin, Lynn Marie Trotti, and Donald L. Bliwise

Contents

Abstract

Sleep disordered breathing (SDB) is a serious medical condition in which there are repeated reductions or cessations of breathing during sleep. Early research suggested that because Parkinson's disease (PD) patients have pulmonary abnormalities while they are awake they may be at increased risk for developing sleep disordered breathing. A large literature now demonstrates that sleep disordered

M.K. Scullin (✉)
Department of Psychology and Neuroscience, Baylor University, Waco, TX, USA
e-mail: michael_scullin@baylor.edu

L.M. Trotti • D.L. Bliwise
Department of Neurology, Emory University School of Medicine, Atlanta, GA, USA
e-mail: lbecke2@emory.edu; dbliwis@emory.edu

© Springer-Verlag Wien 2015
A. Videnovic, B. Högl (eds.), *Disorders of Sleep and Circadian Rhythms in Parkinson's Disease*, DOI 10.1007/978-3-7091-1631-9_7

breathing is common in Parkinson's disease patients, but no different than age-matched controls from the general population. In the general population, sleep disordered breathing often correlates with excessive daytime sleepiness, but this correlation is not typically observed within Parkinson's disease patients. However, sleep disordered breathing in Parkinson's disease has been preliminarily linked to impaired sleep-dependent memory consolidation, blunted sympathetic responses, and worsening motor function Unified Parkinson's Disease Rating Scale (UPDRS). Parkinson's disease patients who have sleep disordered breathing may benefit from positive airway pressure or mandibular advancement treatments, and an exciting avenue for future research is determining whether such treatment also positively affects disease progression and quality of life.

7.1 An Introduction to Sleep Disordered Breathing

Sleep disordered breathing (SDB) is a medical condition in which breathing repeatedly ceases (apnea) or is reduced (hypopnea) during sleep. This condition affects more than 40 million Americans and approximately 75 % of severe cases are undiagnosed [1, 2]. In this chapter, we first discuss SDB in the context of individuals without neurological disease. Then we turn our attention to why SDB might be particularly relevant to Parkinson's disease (PD), and we evaluate the literature with regard to two questions. First, is SDB more common in PD than in the general community? Second, in PD patients, what are the clinically relevant correlates of SDB?

7.1.1 Definitions, Detection, and Diagnosis

SDB is a general term that includes several distinguishable subtypes of poor breathing during sleep. Obstructive sleep apnea is characterized by the cessation of breathing due to an occluded upper airway. By contrast, in central sleep apnea there is an unstable ventilatory control system, which results in periods of absent respiration despite an open airway [3]. Complex sleep apnea syndrome is diagnosed when an individual demonstrates both central and obstructive events.

A variety of questionnaires are used in the clinical assessment of SDB (e.g., Berlin Questionnaire [4], STOP-BANG Questionnaire [5]). Some of the most important screening questions involve the frequency of snoring and bed partner reports of the patient gasping for air, because these signs indicate obstructed breathing. In addition, SDB is more likely in obese individuals [6] and in those who have an enlarged neck circumference, retrognathia, or other craniofacial morphologies that reduce airflow [7]. The gold standard for detecting SDB, however, is nocturnal polysomnographic recordings of electroencephalography, electrooculography, electromyography, respiratory effort, airflow, and oxygen saturation levels. Apneas are scored when there is a $\geq$90 % reduction in airflow for $\geq$10 s and hypopneas are scored when there is a 30–90 % reduction in airflow for $\geq$10 s accompanied by a 4 % reduction in oxygen saturation levels [8]. An apnea-hypopnea index (AHI), which is the total combined number of apneas and hypopneas per hour of sleep, is normal when less than 5; however, an AHI from 5 to 14.9 indicates mild SDB, an AHI from 15 to 29.9 indicates moderate SDB, and an AHI greater than 30 indicates severe SDB.

7.1.2 Correlates of Sleep Disordered Breathing in the General Population

In the general population, the prevalence of SDB increases with age and is more prevalent in men than women [9]. Independent of these demographic factors, SDB has been linked to several poor health outcomes. First, SDB can lead to daytime sleepiness, moodiness, and poor vigilance. Such outcomes may have implications for workplace performance and vehicle accidents [10]. Second, sleep apnea has been implicated to cause poorer cognitive performance on executive control tasks [11], and may increase risk for developing mild cognitive impairment or dementia [12]. Third, SDB is strongly associated with hypertension [13], and may also predispose individuals to cardiac ischemia, congestive heart failure, cardiac arrhythmias, and cerebrovascular disease [14]. Fourth, at least in rodent models, SDB has been implicated in the loss of catecholamine neurons [15], with hypoxia contributing to a reduction in extracellular dopamine [16].

7.2 Relevance of Sleep Disordered Breathing in Parkinson's Disease

There are several reasons why SDB might be particularly important in PD patients. Mortality rates may be elevated in PD patients in the early morning hours relative to other neurological diseases [17], and some have interpreted this result as evidence for respiratory insufficiency during sleep [18]. Moreover, beyond neuropathology in the nigrostriatal pathways, PD may also be associated with neurodegeneration in other brainstem regions [19, 20], which may contribute to SDB by disrupting respiratory and autonomic functions [21].

SDB is also implicated in PD because waking pulmonary function abnormalities are associated with this disease [22]. Such abnormalities may be due to degeneration of dopaminergic neurons or to medication side effects including dyskinesias or wearing-off [23]. Pulmonary abnormalities may include upper airway obstruction as well as chest wall rigidity and hypokinesia, each of which might be expected to result in breathing abnormalities during sleep [23–26].

Another reason why SDB might be particularly important in PD patients is that one of the most common symptoms of SDB in the general population—excessive daytime sleepiness—is also a major concern in PD patients. Hobson et al. [27] found that excessive daytime sleepiness was present in 51 % of a sample of 638 PD patients, even in patients who were living independently and still driving. Though some of the excessive daytime sleepiness in PD patients may be attributable to the usage of dopaminergic medications [28], the relationship between sleepiness and medication class may be complex. Using the objective Maintenance of Wakefulness

Test (MWT) to determine alertness, Bliwise et al. [29] found that higher dosages of dopamine agonists were associated with greater daytime sleepiness (lower alertness) whereas higher dosages of levodopa were associated with lower daytime sleepiness (higher alertness). Additional research has shown that daytime sleepiness is not solely attributable to dopaminergic medications, but appears to be an integral part of the disease [30, 31].

7.3 Prevalence of Sleep Disordered Breathing in Parkinson's Disease

Given the prevalence of symptoms of sleep apnea in PD patients (especially daytime sleepiness) as well as possible mechanisms for its predisposition in PD (chest wall rigidity), a pertinent question is whether SDB is more common in PD patients relative to age-matched controls. There have been two approaches to address this question: one relying on questionnaires and the other relying on in-laboratory polysomnography.

7.3.1 Questionnaires

Chotinaiwattarakul et al. [32] found that high risk for SDB, as assessed by the Berlin Questionnaire [4], was suggested in nearly 50 % of their 134 PD patients whereas only approximately 35 % of non-blood relative controls. Similarly, Rongve et al. [33] compared 39 patients with a diagnosis of PD dementia or Lewy body dementias to 420 healthy controls using the Mayo Sleep Questionnaire. This questionnaire uses bed partner report of arrested respiratory episodes during sleep or the reported use of continuous positive airway pressure to determine probable obstructive sleep apnea. Rongve et al. [33] observed a higher rate of probable obstructive sleep apnea in their patient group (25.7 %) than in their healthy control group (15.2 %). However, not all questionnaire studies have suggested differences in SDB across PD and control groups. For example, using the Sleep Questionnaire and Assessment of Wakefulness (SQAW [34]), Happe et al. [35] found a nominally lower rate of SDB symptoms in the PD group than the control group.

7.3.2 Polysomnography

Polysomnographic studies have also yielded some variable findings for prevalence rates. A summary of these studies is shown in Table 7.1. Prior to modern AHI criteria, early research compared the number of apneic episodes in small samples of PD patients and normal controls, with some findings suggesting greater apneic episodes in PD patients than controls [18, 47], and other findings suggesting no differences [48]. Using more contemporary AHI cutoff scores, 7 out of 12 studies have observed high prevalence of SDB in PD patients. These studies generally observed AHIs

Table 7.1 Overview of polysomnographic studies that assessed the prevalence of sleep disordered breathing (SDB) in Parkinson's disease (PD)

Reference (chronological)	PSG nights	PD group	Control group	No SDB (0–4.9)	Mild SDB (5–15)	Moderate SDB (15.1–30)	Severe SDB (>30)	Author's conclusion
Arnulf [30]	1	N=54	None	50 %	27.8 %	11 %	9.3 %	Higher rate in PD
Maria [36]	1	N=15	Age-matched controls (n=15)	33.3 %		60 %		Higher rate in PD
Baumann [37]	1	N=10	None	0 %	80 %	10 %	10 %	Higher rate in PD
Diederich [38]	1	N=49	AHI-matched controls (n=49)	57.1 %	20.4 %	8.2 %	14.3 %	Lower rate in PD
Shpirer [39]	1	N=46	Age-matched controls (n=30)	78.3 %[a]	21.7 %[a]			AHI was higher in PD
Monaca [40]	1	N=36	None	44.4 %[a]	44.4 %[a]		11.1 %	No commentary
Sixel-Döring [41]	2	N=20	Progressive supranuclear palsy (n=20)	45 %	55 %			Common, undetected in PD
Norlinah [42]	1	N=44	None	51 %	24.5 %	16.3 %	8.2 %	High SDB prevalence in PD
Cochen De Cock [43]	1	N=100	In-hospital controls (n=50)	73 %	6 %	11 %	10 %	Lower rate in PD
Trotti and Bliwise [44]	3	N=55	Sleep Heart Health Study	56.3 % (53.7 %)	29.1 % (28.6 %)	10.9 % (11.7 %)	3.6 % (6.1 %)	No difference
Yong [45]	1	N=56	Age-matched controls (n=68)	50.9 % (34.3 %)	15.1 % (37.3 %)	18.9 % (19.4 %)	15.1 % (9 %)	No difference
Nomura [46]	1	N=107	Non-PD sleep apnea controls (n=31)	77.6 %		22.4 %		No difference or milder in PD

Severity of SDB is determined by the apnea-hypopnea index (AHI; number in parentheses). References are listed in chronological order. When available, data from control groups are presented in parentheses. Missing cells and collapsed cells reflect the manner in which data were reported in the original papers

Notes: [a]indicates that AHI cutoff was at 10 (rather than 5 and 15)

>5 in more than 50 % of their patient samples, and one study even observed an AHI >5 in all of their PD patients. Though this might be considered to be strong evidence for an increased prevalence of SDB in PD, there exist at least three important limitations for these studies. One limitation is that these studies may have preferentially selected PD patients for excessive daytime sleepiness or those who were referred to the sleep center for clinical purposes. Either selection criteria could be expected to bias diagnosis of SDB in the PD group. In addition, only one of these studies used more than one night of polysomnographic assessment and two of these studies had very small sample sizes ($Ns \leq 15$). None of these seven studies included a sample size that exceeded $N = 54$. Furthermore, scoring criteria for apneas and hypopneas vary widely, which is a limitation for studies that did not test (healthy) control groups with blinded scoring. Only two of the six studies that concluded an increased prevalence of SDB in PD patients supported that conclusion by demonstrating significantly greater AHI relative to an age-matched control group.

Several studies have failed to observe significantly higher SDB in PD patients (Table 7.1). For example, Trotti and Bliwise [44] measured AHI in 55 idiopathic PD patients across three nights of in-laboratory polysomnographic testing, and compared prevalence rates against those observed in the Sleep Heart Health Study [13], which is the largest epidemiological study of SDB in the general population. They found no difference in the prevalence of mild, moderate, or severe sleep apnea in their PD patients. Yong et al. [45] also observed no difference between 56 PD patients and 68 age- and sex-matched controls in an Asian population. Our most recent work—the Emory 48-h protocol [29]—also suggests no increased risk of SDB in PD patients. We had 84 idiopathic PD patients undergo at least one night of polysomnographic testing ($N = 74$ completed two nights). Most patients (59.5 %) showed a mean AHI <5, and 32.1 % of patients showed mild sleep apnea (AHI 5–14.9). Only 4.8 % and 3.6 % of patients showed moderate (AHI 15–29.9) or severe (AHI ≥ 30) signs of sleep apnea, respectively. When compared with prevalence estimates from the Sleep Heart Health Study [13], our results suggest that the prevalence rate of AHI is similar for mild sleep apnea, and possibly lower for moderate and severe sleep apnea, in PD patients than in the general population.

Three additional studies have suggested either lower rates, or less severe, SDB in PD patients than in controls. Cochen De Cock et al. [43] found a lower prevalence of mild or greater SDB in a sample of 100 PD patients (27 %) relative to 50 non-neurological in-hospital control patients (40 %). Diederich et al. [38] conducted a case-control study in which 49 idiopathic PD patients were matched to 49 controls based on age, gender, and AHI. They observed fewer obstructive sleep apneas and higher oxygen saturation levels in the PD patients than in the AHI-matched controls. Most recently, Nomura et al. [46] concluded that SDB in their sample of 107 PD patients was very similar to that of the elderly general population; furthermore, relative to a sample of 31 non-PD patients with obstructive sleep apnea, the PD patients who showed an AHI ≥ 15 had a lower respiratory arousal index and a less severe decrease in oxygen saturation.

In sum, though there are reports of a higher prevalence of SDB in PD patients than the general population, several of these studies are based on small sample sizes and may have been confounded by selection biases (referral for sleepiness). Our interpretation of the literature is consistent with Peeraully et al.'s [49] recent review of case-control polysomnographic studies that there is no increased prevalence of SDB in PD. Nevertheless, SDB is still common in PD patients and may have important clinical implications for this population.

7.4 Clinical Implications of Sleep Disordered Breathing

One important clinical consideration for SDB in PD may be poorer quality of life [32]. We next consider the clinical correlates of SDB that might explain why quality of life is dampened in PD patients with probable sleep apnea.

7.4.1 Excessive Daytime Sleepiness

First, because excessive daytime sleepiness greatly affects quality of life in PD patients [50], and because this is a primary symptom of SDB [51], one might expect that some sleepiness in this patient group is due to SDB [37]. Some findings support this association. For example, Shpirer et al. [39] found that PD patients who had an Epworth Sleepiness Scale (ESS) score greater than 10 had a higher AHI than those with scores below 10 (see also [42, 52]). However, when measured as continuous variables, AHI and ESS did not correlate significantly [39]. Other studies have reported no significant correlation between AHI and ESS [43, 44], and we did not observe a correlation in our 48-h protocol [29].

When sleepiness has been measured objectively using the Mean Sleep Latency Test, with few exceptions [53], there is typically no correlation between AHI and mean sleep latency [30, 40]. In the 48-h protocol, we incorporated up to eight Maintenance of Wakefulness Tests (MWTs) in which PD patients were instructed to stay awake while lying in bed for 40 min [29]. In this study, we did not observe a relationship between AHI and MWT scores. Therefore, the relationship between SDB and quality of life in PD [32] does not appear to be mediated by excessive daytime sleepiness. However, the causes of sleepiness are multifactorial (e.g., the presence of dopaminergic medications), which may explain why SDB is a weaker predictor of sleepiness in PD patients.

7.4.2 Cardiovascular Risk

As previously described, common correlates of SDB in healthy controls include hypertension, cardiovascular events, and higher body mass index [13, 14]. Though studies of SDB in PD are not as well powered as those in the general community, it is still surprising that the typical (aforementioned) correlates of SDB have not been observed in studies of PD patients [42, 43, 46]. Valko et al. [54] evaluated the association between heart rate variability and presence or absence of obstructive sleep apnea syndrome in 62 PD patients and 62 age-matched controls. Their control group demonstrated several significant associations between obstructive sleep apnea syndrome and heart rate variability, particularly for the low-frequency power band and the low-frequency/high-frequency power band ratio. By contrast, heart rate variability did not correlate with SDB in the PD group. The authors suggested that there is a blunted sympathetic response to sleep breathing events in PD.

7.4.3 Cognition and Memory Consolidation

SDB has also often been connected to the development of dementia, mild cognitive impairment, or subtle cognitive effects in the general population [12]. It should be noted, however, that this literature has produced variable results, and in the large-scale, multicenter Apnea Positive Pressure Long-Term Efficacy Study (APPLES), few associations were observed [11]. Few studies have examined SDB in relation to cognition in idiopathic PD patients (though much work has been done for REM sleep behavior disorder [55]). Cochen De Cock et al. [43] found no correlation between SDB and Mini-Mental State Examination scores in PD patients. However, more recently, Stavitsky et al. [56] observed a positive correlation between actigraphy-defined sleep efficiency and an executive function composite. Though not necessarily implicating SDB, it is possible that some of the actigraphy-defined poor sleep efficiency might be due to breathing events due to breathing events or periodic limb movements [57].

There is an important distinction to be made between impaired cognition as assessed by neuropsychological testing (as a stable trait feature of PD), versus an emerging "memory consolidation" literature that connects cognitive test performance improvements to the sleep obtained between repeated cognitive tests (for review, see [58]). In the 48-h protocol, we gave PD patients eight digit span backward (executive function) tests across 2 days [59]. As illustrated in Fig. 7.1, PD patients taking dopaminergic medications demonstrated significant digit span backward improvements across the 48-h study. The improvement was not simply due to practice effects because no performance improvements were observed across the repeated daytime tests. Instead, performance improvements were localized to the nocturnal sleep interval (Fig. 7.1). The degree of digit span backward improvement was significantly associated with higher levels of slow-wave sleep and higher oxygen saturation *during the night that constituted the training interval*, and not during the pre-experimental night (laboratory adaptation night). PD patients who demonstrated 5 or more minutes of oxygen saturation below 90 % during the training interval night did not show significant digit span improvements. Though this (sleep) effect appears robust for repeated executive function testing, it has not been observed for motor memory testing in PD patients [60, 61]. We suggest that correcting SDB might improve the ability to acquire some new skills (as suggested by digit span backward training), which could have a positive impact on PD patients' quality of life on a day-to-day basis (cf. [32]).

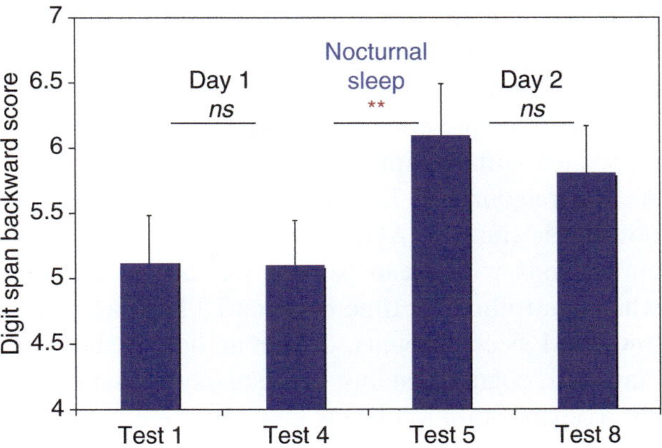

Fig. 7.1 Improvement on the digit span backward test across an interval that included nocturnal sleep, but not daytime wake, in dopamine-treated Parkinson's disease patients [59]. ** indicates $p < .01$

7.4.4 Motor Symptoms

SDB might also be associated with poorer quality of life because nocturnal hypoxia could potentially exacerbate certain aspects of PD neuropathology. Basic science studies have shown experimentally that sleep apnea could cause the loss of catecholamine neurons [15] or reduce extracellular dopamine [16]. Furthermore, oxidative stress has been implicated in dopamine cell degeneration, mitochondrial dysfunction, excitotoxicity, and inflammation in PD [62, 63]. Therefore, one might expect that higher AHI or indices of nocturnal hypoxia would correlate with measures of disease severity in PD. Consistent with this idea, Efthimiou et al. [47] observed more apneas in PD patients with more severe disease (Hoehn and Yahr scale). Moreover, Maria et al. [36] found significant correlations between log-transformed UPDRS motor scores and log-transformed AHI as well as median oxygen saturation levels, even after controlling for age. Cochen De Cock et al. [43] also observed a significant correlation between AHI and UPDRS motor scores, with SDB being more frequent and severe in the most disabled PD patients. One additional study [32] observed a nonsignificant trend for higher SDB risk (Berlin Questionnaire [4]) in PD patients at more severe disease stages, and another study [42] observed significant correlations for greater sleep fragmentation and more severe disease stages, but three studies have reported no significant correlations between *SDB variables* and either UPDRS or Hoehn Yahr scores [41, 42, 64].

We contend that a limitation in prior studies of the clinical correlates of SDB in PD patients is that most studies have examined polysomnography in relation to disease severity in PD patients at a single time point in the course of disease. A current direction of our research is examining the association between polysomnographic variables and change in motor disease severity over the course of disease. We recently evaluated whether change in motor disease severity (UPDRS motor subscale) in 29 idiopathic PD patients was associated with SDB variables [65]. The two time points (Time 1 [T1] and Time 2 [T2]) were separated by an average interval of 265 days, and at T2 patients underwent 2 nights of polysomnographic recording. Variables derived from overnight polysomnography were not associated cross-sectionally with UPDRS motor scores at T1 or T2 in our data. Similar absence of significant findings with cross-sectional analyses has been observed previously [41, 64]. However, in our data poorer sleep was strongly associated with declining function in UPDRS motor scores (i.e., from T1 to T2). As illustrated in Fig. 7.2, there were strong correlations with mean oxygen saturation levels (but not AHI), particularly during REM sleep. The UPDRS-change correlations with mean oxygen saturation during REM sleep was not negated when controlling for time between UPDRS assessments, overt dream enactment, low REM sleep amounts, dopamine dosage, age, gender, education, years since diagnosis, cognitive status, or mean oxygen saturation while awake. Thus, nocturnal oxygen saturation levels may represent an important biomarker of change in disease severity.

7.5 Treatment Options

There are several treatment options for SDB in PD patients. First, breathing problems might be treated by normal antiparkinsonian medications to reduce rigidity [66]. SDB may also be treated using positive airway pressure therapy (e.g., CPAP), which is the most typical treatment for non-PD patients who have obstructive sleep apnea. However, controversy exists over the efficacy of CPAP treatment in PD patients, because some work has suggested that not all PD patients tolerate CPAP [67]. CPAP tolerance might be a particular limitation in PD because these patients often may not be amenable to the restrictive nature of the CPAP mask. Despite these potential issues, at least in severe cases of SDB, CPAP must be considered as a treatment option [68, 69]. In patients who are intolerant of CPAP or have milder SBD, mandibular advancement devices may be a useful second line of treatment [70].

7.6 Future Directions

We believe that an exciting avenue for future research will be in determining whether relatively mild levels of nocturnal hypoxia are associated with motor and nonmotor symptom progression. SDB is very common in PD (but the prevalence does not differ from the general population; Table 7.1), and nocturnal hypoxia might cause the loss of dopamine [15, 16] and result in additional cellular dysfunction [62, 63]. It therefore remains possible that even mild SDB could accelerate disease progression [65], and, conversely, that ameliorating nocturnal hypoxia in PD patients might be a viable target for improving longevity and quality of life.

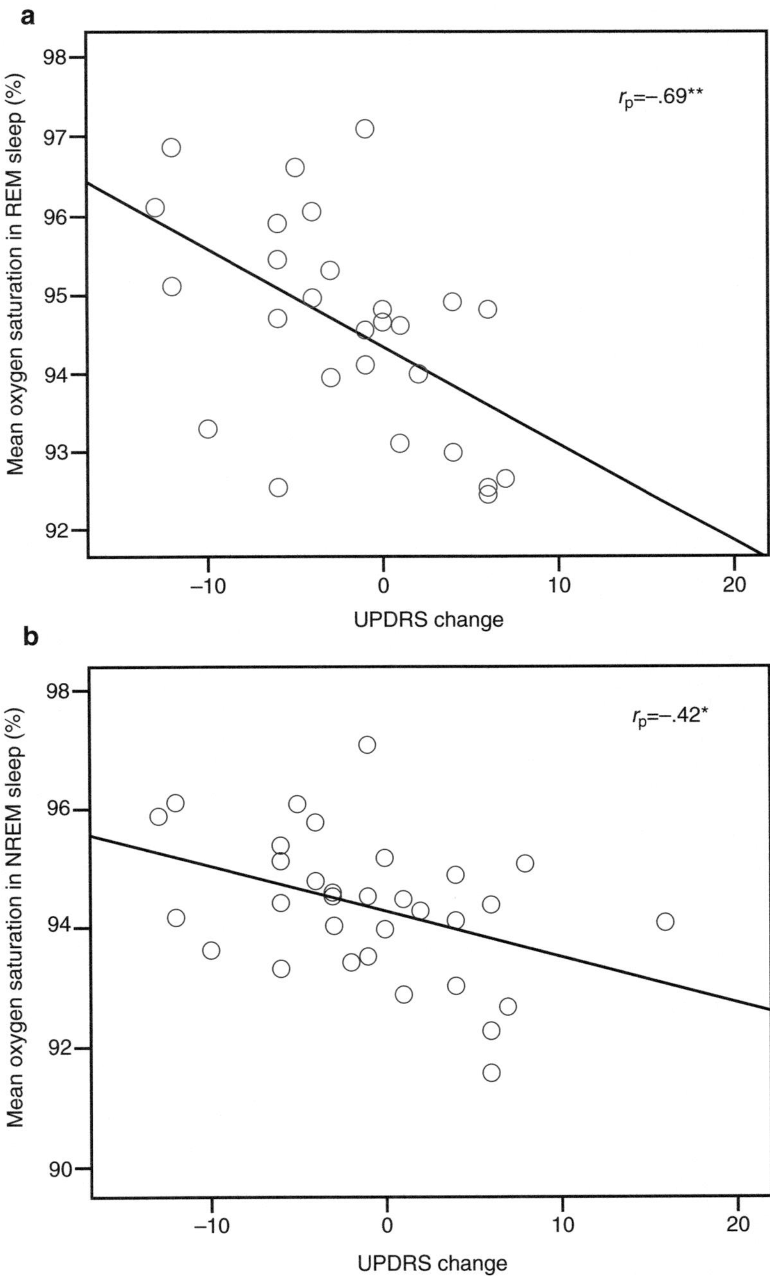

Fig. 7.2 Change in motor symptom severity across approximately 9 months (assessed as UPDRS motor symptom score) correlates with level of oxygen saturation during REM sleep (**a**) and NREM sleep (**b**) in idiopathic Parkinson's disease patients Positive numbers indicate worsening severity of motor symptoms [65]. * indicates $p < .05$, ** indicates $p < .01$

Acknowledgments Preparation of this chapter was supported by funding from the National Institute on Health (grant numbers 1P50NS071669 and F32AG041543). M.K.S. was partially supported by an Emory University School of Medicine Cottrell Fellowship.

References

1. Young T, Palta M, Dempsey J, et al. The occurrence of sleep-disordered breathing among middle-aged adults. N Engl J Med. 1993;328:1230–5.
2. Young T, Evans L, Finn L, et al. Estimation of the clinically diagnosed proportion of sleep apnea syndrome in middle-aged men and women. Sleep. 1997;20:705–6.
3. White DP. Pathogenesis of obstructive and central sleep apnea. Am J Respir Crit Care Med. 2005;172:1363–70.
4. Netzer NC, Stoohs RA, Netzer CM. Using the Berlin Questionnaire to identify patients at risk for the sleep apnea syndrome. Ann Intern Med. 1999;131:485–91.
5. Chung F, Yegneswaran B, Liao P, et al. STOP Questionnaire: a tool to screen patients for obstructive sleep apnea. Anesthesiology. 2008;108:812–21.
6. Strobel RJ, Rosen RC. Obesity and weight loss in obstructive sleep apnea: a critical review. Sleep. 1996;19:104–15.
7. Ferguson KA, Ono T, Lowe AA, et al. The relationship between obesity and craniofacial structure in obstructive sleep apnea. Chest. 1995;108:375–81.
8. Iber C, Ancoli-Israel S, Chesson AL, et al. The AASM manual for the scoring of sleep and associated events: rules, terminology and technical specifications. Westchester: American Academy of Sleep Medicine; 2007.
9. Young T, Shahar E, Nieto FJ, et al. Predictors of sleep-disordered breathing in community-dwelling adults: the Sleep Heart Health Study. Arch Intern Med. 2002;162:893–900.
10. Teran-Santos J, Jimenez-Gomez A, Cordero-Guevara J. The association between sleep apnea and the risk of traffic accidents. N Engl J Med. 1999;340:847–51.
11. Kushida CA, Nichols DA, Holmes TH, et al. Effects of continuous positive airway pressure on neurocognitive function in obstructive sleep apnea patients: the Apnea Positive Pressure Long-term Efficacy Study (APPLES). Sleep. 2012;35:1593–602.
12. Yaffe K, Laffan AM, Harrison SL, et al. Sleep-disordered breathing, hypoxia, and risk of mild cognitive impairment and dementia in older women. JAMA. 2011;306:613–9.
13. Nieto FJ, Young TB, Lind BK, et al. Association of sleep-disordered breathing, sleep apnea, and hypertension in a large community- based study. Sleep Heart Health Study. JAMA. 2000;283:1829–36.
14. Shamsuzzaman AS, Gersh BJ, Somers VK. Obstructive sleep apnea: implications for cardiac and vascular disease. JAMA. 2003;290:1906–14.
15. Zhu Y, Fenik P, Zhan G, et al. Selective loss of catecholaminergic wake–active neurons in a murine sleep apnea model. J Neurosci. 2007;27:10060–71.
16. Decker MJ, Jones KA, Solomon IG, et al. Reduced extracellular dopamine and increased responsiveness to novelty: neurochemical and behavioral sequelae of intermittent hypoxia. Sleep. 2005;28:169–76.
17. Riederer P, Wuketich S. Time course of nigrostriatal degeneration in Parkinson's disease: a detailed study of influential factors in human brain amine analysis. J Neural Transm. 1976;38:277–301.
18. Hardie RJ, Efthimiou J, Stern GM. Respiration and sleep in Parkinson's disease. J Neurol Neurosurg Psychiatry. 1986;49:1326.
19. Braak H, Rüb U, Sandmann-Keil D, et al. Parkinson's disease: affection of brain stem nuclei controlling premotor and motor neurons of the somatomotor system. Acta Neuropathol. 2000;99:489–95.
20. Braak H, Tredici KD, Rüb U, et al. Staging of brain pathology related to sporadic Parkinson's disease. Neurobiol Aging. 2003;24:197–211.

21. Probst A, Bloch A, Tolnay M. New insights into the pathology of Parkinson's disease: does the peripheral autonomic system become central? Eur J Neurol. 2008;15 Suppl 1:1–4.
22. Hovestadt A, Bogaard JM, Meerwaldt JD, et al. Pulmonary function in Parkinson's disease. J Neurol Neurosurg Psychiatry. 1989;52:329–33.
23. Shill H, Stacy M. Respiratory complications of Parkinson's disease. Semin Respir Crit Care Med. 2002;23:261–5.
24. Canning CG, Alison JA, Allen NE, et al. Parkinson's disease: an investigation of exercise capacity, respiratory function, and gait. Arch Phys Med Rehabil. 1997;78:199–207.
25. Herer B, Arnulf I, Housset B. Effects of levodopa on pulmonary function in Parkinson's disease. Chest. 2001;119:387–93.
26. Sabate M, Gonzalez I, Ruperez F, et al. Obstructive and restrictive pulmonary dysfunctions in Parkinson's disease. J Neurol Sci. 1996;138:114–9.
27. Hobson DE, Lang AE, Martin WW, et al. Excessive daytime sleepiness and sudden-onset sleep in Parkinson disease. JAMA. 2002;287:455–63.
28. Ferreira JJ, Galitzky M, Montastruc JL, et al. Sleep attacks and Parkinson's disease treatment. Lancet. 2000;355:1333–4.
29. Bliwise DL, Trotti LM, Wilson AG, et al. Daytime alertness in Parkinson's disease: potentially dose-dependent, divergent effects by drug class. Mov Disord. 2012;27:1118–24.
30. Arnulf I, Konofal E, Merino-Andreu M, et al. Parkinson's disease and sleepiness: an integral part of PD. Neurology. 2002;58:1019–24.
31. Rye DB, Bliwise DL, Dihenia B, et al. Daytime sleepiness in Parkinson's disease. J Sleep Res. 2000;9:63–9.
32. Chotinaiwattarakul W, Dayalu P, Chervin RD, et al. Risk of sleep-disordered breathing in Parkinson's disease. Sleep Breath. 2011;15:471–8.
33. Rongve A, Boeve BF, Aarsland D. Frequency and correlates of caregiver-reported sleep disturbances in a sample of persons with early dementia. J Am Geriatr Soc. 2010;58:480–6.
34. Douglass AB, Bornstein R, Nino-Murcia G, et al. The sleep disorders questionnaire I: creation and multivariate structure of SDQ. Sleep. 1994;17:160–7.
35. Happe S, Schrödl B, Faltl M, et al. Sleep disorders and depression in patients with Parkinson's disease. Acta Neurol Scand. 2001;104:275–80.
36. Maria B, Sophia S, Michalis M, et al. Sleep breathing disorders in patients with idiopathic Parkinson's disease. Respir Med. 2003;97:1151–7.
37. Baumann C, Ferini-Strambi L, Waldvogel D, et al. Parkinsonism with excessive daytime sleepiness—a narcolepsy-like disorder? J Neurol. 2005;252:139–45.
38. Diederich NJ, Vaillant M, Leischen M, et al. Sleep apnea syndrome in Parkinson's disease. A case–control study in 49 patients. Mov Disord. 2005;20:1413–8.
39. Shpirer I, Miniovitz A, Klein C, et al. Excessive daytime sleepiness in patients with Parkinson's disease: a polysomnography study. Mov Disord. 2006;21:1432–8.
40. Monaca C, Duhamel A, Jacquesson JM, et al. Vigilance troubles in Parkinson's disease: a subjective and objective polysomnographic study. Sleep Med. 2006;7:448–53.
41. Sixel-Döring F, Schweitzer M, Mollenhauer B, et al. Polysomnographic findings, video-based sleep analysis and sleep perception in progressive supranuclear palsy. Sleep Med. 2009;10:407–15.
42. Norlinah MI, Afidah KN, Noradina AT, et al. Sleep disturbances in Malaysian patients with Parkinson's disease using polysomnography and PDSS. Parkinsonism Relat Disord. 2009;15:670–4.
43. Cochen De Cock V, Abouda M, Leu S, et al. Is obstructive sleep apnea a problem in Parkinson's disease? Sleep Med. 2010;11:247–52.
44. Trotti LM, Bliwise DL. No increased risk of obstructive sleep apnea in Parkinson's disease. Mov Disord. 2010;25:2246–9.
45. Yong MH, Fook-Chong S, Pavanni R, et al. Case control polysomnographic studies of sleep disorders in Parkinson's disease. PLoS One. 2011;6:e22511.
46. Nomura T, Inoue Y, Kobayashi M, et al. Characteristics of obstructive sleep apnea in patients with Parkinson's disease. J Neurol Sci. 2013.

47. Efthimiou J, Ellis SJ, Hardie RJ, et al. Sleep apnea in idiopathic and postencephalitic parkinsonism. Adv Neurol. 1987;45:275–6.

48. Apps MC, Sheaff PC, Ingram DA, et al. Respiration and sleep in Parkinson's disease. J Neurol Neurosurg Psychiatry. 1985;48:1240–5.

49. Peeraully T, Yong MH, Chokroverty S, et al. Sleep and Parkinson's disease: a review of case-control polysomnography studies. Mov Disord. 2012;27:1729–37.

50. Chaudhuri K, Martinez-Martin P, Schapira A, et al. International multicenter pilot study of the first comprehensive self-completed nonmotor symptoms questionnaire for Parkinson's disease: the NMSquest study. Mov Disord. 2006;21:916–23.

51. Johns MW. A new method for measuring daytime sleepiness: the Epworth sleepiness scale. Sleep. 1991;14:540–5.

52. Gama RL, Távora DG, Bomfim RC, et al. Sleep disturbances and brain MRI morphometry in Parkinson's disease, multiple system atrophy and progressive supranuclear palsy–a comparative study. Parkinsonism Relat Disord. 2010;16:275–9.

53. Poryazova R, Benninger D, Waldvogel D, et al. Excessive daytime sleepiness in Parkinson's disease: characteristics and determinants. Eur Neurol. 2010;63:129–35.

54. Valko PO, Hauser S, Werth E, et al. Heart rate variability in patients with idiopathic Parkinson's disease with and without obstructive sleep apnea syndrome. Parkinsonism Relat Disord. 2012;18:525–31.

55. Vendette M, Gagnon JF, Decary A, et al. REM sleep behavior disorder predicts cognitive impairment in Parkinson disease without dementia. Neurology. 2007;69:1843–9.

56. Stavitsky K, Neargarder S, Bogdanova Y. The impact of sleep quality on cognitive functioning in Parkinson's disease. J Int Neuropsychol Soc. 2011;18:108–17.

57. Scullin MK, Fairley JA, Trotti LM, et al. Sleep correlates of trait executive function and memory in Parkinson's disease. J Parkinsons Dis. 2015;5:49–54.

58. Rasch B, Born J. About sleep's role in memory. Physiol Rev. 2013;93:681–766.

59. Scullin MK, Trotti LM, Wilson AG, et al. Nocturnal sleep enhances working memory training in Parkinson's disease but not Lewy body dementia. Brain. 2012;135:2789–97.

60. Marinelli L, Crupi D, Di Rocco A, et al. Learning and consolidation of visuo-motor adaptation in Parkinson's disease. Parkinsonism Relat Disord. 2009;15:6–11.

61. Terpening Z, Naismith S, Melehan K, et al. The contribution of nocturnal sleep to the consolidation of motor skill learning in healthy ageing and Parkinson's disease. J Sleep Res. 2013.

62. Andersen JK. Oxidative stress in neurodegeneration: cause or consequence? Nat Rev Neurosci. 2004;5:S18–25.

63. Jenner P. Oxidative stress in Parkinson's disease. Ann Neurol. 2003;53:S26–38.

64. Young A, Horne M, Churchward T, et al. Comparison of sleep disturbance in mild versus severe Parkinson's disease. Sleep. 2002;25:573–7.

65. Scullin MK, Trotti LM, Goldstein FC et al. PSG-recorded sleep as a possible biomarker of worsening motor function in Parkinson's disease. In: Abstracts of the annual SLEEP meeting, Baltimore, June 2013.

66. Yoshida T, Kono I, Yoshikawa K, et al. Improvement of sleep hypopnea by antiparkinsonian drugs in a patient with Parkinson's disease: a polysomnographic study. Intern Med. 2003;42:1135–8.

67. Schäfer D. Schlafbezogene Atmungsstörungen bei Parkinsonsyndromen: Häufigkeit, Art und Behandlungsansätze [Sleep related breathing disorders in parkinsonism: frequency, nature, and therapeutical approaches]. Somnologie. 2001;5:103–14.

68. Högl B. Sleep apnea in Parkinson's disease: when is it significant? Sleep Med. 2010;11:233–5.

69. Neikrug AB, Liu L, Avanzino JA, et al. Continuous positive airway pressure improves sleep and daytime sleepiness in patients with Parkinson's disease and sleep apnea. Sleep. 2014;37:177–85.

70. Mehta A, Qian J, Petocz P, et al. A randomized, controlled study of a mandibular advancement splint for obstructive sleep apnea. Am J Respir Crit Care Med. 2001;163:1457–61.

Excessive Daytime Somnolence Associated with Parkinson's Disease

8

James Battista, Renee Monderer, and Michael Thorpy

Contents

Abstract

Excessive daytime sleepiness (EDS) occurs in up to 50 % of patients with Parkinson's disease (PD) and is characterized by an inability to maintain full alertness in the daytime and undesirable lapses into sleep. Often overshadowed by the motor symptoms of PD, EDS can contribute to home and automobile accidents and have a negative impact on mood and overall quality of life. Sleep disturbances and EDS can result from the medications used to treat PD, degeneration of neuronal systems involved in the control of the sleep–wake system that occurs as part of the PD disease process, and comorbid conditions including specific sleep disorders and depression. The treatment of EDS in the PD patient requires careful evaluation of the multiple contributing causes and instituting recommendations that can consist of sleep hygiene and behavioral changes, alterations in the dosing and timing of PD medications, treatment of comor-

J. Battista, MD • R. Monderer, MD (✉) • M. Thorpy, MD
Department of Neurology, Montefiore Medical Center,
111 E. 210th St, Bronx, NY 10467, USA
e-mail: rmondere@montefiore.org; michael.thorpy@einstein.yu.edu

© Springer-Verlag Wien 2015
A. Videnovic, B. Högl (eds.), *Disorders of Sleep and Circadian Rhythms
in Parkinson's Disease*, DOI 10.1007/978-3-7091-1631-9_8

bid disorders, and the use of medications that affect nocturnal sleep quality and daytime alertness.

8.1 Introduction

Sleep disturbances are increasingly recognized as impacting on the quality of life of patients with Parkinson's disease (PD). Although the motor features are the most evident aspects of PD, sleep disturbances and excessive daytime sleepiness (EDS) are common manifestations. EDS is characterized by the inability to maintain alertness during the day resulting in unwanted lapses into sleep. Other manifestations of sleep disorders in PD include episodes of falling asleep without warning (sleep attacks), sleep onset and sleep maintenance insomnia, and abnormal movements during sleep. Sleep disturbances and EDS can result from the medications used to treat PD, degeneration of neuronal systems involved in the control of the sleep–wake system that occurs as part of the PD disease process, and comorbid conditions including specific sleep disorders and depression (Table 8.1). It is essential to recognize and evaluate the sleep disturbances and EDS in PD as interventions, both pharmacologic and nonpharmacologic, can improve the patient's general health, mood, and quality of life.

8.2 Epidemiology of EDS in PD

The estimated prevalence of EDS in PD is 29–49 % [1, 2]. In one study investigating the prevalence of EDS and risk factors in a newly diagnosed PD cohort ($n = 126$), it was found at 3-year follow-up that 49 % experienced EDS. Dopamine agonist treatment and non-tremor dominant motor PD phenotype were most strongly associated

Table 8.1 Factors that contribute to daytime sleepiness

Neuronal degeneration
Dopaminergic medications
Anticholinergic medications
MAOB inhibitor medications
Depression
Anxiety
Sleep apnea
Insomnia
Restless legs syndrome/periodic limb movements in sleep
REM sleep behavior disorder
Circadian rhythm disorders
Psychosis, hallucinations, nightmares
Motor symptoms—tremor, dystonia, akinesia, dyskinesias
Pain
Autonomic dysfunction

with EDS [2]. Other studies have shown that male sex, reduced daily activities of living, and a high daily levodopa equivalent dopaminergic dosage are associated with EDS [1, 3]. In addition, the presence of anxiety and baseline postural instability causing gait difficulty are other factors correlated with EDS in PD [3]. Longitudinal studies have shown an increasing trend between the prevalence of EDS in PD and cognitive decline and disease progression [4].

The estimated prevalence of sleep attacks in PD is 1–4 %, and episodes of sudden sleep onset in PD are 7–42 % [5]. Sleep attacks are defined as abrupt episodes of unexpected sleep that occur during normal activities. Patients may or may not be aware of sleepiness prior to the onset of sleep attacks. Older age, male sex, longer disease duration, disturbed nighttime sleep, and dopaminergic medications have been associated with sleep attacks [6]. In those treated with dopamine agonists, there is a two- to threefold increase in sleep attacks when compared to those who are on levodopa [5]. Genetic polymorphisms in the dopamine D2 receptor gene Taq1A and preprohypocretin have also been significantly associated with sleep attacks in PD [7].

Due to the impairment of daytime sleepiness, an important issue for PD patients is whether they should drive a motor vehicle. A study of 6,620 patients with PD found that 15 % had been involved in and 11 % had caused at least one motor vehicle accident in the past 5 years [8]. PD patients who felt moderately impaired by PD, had an increased Epworth Sleepiness Scale (ESS) score or experienced sudden onset sleeping while driving, had an increased risk of causing accidents. Accidents tended to occur in easy driving situations [8]. Another study compared patients with PD to controls on the ability to perform on a simulated driving test [9]. Subjects with PD committed more errors during both baseline and distractions, driving slower with higher speed variability during distraction. Declining driving performance was associated with multiple symptoms including increased daytime sleepiness [9].

8.3 Evaluations of Sleepiness in PD

Subjective questionnaires and objective tests have been designed to evaluate EDS. The Epworth Sleepiness Scale (ESS) is a questionnaire that assesses how likely patients are to doze off in eight everyday situations that vary in the levels of stimulation, immobility, and relaxation. A score of 10 or above out of 24 is considered pathologic sleepiness.

Additional questionnaires that can be used to assess sleepiness in PD are the UPDRS Part II, the Pittsburg Sleep Quality Index (PSQI), the Scales for Outcomes in PD-Sleep Scale (SCOPA), the Parkinson's Disease Sleep Scale (PDSS) and its second edition (PDSS-2). Questions address subjective sleep quality, sleep latency, sleep duration, habitual sleep efficiency, sleep disturbances, use of sleeping medications, and daytime dysfunction. Sleep disturbances are addressed as part of the overall picture of disease impact.

The first version of PDSS is a visual analogue scale that addresses 15 commonly reported symptoms associated with sleep disturbances such as nighttime sleep awakenings, movements in sleep, and daytime sleepiness. This has been further extended in the PDSS-2, which has five categories and addresses other sleep disturbances such as restless legs syndrome, akinesia, pain, and sleep apnea.

The overnight polysomnogram (PSG) is useful to diagnose, or rule out, underlying sleep disorders including sleep apnea, periodic limb movement disorder (PLMD), REM sleep behavior disorder (RBD), and parasomnias. These sleep disorders, often found in PD patients [10–12], can cause a fragmented nighttime sleep resulting in daytime sleepiness. Studies have found deficiencies in total sleep time, sleep latency, slow-wave sleep, REM sleep, and sleep efficiency in patients with PD [13, 14].

The multiple sleep latency test (MSLT), which typically follows overnight polsomnography, assesses the ability or tendency to fall asleep. The MSLT measures the speed at which a subject falls asleep when given the opportunity to sleep, and whether a patient goes into REM sleep. It consists of five 20-min nap opportunities 2 h apart. Studies have shown pathologic sleepiness, defined as a mean sleep latency <5 min, is prevalent in PD. A study of 27 PD patients found a mean sleep latency of <5 min in 40 of the 134 nap opportunities during MSLTs [15].

Actigraphy is a noninvasive method of monitoring human rest/activity cycles. One study of actigraphy demonstrated that PD patients had a 1.5-fold to twofold lower daytime motor activity level than controls, which suggests daytime sleepiness or limited physical activity [16]. Additionally, the study showed a 1.5-fold to twofold higher nighttime motor activity which represents the fragmented sleep often reported in patients with PD.

8.4 Pathophysiology of EDS in PD

The cause of EDS in PD is often multifactorial with the most relevant effects coming from dopaminergic medications and the disease process itself. The progressive cell loss in the dopaminergic and non-dopaminergic neurons and networks that modulate sleep–wake mechanisms in PD is a major contributing factor to the etiology of sleep disturbances in PD. In addition to the nigrostriatal pathway, PD affects areas of the brainstem, such as the pedunculopontine nucleus, the ventrolateral tegmental area, the locus coeruleus, the dorsal raphe nucleus, and thalamic nuclei, which are involved in maintaining alertness [17]. Circadian sleep–wake dysrhythmia in PD may reflect the central nervous system pathophysiology affecting the retinohypothalamic tract and suprachiasmatic nucleus.

Hypocretin (orexin), which is known to be decreased in narcolepsy, is also thought to be related to the EDS seen in PD; however, the data to support this has varied. One study measuring ventricular cerebrospinal fluid levels found an almost 25 % reduction in PD patients [18]. Another study of 16 PD patients with symptoms of narcolepsy found a correlation with increased objective sleepiness and decreased cerebrospinal fluid (CSF) hypocretin. In addition, in two patients with severe disease serial CSF hypocretin levels decreased over time. Overall, the study concluded that dopamine deficiency correlated with poorer sleep quality and hypocretin signaling related to EDS in PD patients [19]. However, not all studies have shown loss of hypocretin in PD. A study measuring hypocretin levels in cerebrospinal fluid collected by lumbar puncture in 62 patients with PD did not find a decreased level [20].

8.5   Effects of PD Treatment on Sleep and Wakefulness

Medications used to treat PD often lead to EDS both through direct pharmacologic effects and/or by disturbing nighttime sleep. Dopaminergic agents, antidepressants, and amantadine can all cause EDS by disturbing nighttime sleep. Withdrawal from benzodiazepines and other sedatives can cause rebound insomnia resulting in EDS. Anticholinergic agents, through M1 muscarinic receptors, increase REM latency and suppress REM sleep and can cause sedating effects during the day. Trihexyphenidyl increases nighttime wakefulness that can result in daytime sleepiness [21].

Levodopa and dopamine agonists can adversely affect nighttime sleep resulting in EDS. A study of PD patients taking levodopa found that 74 % had a disruption of nighttime sleep [22].

Studies have shown that dopamine agonists increase daytime sleepiness [23–26]. Studies comparing dopamine agonists found that both ergot and nonergot dopamine agonists caused EDS [24–26]. Total dopamine dose, rather than the choice of dopamine agonist, was the best predictor of EDS [26]. In one study of 15 patients evaluated before and 8 months after starting dopaminergic medications, the ESS was significantly increased and the mean sleep latency on MSLT was significantly decreased after treatment [25].

Rotigotine resulted in a higher percentage of patients with improvement in all items of the PDSS-2 except distressing dreams and distressing hallucinations at night [27]. There were significant improvements compared with placebo in the categories of wake with painful limb posturing (increase of 25 % vs decrease by 95 %), limb pain causing waking (decrease in 31 % vs decrease by 83 %), and cramps in limbs causes waking (decrease by 47 % vs 78 %) [27]. Another study looking at nocturnal sleep disturbances using the UPDRS Part III and PDSS-2 with an optimized titration of rotigotine found significant improvement in scores on both scales versus placebo [28].

Catechol *O*-methyltransferase inhibitors enhance dopaminergic activity, which can lead to worsening of levodopa-induced adverse effects, including sleep disorders and hallucinations [29]. Selegiline, which is metabolized to amphetamine, is one of the most likely to cause sleep-onset insomnia that can lead to EDS [30]. Rasagiline is not metabolized to amphetamine metabolites; it may not have the same degree of insomnia as selegiline [31].

Deep brain stimulation (DBS), used for treatment of Parkinson's disease refractory to medications, has also been shown to help improve sleep. DBS of the subthalamic nucleus (STN) has been shown to improve nighttime sleep. In a study of five patients 3 months after surgery, there was an increase in total sleep time and slow-wave sleep as well as a reduction of wakefulness after sleep onset and at 1-year follow-up [17].

A similar improvement in sleep quality was found with DBS of the globus pallidus internal (GPi) segment and the pedunculopontine tegmental nucleus (PPTg). However, unlike STN-DBS, stimulation of the PPTg improved not only nighttime sleep but also ameliorated excessive daytime sleepiness [32]. The ESS was reduced by more than 50 % with PPTg-DBS at 1-year follow up. This improvement was seen both with PPTg stimulation only at night or on for 24 h/day. It is hypothesized that stimulation of the PPTg, which is part of the reticular activating pathway, induces a recovery of the activity of this pathway and therefore improves sleep quality and daytime alertness [32].

8.6 Other Sleep Disturbances in PD as Contributors to EDS

In PD different types of insomnia, sleep related breathing disorders, circadian rhythms disorders, parasomnias, RLS, and other sleep related movement disorders have been reported. The associations and impact of each of these sleep disorders on EDS have not been systematically studied and remain controversial. Clinical studies have found controversial results as to whether sleep apnea is increased in PD. Research studies in PD have shown an increased rate of snoring (71.8 %) [33] and sleep apnea (20 %) [34]. Notably, no correlation was found between apnea/hypopnea index (AHI) and the MSLT, and the authors concluded that sleep apnea may not be a major factor contributing to the severity of sleepiness in most patients with PD [34]. Two case reports of patients with PD and OSA found that CPAP clearly restored more daytime activity [35].

Insomnia is found in 54–60 % of PD patients [36]. Sleep fragmentation and early awakenings are the most common types of insomnia symptoms reported with minimal differences in sleep initiation. While insomnia may contribute to tiredness, fatigue, and EDS in PD, several studies found inverse relationship between daytime sleepiness and overnight sleep quality.

The prevalence of RLS has been shown to be significantly higher in the PD population compared to sex-matched controls [37]. Daytime fatigue is commonly reported in patients with RLS. There have been controversial results regarding the incidence of periodic limb movement disorder (PLMD) in PD [38].

RBD is characterized by acting out of vivid dreams in vigorous and often violent ways during REM sleep. RBD appeared to predict subsequent development of dementia, as well as cognitive fluctuations and hallucinations [39].

Circadian rhythm sleep disorders result from the misalignment sleep patterns and normal daytime activities. Excessive daytime sleepiness and nighttime sleep disturbance often lead to irregular sleep–wake patterns in PD.

In PD motor symptoms, depression and pain can affect sleep. Disruptive nighttime motor symptoms include tremor, nocturnal dystonia, and nocturnal akinesia. Depression often adversely affects sleep in PD causing difficulty falling asleep, staying asleep, and early morning awakenings. Pain is noted in about 50 % of patients with PD [40], which may cause difficulty falling asleep and staying asleep. Disruptive nighttime motor symptoms, depression, and pain all fragment nighttime sleep leading to daytime fatigue and EDS.

Hallucinations can disrupt sleep and affect almost 33 % of patients with PD. PD patients with hallucinations have increased awakenings, decreased sleep efficiency, and more daytime sleepiness [41].

8.7 Treatment of EDS in PD

EDS in PD can be related to sleep disruption, sleep deprivation, medication side effects, underlying sleep disorders, or from the primary disease. The clinician must first determine which factors are involved in producing the EDS. Promoting good sleep hygiene and emphasizing the importance of daytime light exposure and daytime activity are crucial. Good sleep hygiene includes maintaining a regular sleep–wake schedule, spending an appropriate amount of time in bed (~8 h), and avoiding caffeine and frequent naps during the day (Table 8.2). Adjusting doses of dopaminergic medication can help promote daytime alertness and increase quality of sleep at night. The physician must determine if the patient has an underlying sleep disorder and treat as appropriate.

Recognition and treatment of primary sleep disorders in PD patients is essential. CPAP has been shown to improve daytime functioning in those patients with OSA. If insomnia is present, proper sleep hygiene and the possible use of an appropriate hypnotic medication are the main treatments. Levodopa or dopamine agonists improve symptoms of RLS, especially with a nighttime dose of levodopa or dopamine agonists. Gabapentin, opioids, or benzodiazepines are other options. If RBD is present, clonazepam is the most effective treatment for RBD; however, this medication may contribute to daytime sleepiness because it is long-acting and sedating. Melatonin is an alternative treatment for RBD. Melatonin is also useful in treating circadian rhythm disorders.

Bupropion, an antidepressant that increases synaptic dopamine by blocking the dopamine transporter, may be useful not only in improving depression in patients with PD but also in improving daytime alertness [42]. Quetiapine, an antipsychotic drug that has fewer extrapyramidal effects than older antipsychotics, is effective for treating psychosis and hallucinations allowing more restful nocturnal sleep [43].

Table 8.2 Sleep tips to improve sleep and daytime functioning in PD

Avoiding daytime naps
Exposure to bright lights or sunlight in the daytime
Increasing daytime activity level
Obtaining adequate amount of time in bed at night
Avoiding caffeine or nicotine several hours before bedtime
Avoiding alcohol around bedtime that fragments sleep
Avoiding spicy, heavy, or sugary foods before bedtime
Limiting liquids after 8 pm to avoid nighttime urination
Maintaining a regular sleep schedule
Keeping the bedroom quiet, dark, and comfortable

Treatment with modafinil may be helpful for EDS in PD. Several studies have shown that modafinil at doses of 100–200 mg/day showed significant improvements in the ESS and the clinical global impression of change without any major PD symptom adverse effects [44]. Alternatively, one study found that treating patients with modafinil was only partially helpful, and adding sodium oxybate or antihistamine receptor-3 drugs seem to be more activating [45]. However, results have varied as larger study found no significant improvement in the ESS or MSLT with modafinil (200–400 mg/day) [45].

Cognitive behavior therapy has been helpful in those with PD. A recent study found improved scores on the PDSS after cognitive behavior therapy [46].

Conclusions

Excessive daytime sleepiness is common in PD and multifactorial, resulting from medications used to treat PD, mood or anxiety disorders, specific sleep disorders, PD motor symptoms, and primary effects of the disease process of PD on neuronal sleep wake centers. A systematic evaluation should be conducted to assess for the presence of sleep disturbances and daytime sleepiness. Several questionnaires have been developed to assess for the presence of daytime sleepiness and sleep disruption including the ESS, PDSS-2, SCOPA, UPDRS Part II, and the PSQI. These tools should be used to help guide treatment. Sleep studies will determine if a sleep disorder such as obstructive sleep apnea, periodic limb movements, or narcolepsy are contributing disorders.

If nocturnal sleep and daytime alertness are not well controlled, social interactions, work performance, and quality of life can be affected and result in feelings of insecurity, anxiety, and depression. Various therapeutic strategies are available to help with nocturnal sleep including adjusting medications used to treat motor symptoms, treating underlying sleep disorders, encouraging good sleep hygiene, avoiding daytime naps, and increasing daytime activity and light exposure. Alerting medications in the daytime and sedating medications at night can be used when needed. Recognizing and addressing daytime sleepiness and disturbed nocturnal sleep in PD will improve mood, activities of daily living, and quality of life for the patient.

References

1. Ghorayeb I, Loundou A, Auquier P, et al. A nationwide survey of excessive daytime sleepiness in Parkinson's disease in France. Mov Disord. 2007;22:1567–72.
2. Breen DP, Williams-Gray CH, Mason SL, et al. Excessive daytime sleepiness and its risk factors in incident Parkinson's disease. J Neurol Neurosurg Psychiatry. 2013;84:233–4.
3. Boddy F, Rowan EN, Lett D, et al. Subjectively reported sleep quality and excessive daytime somnolence in Parkinson's disease with and without dementia, dementia with Lewy bodies and Alzheimer's disease. Int J Geriatr Psychiatry. 2007;22:529–35.
4. Ondo WG, Dat Vuong K, Khan H, et al. Daytime sleepiness and other sleep disorders in Parkinson's disease. Neurology. 2001;57:1392–6.
5. Arnulf I, Leu-Semenescu S. Sleepiness in Parkinson's disease. Parkinsonism Relat Disord. 2009;15 Suppl 3:S101–4.

6. Manni R, Terzaghi M, Sartori I, et al. Dopamine agonists and sleepiness in PD: review of the literature and personal findings. Sleep Med. 2003;5:189–93.
7. Rissling I, Körner K, Geller F, et al. Preprohypocretin polymorphism in Parkinson's disease patients reporting "sleep attacks". Sleep. 2005;28:871–5.
8. Meindorfner C, Korner Y, Moller JC, et al. Driving in Parkinson's disease: mobility, accidents, and sudden onset of sleep at the wheel. Mov Disord. 2005;20:832–42.
9. Uc EY, Rizzo M, Anderson SW, et al. Driving with distraction in Parkinson's disease. Neurology. 2006;67:1774–80.
10. Brunner H, Wetter TC, Hogl B, et al. Microstructure of the non-rapid eye movement sleep electroencephalogram in patients with newly diagnosed Parkinson's disease: effects of dopaminergic treatment. Mov Disord. 2002;17:928–33.
11. Friedman A. Sleep pattern in Parkinson's disease. Acta Med Pol. 1980;21:193–9.
12. Scaglione C, Vignatelli L, Plazzi G, et al. REM sleep behavior disorder in Parkinson's disease: a questionnaire-based study. Neurol Sci. 2005;25:316–21.
13. Wetter TC, Trenkwalder C, Gershanik O, et al. Polysomnographic measures in Parkinson's disease: a comparison between patients with and without REM sleep disturbances. Wien Klin Wochenschr. 2001;113:249–53.
14. Shpirer I, Minovitz A, Klein C, et al. Excessive daytime sleepiness in patients with Parkinson's disease: a polysomnography study. Mov Disord. 2006;21:1432–8.
15. Rye D, Bliwise DL, Dihenia B, et al. Daytime sleepiness in Parkinson's disease. J Sleep Res. 2000;9:63–9.
16. Nass A, Nass RD. Actigraphic evidence for night-time hyperkinesias in Parkinson's disease. Int J Neurosci. 2008;118:291–310.
17. Amara A, Ray R, Walker H. The effects of deep brain stimulation on sleep in Parkinson's disease. Ther Adv Neurol Disord. 2011;4(1):15–24.
18. Fronczek R, Overeem S, Lee SY, et al. Hypocretin (orexin) loss in Parkinson's disease. Brain. 2007;130:1577–85.
19. Wienecke M, Werth E, Poryazove R, et al. Progressive dopamine and hypocretin deficiencies in Parkinson's disease: is there an impact on sleep and wakefulness? J Sleep Res. 2012;21:710–7.
20. Yasui K, Inoue Y, Kanbayashi T, et al. CSF orexin levels in Parkinson's disease, dementia with Lewy bodies, progressive supranuclear palsy and corticobasal degeneration. J Neurol Sci. 2006;250:120–3.
21. Zoltoski RK, Velazquez-Moctezuma J, Shiromani PJ, et al. The relative effects of selective M1 muscarinic antagonists on rapid eye movement sleep. Brain Res. 1993;608:186–90.
22. Garcia-Borreguero D, Caminero AB, de la Llave Y, et al. Decreased phasic EMG activity during rapid eye movement sleep in treatment of naive Parkinson's disease: effects of treatment with levodopa and progression of illness. Mov Disord. 2002;17:934–41.
23. Rye DB. Parkinson's disease and RLS: the dopaminergic bridge. Sleep Med. 2004;5:317–28.
24. Gjerstad MD, Alves G, Wentzel-Larsen T, et al. Excessive daytime sleepiness in Parkinson's disease: is it the drugs or the disease? Neurology. 2006;6:853–8.
25. Kaynak D, Kiziltan G, Kaynak H, et al. Sleep and sleepiness in patients with Parkinson's disease before and after dopaminergic treatment. Eur J Neurol. 2005;12:199–207.
26. Razmy A, Lang AE, Shapiro CM. Predictors of impaired daytime sleep and wakefulness in patients with Parkinson's disease treated with older (ergot) vs newer (nonergot) dopamine agonists. Arch Neurol. 2004;61:97–102.
27. Ghys L, Surmann E, Whitesides J, et al. Effect of rotigotine on sleep and quality of life in Parkinson's disease patients: post hoc analysis of RECOVER patient who were symptomatic at baseline. Expert Opin Pharmacother. 2011;12(13):1985–98.
28. Trenkwalder C, Kies B, Rudzinska M, et al., Recover Study Group. Rotigotine effects on early morning motor function and sleep in Parkinson's disease: a double-blind, randomized, placebocontrolled study (RECOVER). Mov Disord. 2011;26(1):90–9.
29. Kurth MC, Adler CH, Hilaire MS, et al. Tolcapone improves motor function and reduces levodopa requirement in patients with Parkinson's disease experiencing motor fl uctuations: a

multicenter, double-blind, randomized, placebo-controlled trial. Tolcapone Fluctuator Study Group I. Neurology. 1997;48:81–7.
30. Hublin C, Partinen M, Heinonen EH, et al. Selegiline in the treatment of narcolepsy. Neurology. 1994;44:2095–101.
31. Hoy S, Keating G. Rasagiline: a review of its use in the treatment of idiopathic Parkinson's disease. Drugs. 2012;72(5):643–69.
32. Peppe A, Pierantozzi M, Alamonte V, et al. Deep brain stimulation of pedunculopontine tegmental nucleus: role in sleep modulation in advanced Parkinson's disease patients: one-year follow-up. Sleep. 2012;35(12):1637–42.
33. Braga-Neto P, da Silva-Junior FP, Sueli Monte F, et al. Snoring and excessive daytime sleepiness in Parkinson's disease. J Neurol Sci. 2004;217:41–5.
34. Arnulf I, Konofal E, Merino-Andreu M, et al. Parkinson's disease and sleepiness; an integral part of PD. Neurology. 2002;58:1019–24.
35. Steffen A, Hagenah J, Graefe H, et al. Obstructive sleep apnea in patients with Parkinson's disease – report of two cases and review. Laryngorhinootologie. 2008;87:107–11.
36. Gjerstad MD, Wentzel-Larsen T, Aarsland D, et al. Insomnia in Parkinson's disease: frequency and progression over time. J Neurol Neurosurg Psychiatry. 2007;78:476–9.
37. Nomura T, Inoue Y, Miyake M, et al. Prevalence and clinical characteristics of restless legs syndrome in Japanese patients with Parkinson's disease. Mov Disord. 2006;21:380–4.
38. Happe S, Pirker W, Kloch G, et al. Periodic leg movements in patients with Parkinson's disease are associated with reduced striatal dopamine transporter binding. J Neurol. 2003;250:83–6.
39. Postuma RB, Bertand JA, Montplaisir J. Rapid eye movements sleep behavior disorder and risk of dementia in Parkinson's disease: a prospective study. Mov Disord. 2012;27:720–6.
40. Shulman LM, Taback RL, Rabinstein AA, et al. Non-recognition of depression and other non-motor symptoms in Parkinson's disease. Parkinsonism Relat Disord. 2002;8:193–7.
41. Barnes J, Connelly V, Wiggs L, et al. Sleep patterns in Parkinson's disease patients with visual hallucinations. Int J Neurosci. 2010;120(8):564–9.
42. Rye D. Excessive daytime sleepiness and Unintended sleep in parkinson's disease. Curr Neurol Neurosci Rep. 2006;6:169–76.
43. Fernandez HH, Trieschmann ME, Burke MA, et al. Long-term outcome of quetiapine use for psychosis among parkinsonian patients. Mov Disord. 2003;18:510–4.
44. Lokk J. Daytime sleepiness in elderly PD patients and treatment with the psychostimulant modafinil: a preliminary study. Neuropsychiatr Dis Treat. 2010;6:93–7.
45. Ondo WG, Fayle R, Atassi F, et al. Modafi nil for daytime somnolence in Parkinson's disease: double blind, placebo controlled prallel trial. J Neurol Neruosurg Psychiatry. 2005;76:1636–9.
46. Yang H, Petrini M. Effect of cognitive behavior therapy on sleep disorder in Parkinson's disease in China: a pilot study. Nurs Health Sci. 2012;14(4):458–63.

Dysregulation of Circadian System in Parkinson's Disease

9

Aleksandar Videnovic

Contents

Abstract

Circadian rhythms are physiological and behavioral cycles with a periodicity of approximately 24 h, generated by the endogenous biological clock, the suprachiasmatic nucleus (SCN). These rhythms influence most physiological processes, including the sleep–wake cycle. The exact pathophysiology of sleep–wake disturbances in Parkinson's disease (PD) remains largely unknown, but the etiology is likely to be multifactorial, including influence of motor PD symptoms on sleep, adverse effects of antiparkinsonian medications, and neurodegeneration of

A. Videnovic, MD, MSc
Department of Neurology, Neurological Clinical Research Institute,
Massachusetts General Hospital, Harvard Medical School,
165 Cambridge Street, Suite 600, Boston, MA 02114, USA
e-mail: avidenovic@mgh.harvard.edu

© Springer-Verlag Wien 2015
A. Videnovic, B. Högl (eds.), *Disorders of Sleep and Circadian Rhythms
in Parkinson's Disease*, DOI 10.1007/978-3-7091-1631-9_9

central sleep regulatory areas. The circadian system and its main central pacemaker, the SCN, have a major influence on sleep–wake homeostasis. A growing body of evidence points to significant alterations of the circadian system in PD. Despite this, little is known about the role of the circadian system in the regulation of sleep–wake cycles in PD. In this chapter, we discuss the role of the circadian system in the regulation of the sleep–wake cycle and outline implications of circadian timekeeping in PD.

9.1 Introduction

The human circadian system regulates numerous biological rhythms. The daily sleep–wake cycle is the most notable human behavior that is regulated by the circadian system. The two-process model of sleep regulation has been proposed to explain the relationship between the circadian system and sleep. This model proposes a sleep homeostatic process (process S) that interacts with the circadian process (process C), which is independent of sleep. Thus, process S, which is described in detail in Chap. 1 of this book, represents an internal homeostatic requirement for sleep that increases during wakefulness and decreases with sleep. The sleep homeostatic process regulates the amount and depth of sleep. Although the precise mechanisms of circadian regulation of sleep and alertness are not fully elucidated, it appears that the circadian system functions to consolidate wakefulness and regulate the timing of sleep. In this chapter, we discuss the role of the circadian system in the regulation of the sleep–wake cycle and outline implications of circadian timekeeping in PD.

9.2 Overview of the Human Circadian System

Nearly all physiological and behavioral processes in humans exhibit daily rhythms, regulated by the endogenous circadian timing system. These rhythms recur with a periodicity of approximately 24 h, under the governance of the suprachiasmatic nucleus (SCN) located in the anterior hypothalamus [1]. The timing of human biological rhythms is synchronized to the rotation of earth and is under the influence of numerous external and internal time clues. This synchronization may become disrupted leading to misalignment or *internal desynchronization*. This loss of coordination of rhythms may have negative consequences on sleep–wake cycles and numerous other biological functions.

9.2.1 Neuroanatomy and Neurochemistry of the Circadian System

The circadian timing system has three distinct components: a circadian pacemaker – SCN, afferent pathways for light and other stimuli that synchronize the pacemaker to the environment, and efferent output rhythms that are regulated by the SCN.

The SCN is composed of "core" and "shell" subnuclei. Each of the subnuclei has distinct neurochemical properties [1]. Gamma-aminobutyric acid (GABA) is the dominant neurotransmitter in the SCN, present in nearly all SCN neurons. The SCN core contains high density of vasoactive intestinal polypeptide (VIP), gastrin-releasing peptide (GRP), and bombesin-containing neurons. Somatostatin and neurophysin are dominant neurochemicals within the SCN shell.

The main afferent pathways to the SCN emerge from the retina and reach the SCN directly via the retinohypothalamic tract, or indirectly via retinogeniculate pathways [2]. The melanopsin-containing retinal ganglion retinal cells are the primary photoreceptors for the circadian system. The SCN also receives nonphotic information from the raphe nuclei, basal forebrain, pons, medulla, and posterior hypothalamus.

The major efferents from the SCN project to the subparaventricular zone and the paraventricular nucleus of the hypothalamus, dorsomedial hypothalamus, thalamus, preoptic and retrochiasmatic areas, stria terminalis, lateral septum, and the intergeniculate nucleus. In addition to these distinct neuroanatomical networks, the SCN also communicates via diffusion of humoral signals such as transforming growth factor (TGF)-α, cardiotrophin-like cytokine (CLC), and prokineticin 2 (PK2).

The SCN represents the main clock of the circadian system. Almost all peripheral tissues as well as brain regions outside the SCN contain circadian clocks influenced by the SCN in addition to their own distinct circadian synchronizers [3] (Fig. 9.1).

9.2.2 Genetic Regulation of the Circadian System

Circadian rhythms are generated by a core set of clock genes, including three Period genes (Per1, Per2, Per3), Clock, Bmal1, and two plant cryptochrome gene homologues (Cry1 and Cry2) [4]. The proteins encoded by these genes interact to create a self-sustaining negative transcription–translation feedback loop that drives the timing system. The intracellular levels of CLOCK remain steady during the 24-h period. BMAL1 levels, which are high at the beginning of the day, promote the formation of BMAL1-CLOCK heterodimers. These proteins activate transcription of the PER and CRY genes resulting in high levels of these transcripts. As PER accumulates in the cytoplasm, it becomes phosphorylated and degraded by ubiquitination. Cry accumulates in the cytoplasm late in the subjective day and translocates to the nucleus to inhibit Clock-Bmal1-mediated transcription. During the night, the PER-CRY complex is degraded, and the cycle starts again. This feedback loop ensures a high level of BMAL1 and low levels of PER and CRY at the beginning of a new circadian day.

Circadian clock genes control a significant proportion of genome. It is estimated that approximately 10 % of all expressed genes are under regulation of the clock genes. Furthermore, peripheral tissues contain independent clocks. It is likely that peripheral clocks are synchronized by an input directly from the SCN or SCN-mediated messages. For a detailed overview of the molecular regulation of the circadian system, please see the excellent review by Dardente and Cermakian [2].

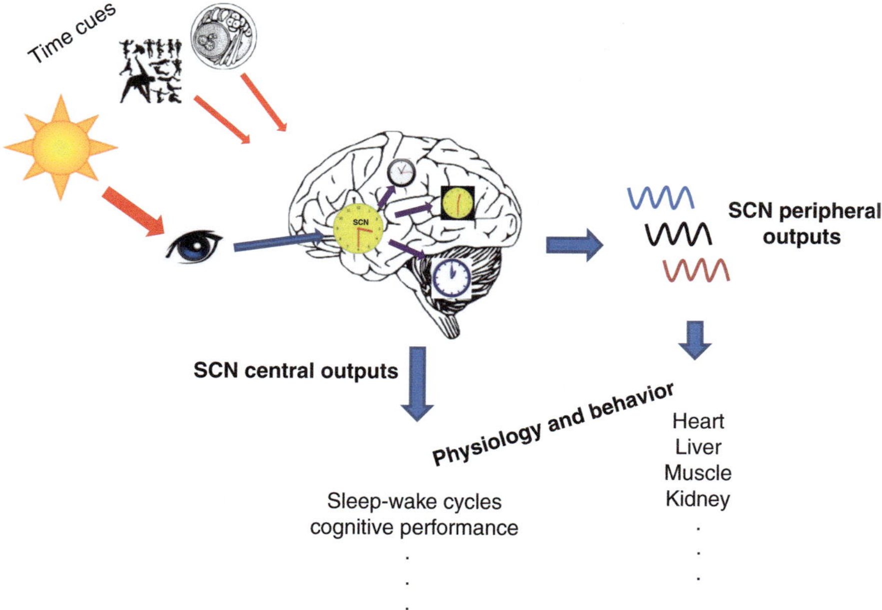

Fig. 9.1 A simplified scheme of the circadian system. The environmental photic (light) and non-photic (feeding schedules, physical activity) zeitgebers synchronize the central circadian pacemaker (*SCN*) to daily light–dark and social rhythms. The SCN synchronizes other central and peripheral clocks via neuronal and humoral efferents. This internal synchronization is important for optimal physiologic function and behavior

9.2.3 Circadian Entrainment and Markers of Circadian Rhythmicity

Circadian rhythms are synchronized with the solar day by daily adjustments in the timing of the SCN, following the exposure to stimuli that signal the time of day. These stimuli are known as "zeitgebers" (German for "time-giver"). Light is the most important and potent zeitgeber. In addition to light, feeding schedules, activity, and the hormone melatonin also influence the circadian timing [1].

Circadian rhythms can be described by their phase and amplitude. Circadian output rhythms are used to estimate the time (the phase) of the clock [5]. In humans, timing of the circadian core body temperature and hormonal rhythms are the most commonly used phase markers. The hormone melatonin is one of the best understood output rhythms of the SCN. The timing of melatonin secretion by the pineal gland is regulated by the SCN, with the onset of secretion being approximately 2 h before natural sleep time and being highest during the middle of the night [1]. Melatonin onset measured in dim light melatonin onset (DLMO) is a stable marker of circadian phase and is used in research as well as clinical practice to determine the timing of the endogenous circadian rhythm. The amplitude of a circadian rhythm refers to the half-distance from the maximum to the minimum of the observed rhythm. Plasma melatonin has been proven reliable as a marker of the amplitude of the circadian clock [6–8]. Since markers of circadian rhythms may be influenced by environmental stimuli and behavior (light–dark, rest–activity, meals), the underlying endogenous circadian rhythms are best assessed under the protocols that minimize exposure to stimuli that evoke responses in the physiological variables being monitored. The constant routine and forced desynchrony are prototypes of protocols used to assess endogenous circadian rhythms. The detailed description of these protocols is beyond the scope of this chapter.

9.3 Dopamine in the Circadian Timing System

Dopaminergic neurotransmission has been implied at several levels in the circadian system, starting with the photic afferent connection with the SCN. In the retina, dopamine (DA) plays an important role in light adaptation [9], and regulates the rhythmic expression of melanopsin, a photopigment of photosensitive retinal ganglion cells which has been implied in circadian entrainment [10]. Dopaminergic retinal cells express circadian rhythms in core clock genes Per, Cry, Clock, and Bmal1 [11]. In addition, DA modulates rhythms in retinal second messengers like cAMP, therefore interacting directly with retinal physiology and sensitivity [12]. Dopamine also affects the phase and amplitude of specific clock genes presumably through dopaminergic D1 receptors in the retina [13]. In the SCN, dopaminergic D1 receptors are present in both fetuses and adults [14, 15].

Several lines of evidence suggest that clock genes play a role in DA metabolism. The *clock* gene regulates dopaminergic activity in the ventral tegmental area (VTA) [16]. Several genes involved in dopaminergic signaling are differentially regulated in the VTA of *Clock* mutant mice, which also exhibits altered circadian rhythmicity, indicating a role of this gene in DA-related transcription in the VTA [16]. Circadian fluctuations in extracellular DA levels have been reported in the striatum and nucleus accumbens [17]. DA also regulates clock gene expression in the dorsal striatum [18, 19]. Promoter regions of the DA active transporter (DAT), D1A receptor, and tyrosine hydroxylase (TH) genes include an E-Box element, which is the target of the canonical molecular clock.

Dopaminergic activity and metabolism can also be considered an output of the circadian clock. DA and its metabolites and receptors exhibit daily fluctuations in their levels in different brain regions [20]. In particular, DA metabolism exhibits a diurnal rhythm in striatal regions, related to cyclic variations in the expression of DAT, D1A receptors, and TH [21]. There is a clear interaction between DA and melatonin, a well-known circadian output, which acts as a marker for both daily and seasonal variations in physiology and behavior, in several areas of the central nervous system [22]. Seasonal variations of DA have also been described in humans, although its importance and consequences remain to be established [23].

In summary, DA exhibits a two-way interaction with the circadian system at several levels. It has been hypothesized that diurnal and circadian changes in dopaminergic neurotransmission influence mood-related behavior [24] as well as addiction-related behavior [21, 25].

9.4   Circadian Rhythm Dysfunction in PD

Circadian biology of PD has not been systematically studied. Exciting emerging evidence suggests that circadian dysregulation plays an important role in PD. Answers to the question "Is PD affected by chronobiology?" require a multidirectional approach that includes a better understanding of common diurnal variations of symptoms and signs in PD as well as the assessment of physiologic and molecular markers of circadian rhythmicity in the PD population. Further, our understanding of circadian regulation in PD will be substantially enriched by examining the effects of potent modulators of the circadian system, such as light and other nonphotic zeitgebers, on PD symptoms and disease progression.

9.4.1   Diurnal Clinical Fluctuations in PD: Are they Driven by Circadian Dysregulation?

Diurnal rhythms of symptoms and signs associated with PD have been reported in numerous studies. Examples include fluctuations in daily motor activity [26–29], autonomic function [30–35], sleep–wake cycles [36–40], visual performance [41], as well as responsiveness to dopaminergic treatments [26, 42]. These observations are suggestive of possible circadian influences on the expression of clinical features of PD.

Fluctuations of motor symptoms in PD are very common. An actigraph, a wrist-worn monitor that detects movements, has been employed in numerous studies that assessed rest–activity rhythms in PD population. These actigraphy studies demonstrate lower peak activity levels and lower amplitude of the rest–activity cycle in PD patients compared to healthy older adults [36–40]. Increased levels of physical activity and shorter periods of immobility during the night result in an almost flat diurnal pattern of motor activity in PD [43, 44]. In addition, PD patients have a more fragmented pattern of activity with transitions from high to low activity periods, leading to less predictable rest–activity rhythm [45]. Motor symptoms tend to be more prominent in the afternoon and evening, both in stable patients and in those with wearing off symptoms [26, 42]. This daily pattern appears to be independent of the timing of dopaminergic medications and may be related to circadian regulation of dopaminergic systems. Furthermore, responsiveness of PD motor symptoms to dopaminergic treatments declines throughout the day, despite the absence of significant changes in levodopa pharmacokinetics [26]. While the presence of motor artifact in PD poses challenges to the interpretation of actigraphy studies in this population, actigraphy can be used in conjunction with PD sleep–wake diaries and newer nonparametric circadian rhythm analysis in order to minimize shortcoming of the actigraphy recordings of the rest–activity cycles in the PD population.

Output rhythms of the autonomic nervous system are influenced by circadian timekeeping. Alterations in the circadian regulation of the autonomic system in PD have been reported. Twenty-four hour ambulatory blood pressure monitoring in patients with PD demonstrates reversal of circadian rhythm of blood pressure, increased diurnal blood pressure variability, postprandial hypotension, and a high nocturnal blood pressure [32, 46–48]. Holter electrocardiographic monitoring in PD patients reveals a decrease of sympathetic activity during the day with a loss of the circadian heart rate variability and a disappearance of the sympathetic morning peak [31]. The spectral analysis of heart rate variability reveals a significant decrease of the daytime low frequency power, decreased daytime low–high frequency ratio, and decreased nighttime high frequency power [31, 35, 49, 50]. These abnormalities, more prominent in advanced PD, are also present in untreated patients with early PD [49]. The prognostic significance and pathophysiological mechanisms leading to altered autonomic circadian variability in PD remain to be determined. While observed abnormalities may arise within the peripheral autonomic ganglia, the influence of central networks including hypothalamus may be significant as well [51–53].

Similarly to motor performance and autonomic function, circadian fluctuations of sensory systems have been reported in PD. For example, visual performance, measured by contrast sensitivity, is altered in PD [41]. Impairment of retinal DA, which exhibits an endogenous circadian rhythm independent of light–dark cycles, is most likely responsible for these changes [54]. Since circadian changes in contrast sensitivity may occur independently of circadian oscillations in motor symptoms, it is possible that various anatomical networks (retina, striatum, and cortex) may have differential threshold to the circadian signaling of DA [55].

The sleep–wake cycle is a prototype of a biological rhythm strongly influenced by circadian system. Disruption of sleep and impaired daytime alertness are common manifestations of PD, affect majority of PD patients, and may emerge early in the course of the disease. Sleep fragmentation and excessive daytime sleepiness are the most common abnormalities of the sleep–wake cycle in PD. While the etiology of insomnia and hypersomnia associated with PD is multifactorial, circadian disruption should be considered as one of the contributing factors. Several lines of evidence stemming from research on animal models of PD support this hypothesis. Transgenic mice overexpressing human alpha-synuclein (Thy1-aSyn) exhibits disrupted circadian behaviors including the temporal distribution of sleep and activity. Furthermore, the firing rate of SCN neurons early in the progression of experimentally induced parkinsonism in the Thy1-aSyn mice may result in impairments of neural and hormonal output rhythms of the SCN.

9.4.2 Circadian Markers in PD

Physiologic and molecular markers of the circadian system may provide insight into the function of circadian timekeeping in PD. Only a few studies attempted to characterize profiles of circadian markers in PD. In a cohort of 26 PD patients, the amplitude of melatonin rhythm was decreased, and the phase was advanced in treated patients with and without motor complications compared to de novo patients [56]. These results suggest a trend toward advanced melatonin phase and amplitude reduction during the evolution of PD. Circadian rhythms of temperature and plasma cortisol did not differ between the groups in this study. In a separate study, nine patients with de novo PD had a preserved melatonin rhythm compared with healthy controls [57]. In a study of 12 PD patients, 24-h mean cortisol production rate was significantly higher and the mean secretory cortisol curve was flatter, leading to significantly reduced diurnal variation in the PD group relative to controls [58]. Body temperature is an excellent marker of endogenous circadian rhythmicity. While 24-h rhythms of core body temperature remain similar in PD relative to healthy controls [59], basal body temperature is significantly lower in parkinsonian patients [60]. PD patients with coexistent depression have altered circadian rhythms of rectal temperature and lower amplitudes of core body temperature [61]. These circadian modifications of temperature regulation have been confirmed in the 6-hydroxydopamine (6-OHDA) animal model of parkinsonism where a significant decrease of the mesor and a phase advance of temperature rhythm have been reported [62]. Although these investigations suggest modifications of circadian rhythmicity in PD, results are to be interpreted with caution due to small sample sizes and study designs that reflect influences of both endogenous circadian and exogenous (e.g., light exposure, physical activity, meals, social schedules) rhythms on PD. In a recent study of 20 patients with mild to moderate PD and 12 age-matched controls that employed modified constant routine experimental protocol that minimize exogenous influences on circadian rhythms, significant blunting of circadian rhythm of melatonin secretion and reduced amplitude of melatonin rhythm was observed [63]. PD patients with excessive daytime somnolence had a more prominent reduction in the amplitude of their melatonin rhythm compared to PD patients without EDS. Significant reductions in the amplitude of melatonin secretion was also demonstrated in de novo PD patients [64]. In contrast to these findings, Bolitho et al. recently reported a threefold increase in melatonin secretion in a cohort of PD patients [65]. While further investigations are needed, these observations provide a rationale for the role of circadian disruption in excessive sleepiness associated with PD.

Several studies have demonstrated strong oscillatory expression patterns of core clock genes in human whole blood and peripheral blood mononuclear cells (PBMCs) [66–68], demonstrating the feasibility of using clock gene expression as a circadian marker. Time-related variations in the expression of circadian clock genes have been recently reported in patients with PD [69]. In a study of 17 individuals with PD and 16 age-matched controls, the relative abundance of the clock gene *Bmal1* was significantly lower during the night in PD patients versus controls. Expression levels of *Bmal1* in PD patients correlated with PD severity as assessed by the UPDRS [69]. A lack of time-dependent variation in Bmal1 expression in PD patients was recently confirmed in another study [64]. Exciting emerging evidence suggests alterations in molecular regulation of circadian timekeeping in animal models of PD. Depletion of striatal DA by 6-OHDA or blockade of D2 DA receptors by raclopride blunts the circadian rhythm of striatal Per2. Furthermore, timed daily activation of D2 DA receptors restores and entrains the Per2 rhythm in DA-depleted striatum. These observations suggest a role of dopaminergic stimulation of D2 DA receptors in the maintenance of circadian molecular oscillations in the striatum.

9.4.3 Light Exposure and Nonphotic Circadian Entrainment in PD

Light, the main synchronizer for the human circadian system, is increasingly applied as therapy in a variety of sleep and neuropsychiatric conditions including circadian rhythm disorders, seasonal affective disorder, and dementia [70]. Light therapy is usually a well tolerated and easily applied nonpharmacological treatment modality. Numerous studies have demonstrated beneficial effects of light therapy on sleep quality, daytime sleepiness, mood, and quality of life in healthy elderly and in patients with dementia. Several lines of evidence support the rationale for exploring supplemental light exposure in PD. For example, DA is likely a mediator of light signaling to the retinal circadian clock which provides direct input to the SCN [9]. Exposure to light facilitates the recovery of motor function in a chronic experimental model of PD [71]. Only a few exploratory studies, however, examined the effects of bright light in patients affected by PD.

In a case series of 12 PD patients, daily exposure to supplemental bright light of 1,000–1,500 lux prior to habitual bedtime resulted in improved sleep quality and mood [72]. Evening exposure to bright light was also associated with improvements in bradykinesia and rigidity. Beneficial effects of supplemental light exposure emerged several days after initiating the treatment. Similar beneficial effects of supplemental bright light on sleep, mood anxiety, and motor performance were reported in an open-label retrospective study of 129 levodopa-treated PD patients followed up to 8 years [73]. In another study, 36 PD patients were randomized to receive treatment with bright light therapy of 7,500 lux (active arm) or 950 lux (placebo arm) in 30-min sessions every morning for 2 weeks [74]. Exposure to bright light of 7,500 lux was associated with improvements in UPDRS part I, II, IV scores, and daytime sleepiness. While these studies demonstrated good feasibility and positive effects of bright light therapy on nonmotor and motor manifestations of PD, further validation studies involving larger cohorts and employing objective outcome measures are needed. The timing, duration, intensity, and spectral qualities of light therapy will need to be optimized for use in the PD population.

9.4.4 Circadian Disruption in PD: Potential Mechanisms

Mechanisms underlying circadian dysregulation in PD are not fully elucidated. Primary neurodegenerative processes of PD leading to progressive depletion of DA likely have negative consequences on circadian timekeeping as dopaminergic transmission is an integral part of circadian homeostasis. Fluctuations in DA metabolism, overnight DA accumulation, or diurnal receptor downregulation may be in part driving diurnal fluctuations of PD clinical features [75–77]. Neuroanatomical sites of circadian disruption in PD may be along the afferent pathways to the SCN, within the SCN itself, or within the downstream peripheral efferents of the SCN. Circadian entrainment may be compromised in the population as PD patients tend to be less active and spend more time indoors. For example, reduced light exposure and/or impaired light transmission, partly due to dopaminergic retinal degeneration [78], may affect circadian timekeeping in the PD population. While the structure and function of the SCN in PD has not been rigorously examined to date, degeneration of this central circadian pacemaker may be yet another possible mechanism of impaired circadian rhythmicity in PD. Hypothalamic dopaminergic neurons, however, do not appear to be involved in the disease [79]. Finally, alterations in SCN output may be primarily responsible for fluctuations in biological rhythms and symptoms of PD.

Conclusion

Increasing evidence suggests disruptions of the circadian system in PD. Further, systematic investigations directed at circadian timekeeping may provide additional insight into the pathogenesis of daytime sleepiness and sleep dysfunction, and may possibly shed new insights into the neurodegenerative processes of PD itself. Furthermore, better understanding of the circadian biology of Parkinson's disease may lead to the development of novel, circadian-based treatment approaches for motor and nonmotor manifestations of PD.

References

1. Golombek DA, Rosenstein RE. Physiology of circadian entrainment. Physiol Rev. 2010;90(3):1063–102.
2. Dardente H, Cermakian N. Molecular circadian rhythms in central and peripheral clocks in mammals. Chronobiol Int. 2007;24(2):195–213.
3. Cermakian N, Boivin DB. The regulation of central and peripheral circadian clocks in humans. Obes Rev. 2009;10 Suppl 2:25–36.
4. Takahashi JS, Hong HK, Ko CH, McDearmon EL. The genetics of mammalian circadian order and disorder: implications for physiology and disease. Nat Rev. 2008;9(10):764–75.
5. Daan S, Pittendrigh CS. A functuional analysis of circadian pacemakers in nocturnal rodents. II. The variability of phase response curve. J Comp Physiol. 1976;106:253.
6. Lewy AJ. Melatonin as a marker and phase-resetter of circadian rhythms in humans. Adv Exp Med Biol. 1999;460:425–34.
7. Lewy AJ, Cutler NL, Sack RL. The endogenous melatonin profile as a marker for circadian phase position. J Biol Rhythms. 1999;14(3):227–36.
8. Selmaoui B, Touitou Y. Reproducibility of the circadian rhythms of serum cortisol and melatonin in healthy subjects: a study of three different 24-h cycles over six weeks. Life Sci. 2003;73(26):3339–49.
9. Witkovsky P. Dopamine and retinal function. Doc Ophthalmol. 2004;108(1):17–40.
10. Sakamoto K, Liu C, Kasamatsu M, Pozdeyev NV, Iuvone PM, Tosini G. Dopamine regulates melanopsin mRNA expression in intrinsically photosensitive retinal ganglion cells. Eur J Neurosci. 2005;22(12):3129–36.
11. Dorenbos R, Contini M, Hirasawa H, Gustincich S, Raviola E. Expression of circadian clock genes in retinal dopaminergic cells. Vis Neurosci. 2007;24(4):573–80.
12. Jackson CR, Chaurasia SS, Hwang CK, Iuvone PM. Dopamine D receptor activation controls circadian timing of the adenylyl cyclase 1/cyclic AMP signaling system in mouse retina. Eur J Neurosci. 2011;34(1):57–64.
13. Ruan GX, Allen GC, Yamazaki S, McMahon DG. An autonomous circadian clock in the inner mouse retina regulated by dopamine and GABA. PLoS Biol. 2008;6(10):e249.

14. Weaver DR, Rivkees SA, Reppert SM. D1-dopamine receptors activate c-fos expression in the fetal suprachiasmatic nuclei. Proc Natl Acad Sci U S A. 1992;89(19):9201–4.
15. Ishida Y, Yokoyama C, Inatomi T, Yagita K, Dong X, Yan L, et al. Circadian rhythm of aromatic L-amino acid decarboxylase in the rat suprachiasmatic nucleus: gene expression and decarboxylating activity in clock oscillating cells. Genes Cells. 2002;7(5):447–59.
16. Roybal K, Theobold D, Graham A, DiNieri JA, Russo SJ, Krishnan V, et al. Mania-like behavior induced by disruption of CLOCK. Proc Natl Acad Sci U S A. 2007;104(15):6406–11.
17. Castaneda TR, de Prado BM, Prieto D, Mora F. Circadian rhythms of dopamine, glutamate and GABA in the striatum and nucleus accumbens of the awake rat: modulation by light. J Pineal Res. 2004;36(3):177–85.
18. Hood S, Cassidy P, Cossette MP, Weigl Y, Verwey M, Robinson B, et al. Endogenous dopamine regulates the rhythm of expression of the clock protein PER2 in the rat dorsal striatum via daily activation of D2 dopamine receptors. J Neurosci. 2010;30(42):14046–58.
19. Imbesi M, Yildiz S, Dirim Arslan A, Sharma R, Manev H, Uz T. Dopamine receptor-mediated regulation of neuronal "clock" gene expression. Neuroscience. 2009;158(2):537–44.
20. Kafka MS, Benedito MA, Roth RH, Steele LK, Wolfe WW, Catravas GN. Circadian rhythms in catecholamine metabolites and cyclic nucleotide production. Chronobiol Int. 1986;3(2):101–15.
21. McClung CA. Circadian rhythms, the mesolimbic dopaminergic circuit, and drug addiction. ScientificWorldJournal. 2007;7:194–202.
22. Zisapel N. Melatonin-dopamine interactions: from basic neurochemistry to a clinical setting. Cell Mol Neurobiol. 2001;21(6):605–16.
23. Eisenberg DP, Kohn PD, Baller EB, Bronstein JA, Masdeu JC, Berman KF. Seasonal effects on human striatal presynaptic dopamine synthesis. J Neurosci. 2010;30(44):14691–4.
24. Hampp G, Albrecht U. The circadian clock and mood-related behavior. Commun Integr Biol. 2008;1(1):1–3.
25. Hampp G, Ripperger JA, Houben T, Schmutz I, Blex C, Perreau-Lenz S, et al. Regulation of monoamine oxidase A by circadian-clock components implies clock influence on mood. Curr Biol. 2008;18(9):678–83.
26. Bonuccelli U, Del Dotto P, Lucetti C, Petrozzi L, Bernardini S, Gambaccini G, et al. Diurnal motor variations to repeated doses of levodopa in Parkinson's disease. Clin Neuropharmacol. 2000;23(1):28–33.
27. Nutt JG, Woodward WR, Carter JH, Trotman TL. Influence of fluctuations of plasma large neutral amino acids with normal diets on the clinical response to levodopa. J Neurol Neurosurg Psychiatry. 1989;52(4):481–7.
28. van Hilten JJ, Kabel JF, Middelkoop HA, Kramer CG, Kerkhof GA, Roos RA. Assessment of response fluctuations in Parkinson's disease by ambulatory wrist activity monitoring. Acta Neurol Scand. 1993;87(3):171–7.
29. van Hilten JJ, Middelkoop HA, Kerkhof GA, Roos RA. A new approach in the assessment of motor activity in Parkinson's disease. J Neurol Neurosurg Psychiatry. 1991;54(11):976–9.
30. Arias-Vera JR, Mansoor GA, White WB. Abnormalities in blood pressure regulation in a patient with Parkinson's disease. Am J Hypertens. 2003;16(7):612–3.
31. Devos D, Kroumova M, Bordet R, Vodougnon H, Guieu JD, Libersa C, et al. Heart rate variability and Parkinson's disease severity. J Neural Transm. 2003;110(9):997–1011.
32. Ejaz AA, Sekhon IS, Munjal S. Characteristic findings on 24-h ambulatory blood pressure monitoring in a series of patients with Parkinson's disease. Eur J Intern Med. 2006;17(6):417–20.
33. Mihci E, Kardelen F, Dora B, Balkan S. Orthostatic heart rate variability analysis in idiopathic Parkinson's disease. Acta Neurol Scand. 2006;113(5):288–93.
34. Pathak A, Senard JM. Blood pressure disorders during Parkinson's disease: epidemiology, pathophysiology and management. Expert Rev Neurother. 2006;6(8):1173–80.
35. Pursiainen V, Haapaniemi TH, Korpelainen JT, Huikuri HV, Sotaniemi KA, Myllyla VV. Circadian heart rate variability in Parkinson's disease. J Neurol. 2002;249(11):1535–40.
36. Comella CL. Sleep disorders in Parkinson's disease: an overview. Mov Disord. 2007;22(S17):S367–73.

37. Placidi F, Izzi F, Romigi A, Stanzione P, Marciani MG, Brusa L, et al. Sleep-wake cycle and effects of cabergoline monotherapy in de novo Parkinson's disease patients. An ambulatory polysomnographic study. J Neurol. 2008;255(7):1032–7.
38. Porter B, Macfarlane R, Walker R. The frequency and nature of sleep disorders in a community-based population of patients with Parkinson's disease. Eur J Neurol. 2008;15(1):50–4.
39. van Hilten JJ, Weggeman M, van der Velde EA, Kerkhof GA, van Dijk JG, Roos RA. Sleep, excessive daytime sleepiness and fatigue in Parkinson's disease. J Neural Transm. 1993;5(3):235–44.
40. Verbaan D, van Rooden SM, Visser M, Marinus J, van Hilten JJ. Nighttime sleep problems and daytime sleepiness in Parkinson's disease. Mov Disord. 2008;23(1):35–41.
41. Struck LK, Rodnitzky RL, Dobson JK. Circadian fluctuations of contrast sensitivity in Parkinson's disease. Neurology. 1990;40(3 Pt 1):467–70.
42. Piccini P, Del Dotto P, Pardini C, D'Antonio P, Rossi G, Bonuccelli U. Diurnal worsening in Parkinson patients treated with levodopa. Riv Neurol. 1991;61(6):219–24.
43. van Hilten B, Hoff JI, Middelkoop HA, van der Velde EA, Kerkhof GA, Wauquier A, et al. Sleep disruption in Parkinson's disease. Assessment by continuous activity monitoring. Arch Neurol. 1994;51(9):922–8.
44. van Hilten JJ, Hoogland G, van der Velde EA, Middelkoop HA, Kerkhof GA, Roos RA. Diurnal effects of motor activity and fatigue in Parkinson's disease. J Neurol Neurosurg Psychiatry. 1993;56(8):874–7.
45. Whitehead DL, Davies AD, Playfer JR, Turnbull CJ. Circadian rest-activity rhythm is altered in Parkinson's disease patients with hallucinations. Mov Disord. 2008;23(8):1137–45.
46. Kallio M, Haapaniemi T, Turkka J, Suominen K, Tolonen U, Sotaniemi K, et al. Heart rate variability in patients with untreated Parkinson's disease. Eur J Neurol. 2000;7(6):667–72.
47. Plaschke M, Trenkwalder P, Dahlheim H, Lechner C, Trenkwalder C. Twenty-four-hour blood pressure profile and blood pressure responses to head-up tilt tests in Parkinson's disease and multiple system atrophy. J Hypertens. 1998;16(10):1433–41.
48. Senard JM, Chamontin B, Rascol A, Montastruc JL. Ambulatory blood pressure in patients with Parkinson's disease without and with orthostatic hypotension. Clin Auton Res. 1992;2(2):99–104.
49. Haapaniemi TH, Pursiainen V, Korpelainen JT, Huikuri HV, Sotaniemi KA, Myllyla VV. Ambulatory ECG and analysis of heart rate variability in Parkinson's disease. J Neurol Neurosurg Psychiatry. 2001;70(3):305–10.
50. Mastrocola C, Vanacore N, Giovani A, Locuratolo N, Vella C, Alessandri A, et al. Twenty-four-hour heart rate variability to assess autonomic function in Parkinson's disease. Acta Neurol Scand. 1999;99(4):245–7.
51. Mochizuki A, Komatsuzaki Y, Shoji S. Association of Lewy bodies and glial cytoplasmic inclusions in the brain of Parkinson's disease. Acta Neuropathol. 2002;104(5):534–7.
52. Wakabayashi K, Takahashi H. Neuropathology of autonomic nervous system in Parkinson's disease. Eur Neurol. 1997;38 Suppl 2:2–7.
53. Langston J. The hypothalamus in Parkinson's disease. Ann Neurol. 1978;3:129–33.
54. Wirz-Justice A, Da Prada M, Reme C. Circadian rhythm in rat retinal dopamine. Neurosci Lett. 1984;45(1):21–5.
55. Dearry A, Burnside B. Dopaminergic regulation of cone retinomotor movement in isolated teleost retinas: I. Induction of cone contraction is mediated by D2 receptors. J Neurochem. 1986;46(4):1006–21.
56. Bordet R, Devos D, Brique S, Touitou Y, Guieu JD, Libersa C, et al. Study of circadian melatonin secretion pattern at different stages of Parkinson's disease. Clin Neuropharmacol. 2003;26(2):65–72.
57. Fertl E, Auff E, Doppelbauer A, Waldhauser F. Circadian secretion pattern of melatonin in de novo parkinsonian patients: evidence for phase-shifting properties of l-dopa. J Neural Transm. 1993;5(3):227–34.
58. Hartmann A, Veldhuis JD, Deuschle M, Standhardt H, Heuser I. Twenty-four hour cortisol release profiles in patients with Alzheimer's and Parkinson's disease compared to normal controls: ultradian secretory pulsatility and diurnal variation. Neurobiol Aging. 1997;18(3):285–9.

59. Pierangeli G, Provini F, Maltoni P, Barletta G, Contin M, Lugaresi E, et al. Nocturnal body core temperature falls in Parkinson's disease but not in Multiple-System Atrophy. Mov Disord. 2001;16(2):226–32.

60. Cagnacci A, Bonuccelli U, Melis GB, Soldani R, Piccini P, Napolitano A, et al. Effect of naloxone on body temperature in postmenopausal women with Parkinson's disease. Life Sci. 1990;46(17):1241–7.

61. Suzuki K, Miyamoto T, Miyamoto M, Kaji Y, Takekawa H, Hirata K. Circadian variation of core body temperature in Parkinson disease patients with depression: a potential biological marker for depression in Parkinson disease. Neuropsychobiology. 2007;56(4):172–9.

62. Ben V, Blin O, Bruguerolle B. Time-dependent striatal dopamine depletion after injection of 6-hydroxydopamine in the rat. Comparison of single bilateral and double bilateral lesions. J Pharm Pharmacol. 1999;51(12):1405–8.

63. Videnovic A, Noble C, Reid KJ, Peng J, Turek FW, Marconi A, et al. Circadian melatonin rhythm and excessive sleepiness in Parkinson disease. JAMA Neurol. 2014;71(4):463–9.

64. Breen DA, Vuono R, Nawarathna U, Fisher K, Shneerson JM, Reddy AB, et al. Sleep and circadian rhythms regulation in early Parkinson disease. JAMA Neurol. 2014;71(5):589–95.

65. Bolitho SJ, Naismith SL, Rajaratnam SM, Grunstein RR, Hodges JR, Terpering Z, et al. Disturbances of melatonin secretion and circadian sleep-wake regulation in Parkinson disease. Sleep Med. 2014;15(3):324–7.

66. Boivin DB, James FO, Wu A, Cho-Park PF, Xiong H, Sun ZS. Circadian clock genes oscillate in human peripheral blood mononuclear cells. Blood. 2003;102(12):4143–5.

67. Takimoto M, Hamada A, Tomoda A, Ohdo S, Ohmura T, Sakato H, et al. Daily expression of clock genes in whole blood cells in healthy subjects and a patient with circadian rhythm sleep disorder. Am J Physiol. 2005;289(5):R1273–9.

68. Teboul M, Barrat-Petit MA, Li XM, Claustrat B, Formento JL, Delaunay F, et al. Atypical patterns of circadian clock gene expression in human peripheral blood mononuclear cells. J Mol Med (Berl, Germany). 2005;83(9):693–9.

69. Cai Y, Liu S, Sothern RB, Xu S, Chan P. Expression of clock genes Per1 and Bmal1 in total leukocytes in health and Parkinson's disease. Eur J Neurol. 2010;17(4):550–4.

70. Shirani A, St Louis EK. Illuminating rationale and uses for light therapy. J Clin Sleep Med. 2009;5(2):155–63.

71. Harrell LE, Balagura S. The effects of dark and light on the functional recovery following lateral hypothalamic lesions. Life Sci. 1974;15(12):2079–87.

72. Willis GL, Turner EJ. Primary and secondary features of Parkinson's disease improve with strategic exposure to bright light: a case series study. Chronobiol Int. 2007;24(3):521–37.

73. Willis GL, Moore C, Armstrong SM. A historical justification for and retrospective analysis of the systematic application of light therapy in Parkinson's disease. Rev Neurosci. 2012;23(2):199–226.

74. Paus S, Schmitz-Hubsch T, Wullner U, Vogel A, Klockgether T, Abele M. Bright light therapy in Parkinson's disease: a pilot study. Mov Disord. 2007;22(10):1495–8.

75. Bruinink A, Lichtensteiger W, Schlumpf M. Ontogeny of diurnal rhythms of central dopamine, serotonin and spirodecanone binding sites and of motor activity in the rat. Life Sci. 1983;33(1):31–8.

76. Khaldy H, Leon J, Escames G, Bikjdaouene L, Garcia JJ, Acuna-Castroviejo D. Circadian rhythms of dopamine and dihydroxyphenyl acetic acid in the mouse striatum: effects of pinealectomy and of melatonin treatment. Neuroendocrinology. 2002;75(3):201–8.

77. Weber M, Lauterburg T, Tobler I, Burgunder JM. Circadian patterns of neurotransmitter related gene expression in motor regions of the rat brain. Neurosci Lett. 2004;358(1):17–20.

78. Archibald NK, Clarke MP, Mosimann UP, Burn DJ. The retina in Parkinson's disease. Brain. 2009;132(Pt 5):1128–45.

79. Matzuk MM, Saper CB. Preservation of hypothalamic dopaminergic neurons in Parkinson's disease. Ann Neurol. 1985;18(5):552–5.

REM Sleep Behavior Disorder

10

Michael J. Howell and Carlos H. Schenck

Contents

Abstract

REM sleep behavior disorder (RBD), a condition of dream enactment, often predates Parkinson's disease (PD) and is the result of early neurodegenerative

M.J. Howell, MD (✉)
Department of Neurology, University of Minnesota, Minneapolis, USA
e-mail: howel020@umn.edu

C.H. Schenck, MD
Department of Psychiatry, University of Minnesota, Minneapolis, USA
e-mail: schen010@umn.edu

© Springer-Verlag Wien 2015
A. Videnovic, B. Högl (eds.), *Disorders of Sleep and Circadian Rhythms in Parkinson's Disease*, DOI 10.1007/978-3-7091-1631-9_10

processes in the brainstem. Normally, REM sleep is characterized by vivid mentation combined with skeletal muscle paralysis. This REM atonia is diminished or absent in RBD, which enables patients to act out their dreams with violent, injurious nocturnal behaviors. Consistent with an impending neurodegenerative disorder, patients with RBD demonstrate subtle motor, autonomic, and cognitive changes frequently seen in synucleinopathies. These disorders include PD as well as multiple system atrophy (MSA) and dementia with Lewy bodies (DLB). In PD, RBD is linked with the akinetic–rigid predominant subtype, gait freezing, and predicts aggressive cognitive impairment. Clinical management is focused upon decreasing the potential for sleep-related injuries (SRIs), treating comorbid sleep disorders, and eliminating exacerbating agents. High-dose melatonin, low-dose clonazepam, and combined melatonin–clonazepam appear to be effective therapies.

10.1 Historical Perspective

In 1817, James Parkinson wrote "An Essay on the Shaking Palsy" [1]. This first comprehensive description of the disorder that would later bear his name noted that "sleep becomes much disturbed" in patients and hinted at a disorder of agitated dream enactment.

> His (Case VI) attendants observed, that of late the trembling would sometimes begin in his sleep, and increase until it awakened him: when he always was in a state of agitation and alarm.
>   …when exhausted nature seizes a small portion of sleep, the motion becomes so violent as not only to shake the bed-hangings, but even the floor and sashes of the room.

Prior to Parkinson's monograph, episodes of dream enactment suggestive of RBD were reported as early by Hippocrates (circa 460–370 BCE), Aristotle (384–322 BCE), and Galen (circa 129–200) and later by Cervantes (1547–1616). By the Renaissance, dream enactment was considered a window into subconscious psychological conflict. In William Shakespeare's Macbeth, the sleepwalking Lady Macbeth admits to being a coconspirator in murder and reveals her subsequent internal torment.

> Out damned spot! Out, I say! …What, will these hands never be clean?

Soon after Aserinsky and Kleitman discovered regularly occurring periods of eye motility during sleep in 1953 [2], investigators began to explore the brainstem mechanisms of REM sleep, including those leading to skeletal muscle paralysis. In 1965, experimental lesions of pontine regions by Jouvet adjacent to the locus coeruleus in cats caused an absence of the expected atonia. These cats demonstrated prominent motor behaviors during REM sleep suspected to be dream mentation ("oneirism") [3].

In 1982, Schenck and Mahowald evaluated a 67-year-old man who presented with a history of violent dream-enactment behavior (DEB). A subsequent polysomnogram demonstrated REM sleep without atonia along with vigorous DEB. In 1986, they published a series of patients and named the condition "REM sleep behavior disorder." By 1996, 38 % of their original series of patients had developed a parkinsonian syndrome and by 2013 the conversion rate reached 81 % [4].

10.2   Clinical Presentation

Prior to developing bradykinesia, cogwheel rigidity, and tremor, many Parkinson's disease (PD) patients will describe a parasomnia or abnormal nocturnal behavior emanating from sleep. The sleep-related movements appear purposeful as if the patient is acting out some internal dream plot and when awoken, vivid dreams are described. The condition typically presents in a middle-aged individual without a history of sleepwalking or other parasomnia. The frequency of incidents ranges from once every few months to multiple nightly episodes. Often, there is a prolonged prodrome lasting years with progressively more prominent nocturnal behaviors occurring over time [5, 6].

The spectrum of dream-enactment behavior (DEB) in RBD varies from small hand movements to violent activities such as punching, kicking, or leaping out of bed. Examples of sleep-related injuries include subdural hematoma, shoulder dislocation, cervical fracture, as well as lacerations severing tendons, arteries, and nerves. As bed partners are frequently the target of violent dream enactment, RBD may have forensic implications, with patients wrongly in the criminal justice system [5, 6].

Patients manifest DEB more often during the second half of the night and sleep-related injury (SRI) is more likely to occur in later REM periods. This is related to the progressive increase in phasic activity, frequency, and duration of REM sleep normally seen throughout a night of sleep.

Importantly, RBD patients may not have more violent dreams than normal individuals. Instead, they merely act them out. Sleep-related vocalizations may be loud and frequently laden with expletives. This is most often discordant from waking personality, and RBD patients do not demonstrate greater daytime aggressiveness.

Patients and families may adopt extraordinary measures to prevent SRI: placing obstacles to hinder exiting the bed or sleeping on a floor mattress in a room devoid of furniture. Prolonged diagnostic delay is common and some families deal with these behaviors for decades prior to seeking medical attention.

Prior to the onset, and early in the course of PD, DEB progresses in frequency and intensity. Then late in the disease state a moderation of RBD occurs, likely secondary to diffuse motor circuit impairment [6].

10.3   Epidemiology

Surveys have revealed that some DEB is nearly universal with 98 % of college-aged students reporting at least one episode of DEB [7]. The vast majority of these cases, however, are transient and nondistressing. Various reports have suggested that the prevalence of RBD is approximately 0.5 % in the general population [5], with higher prevalence among patients with neurodegenerative disease, other sleep disorders, or on antidepressant medications [5, 8]. Thus, there are approximately 35 million patients worldwide; however, the clinical symptoms are frequently dismissed and thus vast majority of cases remain undiagnosed for a long time.

As noted above, RBD is often a heralding manifestation of PD and is common among other alpha-synuclein disorders. According to several studies, approximately one-third to one-half of patients with PD have RBD [6, 9, 10]. Among similar pathologies the frequency is even higher, with 50–80 % of patients with DLB and 80–95 % of patients with MSA [6, 11].

Similar to PD, RBD is associated with various environmental and behavioral risk factors. In particular, RBD patients are more likely to smoke, have a history of traumatic brain injury, farming, pesticide exposure, and fewer years of education [12].

The majority of reported cases are males; however, female RBD is likely underreported. Women present with less injurious dream enactment and thus are less likely to receive medical attention. Further, due to the gender difference in life expectancy, elderly women are less likely to have bed partners than elderly men, and thus less likely to have witnessed parasomnia behaviors [13, 14].

10.4   RBD and Early Features of Alpha-Synuclein Pathology

Patients with RBD demonstrate clinical and subclinical phenomena suggestive of an impending alpha-synuclein CNS pathology. When fully developed, these disorders manifest as either PD, MSA, DLB or rarely pure autonomic failure.

Motor testing in RBD demonstrates slight, often imperceptible parkinsonian abnormalities. In particular, subtle changes are noted on the Purdue Peg Board, alternate tap test, the Unified Parkinson's Disease Rating Scale (UPDRS), and timed evaluation of standing and walking [15]. Further, in a survey of normal elderly individuals, the presence of RBD symptoms was associated with at least mild parkinsonian exam findings [6].

Patients with RBD also have subtle cognitive dysfunction. Studies have demonstrated impairments in visuospatial skills as well as in color and facial expression identification [15, 16]. Other investigations have revealed deficits in attention and executive function [6]. Prospectively, the presence of RBD symptoms confers a greater than twofold risk of developing mild cognitive impairment (MCI) over 4 years [17]. Conversely, among patients with MCI or dementia the presence of RBD helps distinguish DLB from Alzheimer's disease [6, 18].

As in PD, hyposmia/anosmia is frequently noted in RBD. Over half of RBD patients have impairments in smell identification, compared to 10–15 % in age-matched controls [15, 19]. The most common deficit is an inability to identify paint thinner [19]. RBD and hyposmia in combination with impaired color identification place the patient at very high risk of impending PD [16].

In RBD, autonomic dysfunction is consistent with an evolving neurodegenerative disorder. Comorbid enteric neuron pathology manifests as constipation [15] and similar to hyposmia, when combined with impaired color vision predicts progression to PD [20]. Heart rate responses to both orthostasis and arousal are blunted compared to controls and intermediate compared to PD [21]. Cardiac scintigraphy has been used to predict a parkinsonian syndrome. Among RBD patients, reduced uptake of (123) I-metaiodobenzylguanidine, indicating sympathetic denervation, has been demonstrated in PD and DLB but not in MSA [6, 22].

10.4.1 RBD in PD

RBD is associated with the akinetic/rigid subtype of PD and a greater burden of disease. Removal of tremor scores from the UPDRS increases its sensitivity and specificity in diagnosing early PD among RBD patients [23]. Further, RBD in PD is associated with a higher Hoehn and Yahr stage (increased severity), greater motor fluctuations, and increased levodopa dose [9]. Orthostatic hypotension and constipation are both more common in PD with RBD compared to PD alone [9, 24]. In DLB, the presence of RBD is associated with earlier onset of parkinsonism and visual hallucinations [25].

PD patients with RBD are also more likely to have freezing of gait (FOG) and a higher frequency of falls [24]. Interestingly, many of the same brainstem regions implicated in the pathophysiology of RBD mediate the pathogenesis of FOG. Moreover, it was recently demonstrated that PD patients with FOG demonstrate increased tonic REM EMG tone compared to PD patients without FOG [26].

The presence of RBD predicts greater cognitive dysfunction in PD. Neuropsychological testing has demonstrated at least mild cognitive impairment in nearly all (90 %) PD patients with RBD compared to less than half (38 %) of the patients with PD alone [27]. Among PD patients who are without severe cognitive deficit, RBD predicts dementia. In a 4-year prospective study, 48 % of PD patients with RBD developed dementia compared to none of PD patients without RBD [28].

It has been reported that overnight RBD behaviors in PD lack the bradykinesia and hypophonia that characterize daytime motor performance in PD. This phenomenon suggests that RBD motor activity may bypass the basal ganglia regulatory.

10.5 Pathophysiology

Prior to the hallmark destruction of dopamine-producing neurons in the substantia nigra (SN), early alpha-synuclein degeneration occurs in the brainstem nuclei that control REM sleep. Under physiological circumstances the suppression of motor activity during REM is the cumulative result of multiple pathways that ultimately terminate on spinal motor neurons, most notably via the magnocellular reticular formation in the medulla. Multiple areas of the brainstem may influence muscle tone including pontine REM-on (precoeruleus and sublateral dorsal) and REM-off (ventral lateral portion of the periaqueductal gray matter and lateral pontine tegmentum) nuclei [6]. Decreased neuronal fiber integrity is seen in these REM-regulating regions among patients with RBD [29].

By the time PD motor abnormalities develop, the majority of dopaminergic cells in the substantial nigra (SN) are dysfunctional. However, in RBD patients who have not yet manifested parkinsonism, neuroimaging reveals a coincident and progressive reduction in dopamine transporters and innervation [30, 31]. Further, transcranial ultrasound hyperechogenicity of substantial nigra in RBD resembles abnormalities seen in PD [32].

Cholinergic function is impaired in RBD and correlates with cognitive decline. Among PD subjects with RBD compared to PD subjects without RBD positron emission tomography reveals cholinergic denervation [33]. These findings are similar to those seen in transcranial magnetic stimulation studies that demonstrate reduced short latency inhibition, indicating impaired cholinergic activity, in RBD. These cholinergic deficits are linked with deficiencies in episodic verbal memory, executive function, and visuospatial cognitive domains [27].

Cortical abnormalities, similar to those seen in PD and related disorders, are noted in patients with RBD. Voxel-based morphology studies demonstrate gray matter reductions that correlate with decreased regional cerebral blood flow (rCBF) in the parieto-occipital and hippocampal regions [34, 35]. Also, an increase in hippocampal rCBF is noted in RBD patients with MCI and predicts those who will ultimately progress to either PD or DLB [36].

RBD is not associated only with alpha-synuclein neurodegenerative disorders. Other etiologies include other forms of neurodegeneration, side effects of medications, structural CNS lesions, and narcolepsy linked to the orexin dysfunction. RBD has been reported in tauopathy-related parkinsonian syndromes (progressive supranuclear palsy, Guadeloupean parkinsonism, corticobasal degeneration), TDP-43opathies (frontotemporal dementia, amyotrophic lateral sclerosis), trinucleotide repeat disorders (SCA-3, Huntington's disease), and rarely amyloidopathies (Alzheimer's disease) [6]. However, these disorders are not typically preceded by RBD, but instead RBD develops after the onset of other neurological deficits. Medications such as tricyclic antidepressants and serotonin-specific reuptake inhibitors can precipitate or exacerbate RBD [6, 37]. It is uncertain whether these medications cause a de-novo RBD or, unmask latent RBD. Occasionally, various vascular, demyelinating, and traumatic etiologies are linked to development of RBD [38]. In these cases, cranial imaging typically demonstrates pontine tegmentum pathology. Finally, impaired orexin function can precipitate DEB, with up to 50 % of narcolepsy patients having RBD symptoms. This association is strongest among narcolepsy patients with cataplexy [39].

10.6 Clinical Evaluation and Diagnosis

10.6.1 History and Examination

A detailed review of the patient's sleep and circadian rhythm, preferably with the assistance of a bed partner is the first step in the evaluation of all parasomnia behaviors. Recurrent, brief DEB occurring in the later half of the sleep period followed by complete alertness and orientation upon awakening are features that help to distinguish RBD from other similar disorders. This presentation contrasts with sleepwalking where there is often a lifelong history of prolonged, complex, nonviolent activities emanating from the first half of the sleep period with residual confusion [5].

Validated screening surveys are available to help identify RBD and quantify disease burden. These include the RBD Questionnaire-Hong Kong (RBDQ-HK) and the Innsbruck RBD inventory [40, 41]. In addition, two separate groups of investigators have reported one-question instruments to detect RBD. The Mayo Sleep Questionnaire (MSQ) is a comprehensive sleep health survey, filled out by bed partners, that includes the following question: "Have you ever seen the patient appear to 'act out his/her dreams' while sleeping (punched or flailed arms in the air, shouted or screamed)?" [6]. This question is very similar to the RBD Single-Question Screen: "Have you ever been told, or suspected yourself, that you seem to 'act out your dreams' while asleep (for example, punching, flailing your arms in the air, making running movements, etc.)?" [42].

It is important to inquire about alpha-synucleinopathies, when assessing a possible RBD. When chronic unexplained hyposmia and/or constipation coexist with RBD, they are highly suggestive of impending neurodegeneration. Further, it is important to assess early bradykinesia and rigidity. These phenomena are often imperceptible and may be dismissed as routine aging. In particular, a question such as "Does a patient have difficulty turning over in bed, or bradykinesia during routine activities such as eating and dressing, or do they have changes in handwriting?" may be very informative. FOG, commonly present in PD, and can be explored with the question. "Do your feet ever feel as if they are stuck to the floor?"

Among patients with known PD inquiring about DEB is a critical part of a comprehensive evaluation. In the setting of PD falling out of bed during sleep is highly suggestive of RBD and a risk factor for sleep-related injury. Both the Innsbruck RBD inventory and RBDQ-HK are effective screens for RBD among patients with Parkinson's disease.

On examination, careful scrutiny of subtle parkinsonism is essential for accurate longitudinal clinical monitoring. Documentation should contain a patient's affectation, blink rate, volume of voice, speed of articulation, as well as motor tone with distracting maneuvers to elicit subtle cogwheeling rigidity. Important features on gait testing include any freezing of movement, stride length, arm swing, and number of steps to turn 180°. Further, postural instability (loss of righting reflex with sudden retropulsion) is a risk factor for falling and commonly noted in PD patients with RBD. The UPDRS includes these examination features and can be used to prospectively quantify the burden of disease.

10.6.2 Polysomnography

Polysomnography (PSG) with time-synchronized video is necessary for definitive RBD diagnosis and to exclude other conditions [43]. Even when abnormal behavior does not occur during a single night study, the PSG is helpful in documenting the absence of REM atonia. The combination of REM without atonia, a history of DEB, and absence of clinically significant sleep disordered breathing can establish a diagnosis. When RBD behaviors do occur, they are often distinguished from other nocturnal behaviors based on appearance alone. RBD movements more typically appear purposeful, pseudohallucinatory, frequently with hand babbling (limb wrist, flexed fingers—like a baby). Other REM sleep phenomena are often present including snoring and in males, penile tumescence [44].

The American Academy of Sleep Medicine has defined a PSG epoch as either sustained elevation of chin EMG activity (greater than 50 % of the 30-s epoch) or excessive bursts of transient muscle activity (at least half of all 3-s mini epochs). Using this criteria to define RBD epochs, 30 % or greater appears to reliably distinguish RBD from non-RBD patients. Subtle dream enactment often involves only the hands and thus forearm EMG monitoring should be included [6].

PSG is particularly helpful in ruling out conditions such as sleep-disordered breathing, periodic limb movement disorder (PLMD), and nocturnal epilepsy as a source of the reported behaviors. The REM sleep fragmentation of obstructive sleep apnea (OSA) can lead to DEB, but typically resolves with CPAP therapy. PLMD, primarily a NREM sleep phenomena, can be confused with RBD by history if the leg movements are especially prominent, but is easily discernible on PSG. Nocturnal seizures should be evaluated with an expanded EEG montage especially if there is a history of stereotyped, abnormal, and repetitive behaviors.

10.7 Treatment

Modifying the sleeping environment with a focus upon patient safety is the initial step in RBD treatment. The patient should remove any bedside object or furniture that could be injurious. In particular, firearms and windows should not be easily accessible. Bed partners are advised to sleep separately until RBD is brought under control. However, this advice is commonly disregarded as bed partners will describe an ability to pacify DEB with a few firm, but calm words.

RBD inducing or aggravating medications should be eliminated and comorbid sleep disorders treated. Most cases of medication-induced RBD are self-limited following discontinuation of offending medication. DEBs frequently seen in association with OSA typically resolve with treatment of OSA.

When violent nocturnal behaviors persist despite these interventions or in situations with a high probability of injury, pharmacotherapy is appropriate [45]. The most commonly prescribed medications include clonazepam and/or melatonin [6, 46, 47]. As large randomized placebo-controlled therapeutic trials have not yet been performed, consensus treatment has arisen based upon case series and small clinical trials [45, 48].

10.7.1 Clonazepam

Over the last 30 years, clonazepam has been the most widely prescribed agent for RBD and approximately 90 % of patients initially respond well to low doses (0.5–1.0 mg) administered at bedtime [4, 49]. Clonazepam reduces phasic EMG activity during REM sleep with minimal effect on tonic muscle activity. The agent also appears to be effective in cases that have progressed to PD [4, 6].

Long-term follow-up studies revealed mixed results, ranging from sustained benefit without dose escalation to frequent dose escalations and treatment failures [4, 50–52]. In one series, 58 % of patients on clonazepam reported clinically significant adverse effects with 50 % either stopping the medication or reducing the dose [52]. Also, clonazepam may be particularly problematic in the setting of advanced PD where its prolonged duration of action can result in morning sedation, impaired gait, and cognitive side effects [53].

10.7.2 Melatonin

Recently, several studies have suggested that melatonin may be an effective and safe first-line treatment for RBD either in combination with clonazepam or as sole therapy. By uncertain mechanisms, melatonin in high doses at bedtime (6–15 mg) augments REM atonia and improves RBD symptoms. Effects persist for weeks after the agent is discontinued [6, 47].

Importantly, a recent direct comparison study noted that melatonin was equal to clonazepam in treatment efficacy and superior in side effect profile. Patients on melatonin reported fewer adverse effects, in particular less falls and injuries compared to clonazepam [54]. In the setting of advanced PD, melatonin is a particularly intriguing option as it is only mildly sedating.

10.7.3 Pramipexole

Pramipexole may be effective in mild cases of RBD, in particular those associated with frequent PLMs. Compared to clonazepam responsive patients, pramipexole responsive patients have milder disease at baseline as measured by REM atonia. Similar to treating OSA in RBD, pramipexole may decrease nocturnal behaviors by reversing a sleep fragmenting condition. Patients report a decrease in distressing nocturnal behaviors along with a decrease in PLMs; however, pramipexole has no effect upon REM atonia [55].

10.7.4 Rivastigmine

Cholinergic agents may be useful in RBD among patients who have failed conventional therapy. One small placebo-controlled crossover trial noted that the cholinesterase inhibitor rivastigmine reduced the number of DEB episodes as noted by bed partners [56].

10.7.5 Other Medications

Various therapies have been reported at least once to be successful. These include imipramine, carbamazepine, levodopa, donepezil, sodium oxybate, triazolam, zopiclone, quetiapine, and clozapine [45, 46, 52].

10.7.6 Deep Brain Stimulation

Deep brain stimulation (DBS) for PD has thus far not been therapeutic for comorbid RBD. Three case series of PD patients with RBD undergoing DBS noted improvements in subjective sleep quality and sleep architecture on PSG, however, with little to no improvement in DEB or REM atonia [57–59]. These findings were not unexpected as the target of DBS in these studies, the subthalamic nucleus, does not have a known effect upon REM sleep. Other DBS targets for PD include the globus pallidus internus and the paramedian pontine nucleus. The PPN is an REM-modulating nucleus and thus an intriguing target for future RBD investigations.

10.7.7 Bed Alarm Therapy

Medication refractory RBD is a daunting and potentially life-threatening condition. Exiting the bed while acting out a dream is a particularly high-risk behavior and may result in severe traumatic injury.

The low arousal threshold and rapid transition to alert wakefulness from REM sleep offers a therapeutic window to halt behavior prior to SRI. Despite apparent unconsciousness during REM sleep, the brain is readily responsive to complex auditory sound processing. This contrasts with the high arousal threshold of NREM sleep often demonstrated by the inability to redirect or wake up SW patients (a NREM parasomnia). This phenomenon is often noted by bed partners who describe an ability to calm RBD patients with a simple phrase such as, "sweetheart, you are having a dream go back to sleep." A customized bed alarm, delivering such a calming message when a patient attempts to leave the bed can halt potentially injurious dream enactment [53].

10.8   Future Directions

10.8.1 Possible Neuroprotection

At this time, it is uncertain what measures may be taken to prevent or delay the onset of a neurodegenerative disorder such as PD. However, as RBD may help identify patients at high risk for developing PD, it may also be an important target in studies of neuroprotective/disease-modifying therapies.

These preliminary investigations have begun to explore whether compounds can slow, halt, or possibly even reverse alpha-synuclein neurodegeneration. Recently, riluzole, an antiglutamate compound currently used as neuroprotection in amyotrophic lateral sclerosis, has been demonstrated to both prevent RBD and increase the number of surviving dopamine neurons in the marmoset MPTP model of Parkinson's disease [60]. Another intriguing agent, already in use among RBD patients, is melatonin. Recently, melatonin has been demonstrated to have antioxidant properties and to protect mitochondrial function, suggesting it has potential as a neuroprotective agent [61]. Obviously, prospective randomized-controlled trials are needed prior to concluding that any substance may prevent or slow neurodegeneration.

References

1. Parkinson J. An essay on the shaking palsy. London: Sherwood, Neely, and Jones; 1817.
2. Aserinsky E, Kleitman N. Regularly occurring periods of eye motility, and concomitant phenomena, during sleep. Science. 1953;118(3062):273–4.
3. Jouvet D, Vimont P, Delorme F. Study of selective deprivation of the paradoxal phase of sleep in the cat. J Physiol Paris. 1964;56:381.
4. Schenck CH, Boeve BF, Mahowald MW. Delayed emergence of a parkinsonian disorder or dementia in 81 % of older males initially diagnosed with idiopathic REM sleep behavior disorder (RBD): 16year update on a previously reported series. Sleep Med. 2013;14:744–8.
5. American Academy of Sleep Medicine. International classification of sleep disorders: diagnostic and coding manual. 2nd ed. Westchester: American Academy of Sleep Medicine; 2005.
6. Boeve BF. REM sleep behavior disorder: updated review of the core features, the REM sleep behavior disorder-neurodegenerative disease association, evolving concepts, controversies, and future directions. Ann N Y Acad Sci. 2010;1184:15–54.
7. Nielsen T, Svob C, Kuiken D. Dream-enacting behaviors in a normal population. Sleep. 2009;32(12):1629–36.
8. Boeve BF, Silber MH, Parisi JE, Dickson DW, Ferman TJ, Benarroch EE, et al. Synucleinopathy pathology and REM sleep behavior disorder plus dementia or parkinsonism. Neurology. 2003;61(1):40–5.
9. Nihei Y, Takahashi K, Koto A, Mihara B, Morita Y, Isozumi K, et al. REM sleep behavior disorder in Japanese patients with Parkinson's disease: a multicenter study using the REM sleep behavior disorder screening questionnaire. J Neurol. 2012;259(8):1606–12.
10. Poryazova R, Oberholzer M, Baumann CR, Bassetti CL. REM sleep behavior disorder in Parkinson's disease: a questionnaire-based survey. J Clin Sleep Med. 2013;9(1):55–9.
11. Plazzi G, Corsini R, Provini F, Pierangeli G, Martinelli P, Montagna P, et al. REM sleep behavior disorders in multiple system atrophy. Neurology. 1997;48(4):1094–7.
12. Postuma RB, Montplaisir JY, Pelletier A, Dauvilliers Y, Oertel W, Iranzo A, et al. Environmental risk factors for REM sleep behavior disorder: a multicenter case-control study. Neurology. 2012;79(5):428–34.
13. Bodkin CL, Schenck CH. Rapid eye movement sleep behavior disorder in women: relevance to general and specialty medical practice. J Womens Health (Larchmt). 2009;18(12):1955–63.
14. Bjornara KA, Dietrichs E, Toft M. REM sleep behavior disorder in Parkinson's disease–is there a gender difference? Parkinsonism Relat Disord. 2013;19(1):120–2.
15. Postuma RB, Lang AE, Massicotte-Marquez J, Montplaisir J. Potential early markers of Parkinson disease in idiopathic REM sleep behavior disorder. Neurology. 2006;66(6):845–51.

16. Postuma RB, Gagnon JF, Vendette M, Desjardins C, Montplaisir JY. Olfaction and color vision identify impending neurodegeneration in rapid eye movement sleep behavior disorder. Ann Neurol. 2011;69(5):811–8.

17. Boot BP, Boeve BF, Roberts RO, Ferman TJ, Geda YE, Pankratz VS, et al. Probable rapid eye movement sleep behavior disorder increases risk for mild cognitive impairment and Parkinson disease: a population-based study. Ann Neurol. 2012;71(1):49–56.

18. Ferman TJ, Boeve BF, Smith GE, Lin SC, Silber MH, Pedraza O, et al. Inclusion of RBD improves the diagnostic classification of dementia with Lewy bodies. Neurology. 2011;77(9):875–82.

19. Fantini ML, Postuma RB, Montplaisir J, Ferini-Strambi L. Olfactory deficit in idiopathic rapid eye movements sleep behavior disorder. Brain Res Bull. 2006;70(4–6):386–90.

20. Ferini-Strambi L. Does idiopathic REM sleep behavior disorder (iRBD) really exist? What are the potential markers of neurodegeneration in iRBD? Sleep Med. 2011;12 Suppl 2:S43–9.

21. Frauscher B, Nomura T, Duerr S, Ehrmann L, Gschliesser V, Wenning GK, et al. Investigation of autonomic function in idiopathic REM sleep behavior disorder. J Neurol. 2012;259:1056–61.

22. Miyamoto T, Miyamoto M, Suzuki K, Nishibayashi M, Iwanami M, Hirata K. 123I-MIBG cardiac scintigraphy provides clues to the underlying neurodegenerative disorder in idiopathic REM sleep behavior disorder. Sleep. 2008;31(5):717–23.

23. Postuma RB, Lang AE, Gagnon JF, Pelletier A, Montplaisir JY. How does parkinsonism start? Prodromal parkinsonism motor changes in idiopathic REM sleep behaviour disorder. Brain. 2012;135(Pt 6):1860–70.

24. Romenets SR, Gagnon JF, Latreille V, Panniset M, Chouinard S, Montplaisir J, et al. Rapid eye movement sleep behavior disorder and subtypes of Parkinson's disease. Mov Disord. 2012;27(8):996–1003.

25. Dugger BN, Boeve BF, Murray ME, Parisi JE, Fujishiro H, Dickson DW, et al. Rapid eye movement sleep behavior disorder and subtypes in autopsy-confirmed dementia with Lewy bodies. Mov Disord. 2012;27(1):72–8.

26. Videnovic A, Marlin C, Alibiglou L, et al. Increased REM sleep without atonia in Parkinson's disease patients with freezing of gait. Neurology. 2013;81:1030–5.

27. Nardone R, Bergmann J, Brigo F, Christova M, Kunz A, Seidl M, et al. Functional evaluation of central cholinergic circuits in patients with Parkinson's disease and REM sleep behavior disorder: a TMS study. J Neural Transm. 2013;120(3):413–22.

28. Postuma RB, Bertrand JA, Montplaisir J, Desjardins C, Vendette M, Rios Romenets S, et al. Rapid eye movement sleep behavior disorder and risk of dementia in Parkinson's disease: a prospective study. Mov Disord. 2012;27(6):720–6.

29. Scherfler C, Frauscher B, Schocke M, Iranzo A, Gschliesser V, Seppi K, et al. White and gray matter abnormalities in idiopathic rapid eye movement sleep behavior disorder: a diffusion-tensor imaging and voxel-based morphometry study. Ann Neurol. 2011;69(2):400–7.

30. Eisensehr I, Linke R, Tatsch K, Kharraz B, Gildehaus JF, Wetter CT, et al. Increased muscle activity during rapid eye movement sleep correlates with decrease of striatal presynaptic dopamine transporters. IPT and IBZM SPECT imaging in subclinical and clinically manifest idiopathic REM sleep behavior disorder, Parkinson's disease, and controls. Sleep. 2003;26(5):507–12.

31. Iranzo A, Valldeoriola F, Lomena F, Molinuevo JL, Serradell M, Salamero M, et al. Serial dopamine transporter imaging of nigrostriatal function in patients with idiopathic rapid-eye-movement sleep behaviour disorder: a prospective study. Lancet Neurol. 2011;10(9):797–805.

32. Miyamoto M, Miyamoto T, Iwanami M, Muramatsu S, Asari S, Nakano I, et al. Preclinical substantia nigra dysfunction in rapid eye movement sleep behaviour disorder. Sleep Med. 2012;13(1):102–6.

33. Kotagal V, Albin RL, Muller ML, Koeppe RA, Chervin RD, Frey KA, et al. Symptoms of rapid eye movement sleep behavior disorder are associated with cholinergic denervation in Parkinson disease. Ann Neurol. 2012;71(4):560–8.

34. Hanyu H, Inoue Y, Sakurai H, Kanetaka H, Nakamura M, Miyamoto T, et al. Regional cerebral blood flow changes in patients with idiopathic REM sleep behavior disorder. Eur J Neurol. 2011;18(5):784–8.

35. Vendette M, Gagnon JF, Soucy JP, Gosselin N, Postuma RB, Tuineag M, et al. Brain perfusion and markers of neurodegeneration in rapid eye movement sleep behavior disorder. Mov Disord. 2011;26(9):1717–24.
36. Dang-Vu TT, Gagnon JF, Vendette M, Soucy JP, Postuma RB, Montplaisir J. Hippocampal perfusion predicts impending neurodegeneration in REM sleep behavior disorder. Neurology. 2012;79(24):2302–6.
37. Hoque R, Chesson Jr AL. Pharmacologically induced/exacerbated restless legs syndrome, periodic limb movements of sleep, and REM behavior disorder/REM sleep without atonia: literature review, qualitative scoring, and comparative analysis. J Clin Sleep Med. 2010;6(1):79–83.
38. Boeve BF, Silber MH, Saper CB, Ferman TJ, Dickson DW, Parisi JE, et al. Pathophysiology of REM sleep behaviour disorder and relevance to neurodegenerative disease. Brain. 2007; 130(Pt 11):2770–88.
39. Dauvilliers Y, Jennum P, Plazzi G. REM sleep behavior disorder and REM sleep without atonia in narcolepsy. Sleep Med. 2013;14:775–81.
40. Li SX, Wing YK, Lam SP, Zhang J, Yu MW, Ho CK, et al. Validation of a new REM sleep behavior disorder questionnaire (RBDQ-HK). Sleep Med. 2010;11(1):43–8.
41. Frauscher B, Ehrmann L, Zamarian L, Auer F, Mitterling T, Gabelia D, et al. Validation of the Innsbruck REM sleep behavior disorder inventory. Mov Disord. 2012;27(13):1673–8.
42. Postuma RB, Arnulf I, Hogl B, Iranzo A, Miyamoto T, Dauvilliers Y, et al. A single-question screen for rapid eye movement sleep behavior disorder: a multicenter validation study. Mov Disord. 2012;27(7):913–6.
43. Neikrug AB, Ancoli-Israel S. Diagnostic tools for REM sleep behavior disorder. Sleep Med Rev. 2012;16:415–29.
44. Oudiette D, Leu-Semenescu S, Roze E, Vidailhet M, De Cock VC, Golmard JL, et al. A motor signature of REM sleep behavior disorder. Mov Disord. 2012;27(3):428–31.
45. Aurora RN, Zak RS, Maganti RK, Auerbach SH, Casey KR, Chowdhuri S, et al. Best practice guide for the treatment of REM sleep behavior disorder (RBD). J Clin Sleep Med. 2010;6(1):85–95.
46. Gagnon JF, Postuma RB, Montplaisir J. Update on the pharmacology of REM sleep behavior disorder. Neurology. 2006;67(5):742–7.
47. Kunz D, Mahlberg R. A two-part, double-blind, placebo-controlled trial of exogenous melatonin in REM sleep behaviour disorder. J Sleep Res. 2010;19(4):591–6.
48. Seppi K, Weintraub D, Coelho M, Perez-Lloret S, Fox SH, Katzenschlager R, et al. The movement disorder society evidence-based medicine review update: treatments for the non-motor symptoms of Parkinson's disease. Mov Disord. 2011;26 Suppl 3:S42–80.
49. Olson EJ, Boeve BF, Silber MH. Rapid eye movement sleep behaviour disorder: demographic, clinical and laboratory findings in 93 cases. Brain. 2000;123(Pt 2):331–9.
50. Gagnon JF, Petit D, Fantini ML, Rompre S, Gauthier S, Panisset M, et al. REM sleep behavior disorder and REM sleep without atonia in probable Alzheimer disease. Sleep. 2006;29(10):1321–5.
51. Gugger JJ, Wagner ML. Rapid eye movement sleep behavior disorder. Ann Pharmacother. 2007;41(11):1833–41.
52. Anderson KN, Shneerson JM. Drug treatment of REM sleep behavior disorder: the use of drug therapies other than clonazepam. J Clin Sleep Med. 2009;5(3):235–9.
53. Howell MJ, Arneson PA, Schenck CH. A novel therapy for REM sleep behavior disorder (RBD). J Clin Sleep Med. 2011;7(6):639–644A.
54. McCarter SJ, Boswell CL, St Louis EK, Dueffert LG, Slocumb N, Boeve BF, et al. Treatment outcomes in REM sleep behavior disorder. Sleep Med. 2013;14(3):237–42.
55. Sasai T, Matsuura M, Inoue Y. Factors associated with the effect of pramipexole on symptoms of idiopathic REM sleep behavior disorder. Parkinsonism Relat Disord. 2013;19(2):153–7.
56. Di Giacopo R, Fasano A, Quaranta D, Della Marca G, Bove F, Bentivoglio AR. Rivastigmine as alternative treatment for refractory REM behavior disorder in Parkinson's disease. Mov Disord. 2012;27(4):559–61.
57. Arnulf I, Bejjani BP, Garma L, Bonnet AM, Houeto JL, Damier P, et al. Improvement of sleep architecture in PD with subthalamic nucleus stimulation. Neurology. 2000;55(11):1732–4.

58. Iranzo A, Valldeoriola F, Santamaria J, Tolosa E, Rumia J. Sleep symptoms and polysomnographic architecture in advanced Parkinson's disease after chronic bilateral subthalamic stimulation. J Neurol Neurosurg Psychiatry. 2002;72(5):661–4.
59. Cicolin A, Lopiano L, Zibetti M, Torre E, Tavella A, Guastamacchia G, et al. Effects of deep brain stimulation of the subthalamic nucleus on sleep architecture in parkinsonian patients. Sleep Med. 2004;5(2):207–10.
60. Verhave PS, Jongsma MJ, Van Den Berg RM, Vanwersch RA, Smit AB, Philippens IH. Neuroprotective effects of riluzole in early phase Parkinson's disease on clinically relevant parameters in the marmoset MPTP model. Neuropharmacology. 2012;62(4):1700–7.
61. Srinivasan V, Cardinali DP, Srinivasan US, Kaur C, Brown GM, Spence DW, et al. Therapeutic potential of melatonin and its analogs in Parkinson's disease: focus on sleep and neuroprotection. Ther Adv Neurol Disord. 2011;4(5):297–317.

Quality Control for Diagnosis of REM Sleep Behavior Disorder: Criteria, Questionnaires, Video, and Polysomnography

11

Birgit Frauscher and Birgit Högl

Contents

Abstract

The diagnosis of REM sleep behavior disorder (RBD) is based on clinical criteria, which include history and information from video/polysomnography. While probable RBD can be diagnosed from questionnaires, for a definite diagnosis polysomnography demonstrating REM sleep without atonia is necessary. Several studies have provided cut-off values for excessive muscle activity during REM sleep to make an objective and accurate diagnosis of RBD. Recent advances include development of computerized softwares for the automatic quantification of electromyographic (EMG) activity during REM sleep. An exact and accurate quality control in the diagnosis of RBD is necessary to avoid wrong classification.

B. Frauscher • B. Högl, MD (✉)
Department of Neurology, Medical University of Innsbruck,
Anichstrasse 35, Innsbruck A-6020, Austria
e-mail: birgit.frauscher@i-med.ac.at; birgit.ho@i-med.ac.at

© Springer-Verlag Wien 2015
A. Videnovic, B. Högl (eds.), *Disorders of Sleep and Circadian Rhythms in Parkinson's Disease*, DOI 10.1007/978-3-7091-1631-9_11

11.1 Introduction

REM sleep behavior disorder (RBD) has recently attracted major interest from investigators due to the fact that approximately 80 % of those initially diagnosed with idiopathic RBD (iRBD) will convert to a neurodegenerative disorder, mainly a synucleinopathy (for more details please see Chap. 10). As a high-risk population for neurodegeneration, patients with iRBD are candidates to benefit from preventive or disease modification strategies. Early and safe detection of preclinical stages of neurodegeneration, namely RBD, is therefore of paramount importance.

RBD has a prevalence of 0.5–2 % in the general population [1–3], but >50 % in patients with Parkinson syndromes [4, 5]. Beyond the often-dramatic clinical picture with violent dream enactment, leading to potential injury to patients and their bed partners, RBD has recently started to solicit increased attention and to become a major target of neurodegeneration research due to its unique position as a highly predictive indicator of an imminent synucleinopathy.

As outlined above, patients with iRBD have a very high risk of developing an overt neurodegenerative disorder after a decade or more [6]. Belonging to a high-risk population for imminent neurodegenerative disorders, it is expected that patients with RBD would greatly benefit from neuroprotective treatments, once these become available, and they will provide an adequate population for any randomized double-blind controlled study of neuroprotective treatments. First recommendations for such future studies have already been made by the International RBD Study Group [7]. Evaluating potential disease-modifying strategies in such a high-risk group will be more effective than testing an unselected population in which the conversion rate is very low.

In contrast to the potentially outstanding role of iRBD for the development of neuroprotective or curative treatments are the difficulties encountered in making an accurate diagnosis of RBD. For a definite diagnosis of RBD, polysomnography is a requirement (ICSD 3) [8]. However, polysomnography is cost-intensive and not widely available for all patient groups, or in all countries of the world.

11.2 RBD Screening Questionnaires

In light of the difficulty in accessing full polysomnography, especially for screening and first clinical selection purposes, questionnaires have been developed to aid screening for RBD (see also Table 11.1). Nevertheless, questionnaires can only diagnose probable RBD. The first validation studies of these RBD questionnaires have been performed with acceptable results [9–15]. Sensitivity ranged from 74.3 to 96 % and specificity from 56 to 92.9 %. Even single RBD screening questions were initially reported to have a good sensitivity and specificity [13, 14]. Despite these initially encouraging results in detecting probable RBD, more recent work increasingly suggests that beyond the narrow context of a validation study, the diagnostic value of questionnaires in detecting RBD may be lower than previously thought.

Table 11.1 Characteristics and validation results for questionnaires to detect probable RBD

Author	Questionnaire	Characteristics	Sensitivity (%)	Specificity (%)
Stiasny-Kolster et al. [9]	RBD Screening Questionnaire	10 items with 13 questions	96	56
		Yes/no answers		
		Max score =13		
Li et al. [11]	RBDQ-HK	13 questions	82	87
		Assesses for life time and recent (1 year) occurrence		
Boeve et al. [12]	Mayo Sleep Questionnaire	Contains an introductory question about RBD, followed by 5 subsequent questions about RBD symptoms	98	74
Postuma et al. [14]	Single question Screen for RBD	Single question	94	87
Frauscher et al. [13]	Innsbruck RBD Inventory	5 questions	91	86
		Yes/no/do not know answers		
Frauscher et al. [13]	RBD summary question (from Innsbruck RBD Inventory)	Single question	74	93

For example, a recent study demonstrates that even in a Parkinson's disease population, the validity of the RBD questionnaire clearly depends on the setting, and where and how it is administered [16]. Even more importantly, 16 % false positives were obtained with a validated RBD screening questionnaire in healthy sleepers in whom RBD was later definitely excluded both by sleep expert interview and polysomnography [17, 18]. An unexpectedly high rate of RBD screening questionnaire positives, probably reflecting major false positive numbers, was also accumulated in a current research initiative to detect Parkinson's disease progression markers in a Parkinson's disease population versus a control population, in which 20 % of the healthy control group exceeded the RBD cut-off score (http://www.ppmi-info.org). Therefore, using a questionnaire alone must definitely be considered unreliable as a diagnostic instrument, even more so in the context of iRBD without any already diagnosed synucleinopathy, and when they are administered outside a study or hospital setting, or by untrained interviewers or as handouts only. Thus, the application of questionnaires alone without polysomnography can carry a substantial risk to both over- and underestimating RBD. This is of particular relevance in RBD as the clinical differential diagnosis is a challenging one. Patients with obstructive sleep apnea, a highly frequent disorder in the elderly, often exhibit violent limb movements in the arousal at the end of each apnea [19], and patients with RLS/PLM can have intense limb or whole body jerks [20]. Sleep-related seizures, non-REM parasomnias, psychiatric disorders, and drug-induced conditions are among the remaining differential diagnoses which are very difficult, if not impossible, to disentangle without PSG.

## 11.3	Polysomnographic Criteria for REM Sleep Without Atonia

The polysomnographic hallmark of RBD is the electromyographic demonstration of REM sleep without atonia. Current ICSD-criteria require polysomnographic evaluation as mandatory for a definite diagnosis of RBD [8]. It is defined qualitatively as "the EMG finding of excessive amounts of sustained or intermittent elevation of submental EMG tone or excessive phasic submental or (upper or lower) limb EMG twitching" [8]. As the qualitative assessment of REM sleep without atonia is dependent on the individual polysomnographic scorer, the current ICSD-3 criteria cite a normative study reporting that a total of 27 % of 30 s epochs which are positive for any (tonic/phasic or both) EMG activity in the chin or phasic activity detected in the bilateral flexor digitorum superficialis, reliably distinguish RBD patients from controls [21]. Examples of a 30 s epoch of normal REM sleep and of REM sleep without atonia are provided in Fig. 11.1.

11.3.1 Manual Quantification of REM Sleep Without Atonia

Manual quantification of EMG activity during REM sleep was first performed in healthy normals in the mid-seventies and early eighties (for an overview, see [22]) REM sleep without atonia in the context of RBD was first systematically assessed by Lapierre and Montplaisir in 1992 [23], who classified EMG activity as "phasic" and "tonic" EMG activity within 2 s mini-epochs and 20 s epochs. Phasic EMG activity was defined as EMG activity between 0.1 and 5 s with an amplitude exceeding four times the background EMG, and tonic EMG activity was defined as the presence of tonic EMG activity for at least 50 % of the total epoch. This classification system is still the most widely used system for EMG quantification [21, 24–28]. Minor modifications of the original scoring system introduced by the various investigators concern the duration of the evaluated mini-epochs (2 vs. 3 s) and epochs (20 vs. 30 s) depending on historical national differences in polysomnographic recording paper speed, and the amplitude criterion with 4-times vs. 2-times the background EMG activity, as well as the duration of phasic EMG activity with 0.1–5 s vs. 0.1–10 s (for details, see [22]). The latest modification concerns the new introduction of the measure "any" in order to simplify the quantification of EMG activity during REM sleep, as the differentiation between phasic and tonic EMG activity can be challenging in clinical practice [21]. "Any" EMG activity is defined as presence of any EMG activity exceeding 0.1 s with an amplitude of twice the background EMG activity [21]. Apart from the Lapierre & Montplaisir scoring system, two different scoring approaches have been introduced [29–32]. Eisensehr et al. differentiated between short- and long-lasting EMG activity [29]: short-lasting EMG activity is defined as a minimum of 10 bursts of EMG activity between 0.1 and 0.5 s during a 10 s EEG epoch, and long-lasting EMG activity as >0.5 s activity for at least 1 s of the 10 s epoch [29]. Bliwise et al. [30] investigated the phasic electromyographic metric (PEM) which is defined as EMG activity exceeding 0.1 s with an identifiable

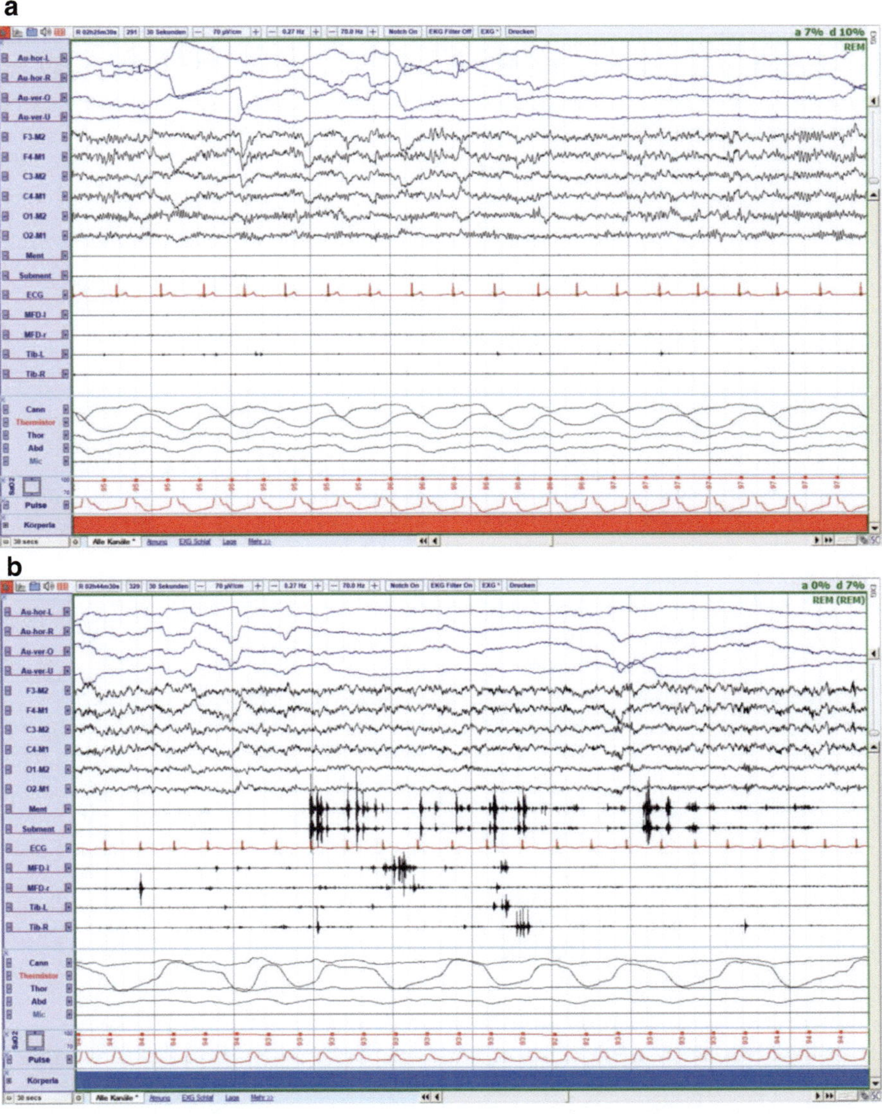

Fig. 11.1 Examples of normal REM sleep and REM sleep without atonia. (**a**) Thirty sepoch of normal REM sleep. Note that few bursts of EMG activity are also present during normal REM sleep. (**b**) Thirty sepoch of REM sleep without atonia. Note increased levels of phasic EMG activity in the chin and the extremities. In the chin, there is in addition an increase of tonic background EMG activity

return to baseline during the respective 2.5 s mini-epochs. In a recent study, the Mayo group introduced phasic burst duration as a new related measure [35]. Higher levels of phasic muscle activity even in nights without behavioral abnormalities have previously been described by Bliwise and Rye [33].

For further details see Table 11.2.

The most obvious advantage of the Lapierre & Montplaisir scoring system is that it is a simple practical method as it does not assess absolute EMG events, but the presence or absence of defined EMG activity in mini-epochs which can thus be positive or negative [23].

Table 11.2 Overview of studies which manually quantified REM sleep-related EMG activity

Authors	EMG measure	Amplitude	Duration (s)	Evaluated muscles	Epoch duration (s)
Lapierre and Montplaisir [23]	Phasic	4× background	0.1–5	Submental	2
	Tonic	N/A	>50 % of epoch		20
Eisensehr et al. [29]	Short-lasting	50 % amplitude increase	>10×0.1–0.5	Mental, submental, TA	10
	Long-lasting	50 % amplitude increase	>0.5 for >1		
Consens et al. [24]	Phasic	>4× background	0.1–5	Chin	3
	Tonic	>4× background	50 % of epoch		30
Bliwise et al. [30–32]	PEM	>2× background	0.1, identifiable return to baseline in the mini-epoch	Mental, brachioradialis, TA	2.5
AASM [34, 35]	Phasic	>4× background	0.1–5 (total >5)	Chin, limbs	30
	Tonic	> the minimum NREM amplitude	>50 % of epoch		30
Zhang et al. [26]	Phasic	>4× background	0.1–5	Chin, extensor forearm, TA	3
	Tonic	>2× background	50 % of epoch		30
SINBAR (Frauscher et al. [25])	Phasic	>2× background	0.1–5	Mental, SCM, deltoid, biceps, FDS, APB, TL paraspinal, RF, GAS, TA, EDB	3
Montplaisir et al. [27]	Phasic	>4× background	0.1–10	Mental, TA	2
	Tonic	>2× background or 10 µV	>50 % of epoch		20
SINBAR (Iranzo et al. [28])	Phasic	>2× background	0.1–5.0 s	Mental, FDS, EDB	3

Table 11.2 (continued)

Authors	EMG measure	Amplitude	Duration (s)	Evaluated muscles	Epoch duration (s)
SINBAR (Frauscher et al. [21]	Phasic	>2× background	0.1–5	Mental, SCM, biceps, FDS, TA, EDB	3
	Tonic	>2× background or 10 μV	>50 % of epoch		30
	Any	>2× background	≥0.1		3
McCarter et al. [33]	Phasic burst	>4× background	≥0.1	Chin, limbs	Single counts
	Phasic	>4× background	0.1–14.9 s		3
	Any	>4× background	≥0.1		3
	Tonic	>2× background or 10 μV	>15 s		30

Legend: *PEM* phasic electromyographic metric, *TA* tibialis anterior, *SCM* sternocleidomastoid, *FDS* flexor digitorum superficialis, *APB* abductor pollicis brevis, *TL* thoracolumbal, *RF* rectus femoris, *GAS* gastrocnemius, *EDB* extensor digitorum brevis

11.3.2 Computer-Assisted Scoring Algorithms for REM Sleep Without Atonia

Due to the time intensity of manual quantitative EMG scoring, six different computer-assisted algorithms for the detection of REM sleep without atonia have been developed [36–44]. For an overview, see Table 11.3.

The best evidence exists for the REM atonia index [41–43]. This index varies between 0 (complete loss of REM atonia) to 1 (complete REM atonia). A score below 0.8 was demonstrated to be highly suggestive for RBD [42, 43]. The REM atonia index was validated against the manual gold standard, and showed a high correlation with a Spearman's rho of at least 0.75. The remaining studies used different measures. A validation against manual quantification was performed by only two of these studies [36, 44]. Of note, for all of the computer-assisted scoring algorithms manual artifact detection and exclusion is necessary.

11.3.3 Manual Versus Computer-Assisted Scoring of REM Sleep Without Atonia

Manual scoring of REM sleep without atonia is still the gold standard in current RBD research, but is often not feasible in clinical practice due to the time required for such a procedure. Therefore, a computer-assisted algorithm for quantitative scoring of EMG activity seems a mandatory requirement for implementation of

Table 11.3 Overview of studies with computer-assisted quantification of REM sleep without atonia

Authors	EMG measure	Definition	Evaluated muscle	Validation	N subjects (patients/ controls)
Burns et al. [36]	STREAM	Variance of the EMG signal per 3 s epochs	Chin	Manual scoring according to Lapierre & Montplaisir: sens 100 %, spec 71 %	17/6
Ferri et al. [41]	REM atonia index	Ratio between the percentage of EMG mini-epochs with average $\leq 1\ \mu V$ and the total mini-epochs	Chin	Manual scoring according to Lapierre & Montplaisir: high correlation (rho >0.75)	31/34
Ferri et al. [42]		Index improvement		Validation against manual scoring: sens 84 %, spec 81 %	49/35 + 5 OSAS
Ferri et al. [43]					74/75
Mayer et al. [37]	Short-and long-lasting muscle activity	Short: 0.1–0.5 s / Long: > 0.5 s	Chin	Not validated against manual scoring	48/25
Shokrollahi et al. [38]	Quantitative EMG analysis	Wavelet analysis	Chin	Not validated against manual scoring, accuracy of classification 94.3 %	4/4
Kempfner et al. [39]	Quantitative EMG analysis	Signal processing and statistical classifier	Chin	Validated against STREAM: sens 100 %, spec 100 %	6/6
Kempfner et al. [40]	Quantitative EMG analysis	One-class support vector machine classifier	Chin + further muscles	Not validated against manual scoring, ROC 0.993 for combination of submentalis + anterior tibialis	16/16 + 16 PLMD
Frauscher et al. [44]	SINBAR	Tonic, phasic, any	Chin, FDS	Validated against manual scoring; sens 89 %, spec 83 %, Spearman rho 0.98.	20/60

Legend: *FDS* flexor digitorum superficialis muscle, *PD* Parkinson disease, *ROC* receiver operating curve, *sens* sensitivity, *SINBAR* Sleep Innsbruck-Barcelona, *spec* specificity, *STREAM* supra-threshold REM EMG activity metric quantitative motor analysis in clinical routine. Such an algorithm will allow for a rater-independent, easy and fast to apply quantification of absolute EMG events and calculation of precise objective indices. Major criticisms of the published algorithms and software focus on the fact that all of them use only the chin muscle activity, and not the extremities, which were shown to be predominantly associated with movements related to RBD [28]. Moreover, none of the previous algorithms was incorporated into the polysomnographic software, which is a mandatory prerequisite for manual artifact elimination. Both disadvantages were recently overcome by a study validating software specifically developed and integrated with polysomnography for RWA detection against the gold standard of manual RWA quantification. The authors found both a high sensitivity and specificity for this software with further improvement of the results when performing manual artifact correction [44].

This automatic scoring system has three major advantages: (1) This algorithm does not only evaluate chin muscle tone as is the case with other algorithms. Chin EMG tone is sensitive, but also highly susceptible to recording artifacts, and a good signal might be difficult to obtain in less specialized clinical conditions. The concomitant recording of the flexor digitorum superficialis muscle, and quantification of EMG activity in that muscle, provides an extra assurance against false positive recordings. (2) The result of computer-based classification into tonic, any or phasic activity in chin and phasic activity in the extremities is readily visible for each epoch of the whole recording on the polysomnographic screen, and a validation and artifact control is easy and feasible. (3) This is the first RWA quantification system already integrated and built into a polysomnographic system, and therefore does not require data export, data transformation, and separate handling, but the quantitative values can be obtained during polysomnographic, similar to apnea indices [44].

11.3.4 Recommended Montage for RBD Detection

The mentalis muscle has been best investigated for RBD detection as it is part of the routine polsomnographic evaluation. Studies on other additional muscles are comparatively scarce, but it has been demonstrated that adding extremity muscles improves the detection of REM-related movements in RBD patients [21]. Furthermore, it has been shown that a combination between the chin and the flexor digitorum superficialis muscles is most suitable for RBD detection [25].

11.3.5 Normative EMG Values for Detection of REM Sleep Without Atonia

Objective polysomnographic demonstration of REM sleep without atonia is essential. However, also during normal REM sleep phasic EMG activity, especially in the context of rapid eye movements can be present. As presence or absence of REM sleep without atonia is therefore not exclusive, quantitative cut-off values are very much needed and should be implemented for both clinical and research purposes.

Up till now, four groups have worked on normative EMG values for a correct diagnosis of RBD [17, 21, 27, 33, 41–43]. Montplaisir et al. manually investigated phasic and tonic chin EMG activity and leg movements in the tibialis anterior muscles in 80 idiopathic RBD subjects and 80 sex- and age-matched normal controls. Another study in 30 RBD patients and 30 controls investigated the area-under-the-curves (AUC) in different muscles of the human body, namely the mentalis, sternocleidomastoid, biceps, flexor digitorum superficialis, tibialis anterior, and extensor digitorum brevis muscles on both sides. The authors demonstrated that although all investigated muscles differentiated well between patients and controls, the chin and muscles of the upper limbs had even better AUCs than the lower limbs which might be explained by overlapping phenomena such as periodic leg movements in sleep or fragmentary myoclonus. Moreover, the authors found that the measure of "any" EMG activity which is a simplified version of phasic and tonic EMG activity discriminates identically between cases and controls. In addition, the 30 s epoch scoring approach as introduced by the AASM in 2007 was also found to be sufficient to differentiate cases from controls [21]. Similar cut-off values were found by investigating healthy normal sleepers between 18 and 80 years of age as well as patients with sleep apnea syndrome [17, 33]. Ferri et al. established normative values for a computer-assisted scoring algorithm for REM sleep without atonia [41–43].

11.4 Conclusions and Outlook

Despite several questionnaires for RBD being available [9–15], and despite solid validation studies with single questions [10, 13] it should be kept in mind that questionnaires can help find probable RBD but are not appropriate to make a definite diagnosis of RBD and rule out the most relevant differential diagnosis. On the other hand, criteria for the polysomnographic diagnosis of RBD are currently under reconsideration and debate, and quantitative cut-off scores have been provided by a few investigators [21, 27, 33, 41]. These cut-off scores await future replication in adequately sized populations of normal sleepers. Whereas manual scoring is still the gold standard, computer-assisted scoring algorithms will gain increasing importance when implementing the scoring of REM-related EMG activity in clinical routine, as traditional manual scoring is very time consuming. *The current drawback of the existing softwares is that no automatic artifact detection algorithm is included.* Therefore, manual artifact correction is crucial when applying one of the existing computer softwares in order to avoid false positive RBD diagnoses. Ambulatory screening instruments to apply to the general population to detect RBD would be a necessary next step to further advance the field.

While diagnosis of RBD is still made on qualitative grounds or without polysomnography for clinical routine and even in many research settings, the authors think that a stringent quality control for the diagnosis of RBD is necessary to provide a good basis for further clinical and research applications. The evidence compiled in this chapter indicates that suitable instruments have been developed to make an objective, and quantitative accurate diagnosis.

References

1. Chiu HF, Wing YK, Lam LC, et al. Sleep-related injury in the elderly–an epidemiological study in Hong Kong. Sleep. 2000;23:513–7.
2. Ohayon MM. Prevalence and comorbidity of sleep disorders in general population. Rev Prat. 2007;57:1521–8.
3. Kang S-H, Yoon I-Y, Lee SD, Han JW, Kim TH, Kim KW. REM sleep behavior disorder in the Korean elderly population: prevalence and clinical characteristics. Sleep. 2013;36:1147–52.
4. Wetter TC, Trenkwalder C, Gershanik O, Hogl B. Polysomnographic measures in Parkinson's disease: a comparison between patients with and without REM sleep disturbances. Wien Klin Wochenschr. 2001;113:249–53.
5. Sixel-Doring F, Trautmann E, Mollenhauer B, Trenkwalder C. Associated factors for REM sleep behavior disorder in Parkinson disease. Neurology. 2011;77:1048–54.
6. Lerche S, Seppi K, Behnke S, et al. Risk factors and prodromal markers and the development of Parkinson's disease. J Neurol. 2014;261:180–7.
7. Schenck CH, Montplaisir JY, Frauscher B, et al. Rapid eye movement sleep behavior disorder: devising controlled active treatment studies for symptomatic and neuroprotective therapy–a consensus statement from the International Rapid Eye Movement Sleep Behavior Disorder Study Group. Sleep Med. 2013;14:795–806.
8. The international classification of sleep disorders: diagnostic and coding manual (ICSD-3). 3rd ed. Westchester: American Academy of Sleep Medicine; 2014.
9. Stiasny-Kolster K, Mayer G, Schäfer S, Möller JC, Heinzel-Gutenbrunner M, Oertel WH. The REM sleep behavior disorder screening questionnaire–a new diagnostic instrument. Mov Disord. 2007;22(16):2386–93.
10. Miyamoto T, Miyamoto M, Iwanami M, et al. The REM sleep behavior disorder screening questionnaire: validation study of a Japanese version. Sleep Med. 2009;10:1151–4.
11. Li SX, Wing YK, Lam SP, et al. Validation of a new REM sleep behavior disorder questionnaire (RBDQ-HK). Sleep Med. 2010;11:43–8.
12. Boeve BF, Molano JR, Ferman TJ, Smith GE, Lin SC, Bieniek K, Haidar W, Tippmann-Peikert M, Knopman DS, Graff-Radford NR, Lucas JA, Petersen RC, Silber MH. Validation of the Mayo Sleep Questionnaire to screen for REM sleep behavior disorder in an aging and dementia cohort. Sleep Med. 2011;12(5):445–53.
13. Frauscher B, Ehrmann L, Zamarian L, et al. Validation of the Innsbruck REM sleep behavior disorder inventory. Mov Disord. 2012;27:1673–8.
14. Postuma RB, Arnulf I, Hogl B, et al. A single-question screen for rapid eye movement sleep behavior disorder: a multicenter validation study. Mov Disord. 2012;27:913–6.
15. Boeve BF, Molano JR, Ferman TJ, et al. Validation of the Mayo Sleep Questionnaire to screen for REM sleep behavior disorder in a community-based sample. J Clin Sleep Med. 2013;9:475–80.
16. Stiasny-Kolster K, Sixel-Döring F, Trenkwalder C, et al. Diagnostic value of the REM sleep behavior disorder screening questionnaire in Parkinson's disease. Sleep Med. 2015;16:186–9.
17. Frauscher B, Gabelia D, Mitterling T, et al. Motor events during healthy sleep: a quantitative polysomnographic study. Sleep. 2014;37:763–73.
18. Frauscher B, Mitterling T, Bode A, et al. A prospective questionnaire study in 100 healthy sleepers: non-bothersome forms of recognizable sleep disorders are still present. J Clin Sleep Med. 2014;10:623–9.
19. Iranzo A, Santamaria J. Severe obstructive sleep apnea/hypopnea mimicking REM sleep behavior disorder. Sleep. 2005;28:203–6.
20. Hogl B, Zucconi M, Provini F. RLS, PLM, and their differential diagnosis–a video guide. Mov Disord. 2007;22 Suppl 18:S414–9.
21. Frauscher B, Iranzo A, Gaig C, et al. Normative EMG values during REM sleep for the diagnosis of REM sleep behavior disorder. Sleep. 2012;35:835–47.
22. Frauscher B, Högl B. REM sleep behavior disorder: discovery of RBD, clinical and laboratory diagnosis, and treatment. In: Walters AS, Allen RP, Chokroverty S, Montagna P, editors. Movement disorders in sleep. Oxford University Press USA; 2012.

23. Lapierre O, Montplaisir J. Polysomnographic features of REM sleep behavior disorder: development of a scoring method. Neurology. 1992;42:1371–4.
24. Consens FB, Chervin RD, Koeppe RA, et al. Validation of a polysomnographic score for REM sleep behavior disorder. Sleep. 2005;28:993–7.
25. Frauscher B, Iranzo A, Hogl B, et al. Quantification of electromyographic activity during REM sleep in multiple muscles in REM sleep behavior disorder. Sleep. 2008;31:724–31.
26. Zhang J, Lam SP, Ho CK, et al. Diagnosis of REM sleep behavior disorder by video-polysomnographic study: is one night enough? Sleep. 2008;31:1179–85.
27. Montplaisir J, Gagnon JF, Fantini ML, et al. Polysomnographic diagnosis of idiopathic REM sleep behavior disorder. Mov Disord. 2010;25:2044–51.
28. Iranzo A, Frauscher B, Santos H, et al. Usefulness of the SINBAR electromyographic montage to detect the motor and vocal manifestations occurring in REM sleep behavior disorder. Sleep Med. 2011;12:284–8.
29. Eisensehr I, Linke R, Tatsch K, et al. Increased muscle activity during rapid eye movement sleep correlates with decrease of striatal presynaptic dopamine transporters. IPT and IBZM SPECT imaging in subclinical and clinically manifest idiopathic REM sleep behavior disorder, Parkinson's disease, and controls. Sleep. 2003;26:507–12.
30. Bliwise DL, Trotti LM, Greer SA, Juncos JJ, Rye DB. Phasic muscle activity in sleep and clinical features of Parkinson disease. Ann Neurol. 2010;68:353–9.
31. Bliwise DL. Periodic leg movements in sleep and restless legs syndrome: considerations in geriatrics. Sleep Med Clin. 2006;1:263–71.
32. Bliwise DL, Rye DB. Elevated PEM (phasic electromyographic metric) rates identify rapid eye movement behavior disorder patients on nights without behavioral abnormalities. Sleep. 2008;31:853–7.
33. McCarter SJ, St Louis EK, Duwell EJ, et al. Diagnostic thresholds for quantitative REM sleep phasic burst duration, phasic and tonic muscle activity, and REM atonia index in REM sleep behavior disorder with and without comorbid obstructive sleep apnea. Sleep. 2014;37:1649–62.
34. Iber C, Ancoli-Israel S, Chesson A, Quan SF for the American Academy of Sleep Medicine. The AASM Manual for the Scoring of Sleep and Associated Events: Rules, Terminology and Technical Specifications, 1st ed.: Westchester, Illinois: American Academy of Sleep Medicine; 2007.
35. Berry RB, Brooks R, Gamaldo CE, Harding SM, Marcus CL, Vaughn BV for the American Academy of Sleep Medicine. The AASM Manual for the Scoring of Sleep and Associated Events: Rules, Terminology and Technical Specifications, Version 2.0. Darien, Illinois: American Academy of Sleep Medicine; 2012.
36. Burns JW, Consens FB, Little RJ, Angell KJ, Gilman S, Chervin RD. EMG variance during polysomnography as an assessment for REM sleep behavior disorder. Sleep. 2007;30:1771–8.
37. Mayer G, Kesper K, Ploch T, et al. Quantification of tonic and phasic muscle activity in REM sleep behavior disorder. J Clin Neurophysiol. 2008;25:48–55.
38. Shokrollahi M, Krishnan S, Jewell D, Murray B. Analysis of the electromyogram of rapid eye movement sleep using wavelet techniques. Conf Proc IEEE Eng Med Biol Soc. 2009;2009:2659–62.
39. Kempfner J, Sorensen G, Zoetmulder M, Jennum P, Sorensen HB. REM behaviour disorder detection associated with neurodegenerative diseases. Conf Proc IEEE Eng Med Biol Soc. 2010;2010:5093–6.
40. Kempfner J, Sorensen GL, Nikolic M, Frandsen R, Sorensen HB, Jennum P. Rapid eye movement sleep behavior disorder as an outlier detection problem. J Clin Neurophysiol. 2014;31:86–93.
41. Ferri R, Manconi M, Plazzi G, et al. A quantitative statistical analysis of the submentalis muscle EMG amplitude during sleep in normal controls and patients with REM sleep behavior disorder. J Sleep Res. 2008;17:89–100.

42. Ferri R, Rundo F, Manconi M, et al. Improved computation of the atonia index in normal controls and patients with REM sleep behavior disorder. Sleep Med. 2010;11:947–9.
43. Ferri R, Gagnon JF, Postuma RB, Rundo F, Montplaisir JY. Comparison between an automatic and a visual scoring method of the chin muscle tone during rapid eye movement sleep. Sleep Med. 2014;15:661–5.
44. Frauscher B, Gabelia D, Biermayr M, et al. Validation of an integrated software for the detection of REM sleep behavior disorder. Sleep. 2014;37:1663–71.

Restless Legs Syndrome and Periodic Limb Movements in Parkinson's Disease

12

William G. Ondo

Contents

Abstract

The symptoms of Parkinson's disease (PD) commonly include a number of sleep disorders, including restless legs syndrome (RLS) and periodic limb movements of sleep (PLMS). RLS occurs in about 20 % of PD patients in most studies, but idiopathic RLS does not seem to precede the development of PD. In fact there is some evidence that idiopathic RLS may prevent the subsequent development of PD. In cases of PD/RLS the PD usually presents first, and RLS may represent one of many non-motor features associated with PD. Although common, RLS is usually not a major contributor to sleep deprivation or functional impairment in the PD population. PLMS are seen in many neurodegenerative disorders, as well as idiopathic RLS. Most studies report higher rates of PLMS in PD, but polysomnography studies suggest relatively little impact of PLMS on other sleep measures. The response of both PD and RLS to dopaminergics is of great interest, especially given the lack of overt dopamine pathology in RLS.

W.G. Ondo, MD
Department of Neurology, University of Texas Health Science Center-Houston,
Houston, TX, USA
e-mail: William.Ondo@uth.tmc.edu

© Springer-Verlag Wien 2015

A. Videnovic, B. Högl (eds.), *Disorders of Sleep and Circadian Rhythms in Parkinson's Disease*, DOI 10.1007/978-3-7091-1631-9_12

12.1 Introduction

Parkinson's disease (PD) is a complex neurodegenerative disorder. Although clinically defined by rigidity, bradykinesia, and tremor, numerous sensory, autonomic, sleep symptoms, and other non-motor symptoms are commonly reported. Some of these symptoms likely result from dopamine cell loss, while others do not.

Restless legs syndrome (RLS) and PD both respond to dopaminergic treatments, both show some dopaminergic abnormalities on functional imaging, and are both variably associated with periodic limb movements of sleep [1]. Therefore, a relationship between the two conditions has long been sought. Earlier results, however, were mixed. Prior to the development of current RLS criteria, some studies [2, 3], but not others [4, 5], reported a higher prevalence of RLS in patients with PD. Diagnostic inconsistency makes these reports difficult to interpret. Most reports employing current criteria do suggest that PD patients have higher rates of RLS than the general population; however, clear pathophysiological connections are lacking.

12.2 Restless Legs Syndrome

A 2003 NIH consensus summit defined Restless legs syndrome by the simultaneous presence of: (1) Desire to move the extremities, often associated with paresthesia/dysesthesia; (2) worsening of symptoms at rest; (3) transient improvement with movement; and (4) worsening of symptoms in the evening or night [6]. No widely available biomarker or test corroborates the diagnosis, which is made exclusively via interview. Patients, however, often have difficulty describing their sensory component of their RLS. The descriptions are quite varied and tend to be suggestible and education dependent. The limb sensation is always unpleasant but not necessarily painful. It is usually deep within the legs. In one study of RLS patients, the most common terms used, in descending order of frequency included: "need to move," "crawling," "tingling," "restless," "cramping," "creeping," "pulling," "painful," "electric," "tension," "discomfort," and "itching" [7]. Patients usually deny any "burning" or "pins and needles" sensations, commonly experienced in neuropathies or nerve entrapments, although neuropathic pain and RLS can coexist. RLS differs from akathisia, also reported in PD, in that (1) the urge to move is isolated in the limbs, rather than the entire body, (2) there is more dramatic relief with ambulation, and (3) there is a more robust worsening at night, with near complete cessation of symptoms in the early morning.

RLS is extremely common, affecting about 10 % of Caucasian populations [8], although it appears less common in Asian and African populations [9]. In roughly 60 % of cases, a family history of RLS can be found, although this is often not initially reported by the patient. Multiple genes and additional loci have been published [10–14].

12.3   Pathophysiology of RLS Compared to PD

The pathology of idiopathic RLS involves CNS iron homeostatic dysregulation. CSF ferritin and other measures of iron are lower in RLS cases [15]. Specially sequenced MRI studies and transcranial ultrasound show reduced iron stores in the striatum and substantia nigra [16, 17]. Most importantly, pathologic data in RLS autopsied brains show reduced ferritin staining, reduced iron staining, increased transferrin stains, reduced iron regulatory protein-1 activity, and also reduced transferrin receptors [18, 19]. The transferrin receptor downregulation is particularly telling, as a simple reduction of iron availability to the area would upregulate these receptors. Therefore, it appears that primary RLS has reduced intracellular iron indices secondary to a perturbation of homeostatic mechanisms that regulate iron influx and/or efflux from the cell. In contrast, PD is associated with increased iron in dopaminergic areas [16].

Two Korean studies have evaluated CNS iron, as measured by sonography, in subjects with both PD and RLS, compared to PD without RLS and idiopathic RLS [20, 21]. Both found that the PD/RLS group had increased CNS iron similar to PD without RLS. Idiopathic RLS showed reduced CNS iron similar to other studies. It should be noted that patient with PD/RLS generally had PD first and later developed RLS. Similar studies on subjects with young onset RLS that later developed PD have not been done.

CNS dopaminergic systems are implicated in RLS; however, pathophysiologic understanding of this is lacking. Dopaminergic medications, especially dopamine agonists robustly improve RLS, even at low doses. Normal circadian dopaminergic variation is also augmented in patients with RLS [22]. Dopamine imaging studies in RLS, however, have been inconsistent and difficult to interpret. PET studies measuring levodopa/dopamine have been normal [23] or shown slight reductions [24, 25]. Imaging of dopamine transporter protein have been normal [26–28] or shown modest reductions [29]. Imaging of dopamine receptors show normal [28] or modestly reduced availability of receptors [25, 26], suggesting either decreased receptors or increased endogenous dopamine occupancy. Explanations for these disparities include different severities of RLS subjects, the variable use of dopaminergic medications as treatments, different times of data acquisition (day vs. night), different ligands, rapid turnover of DAT faster than the fidelity of slower acting ligands, and other technical considerations. They are difficult to reconcile but may be limited by only assessing nigrostriatal dopamine. Some models and theories of RLS suggest that spinal dopaminergic areas are culpable [30]. These areas, however, are too small to image.

Pathologic data does not suggest reduced dopamine in RLS. CSF studies and human brain studies of the nigrostriatal system generally suggest normal or even increased dopaminergic turnover [31–33]. Specifically, substantia nigra dopaminergic cells are not reduced in number, nor are there markers associated with neurodegenerative diseases, such as tau or alpha-synuclein abnormalities [19, 34]. PD, of course, exhibits reduced dopamine cells and multiple neurodegenerative markers.

In RLS, the relationship between reduced iron pathology and the effective treatment with dopaminergics is not clearly understood, and beyond the scope of this text. However, some evidence suggests that the bridge is Thy1. This cell adhesion molecule, which is robustly expressed on dopaminergic neurons, is reduced in brain homogenates in iron-deprived mice [35] and in brains of patients with RLS [36]. Thy1 regulates vesicular release of monoamines, including dopamine [37]. A leading theory suggests that reduced iron stores decrease Thy1, which is necessary for the transmission of dopamine across the synapse. Thy1 status in PD has not been explored.

Both conditions, especially RLS, have a genetic contribution. Genes associated with RLS do not seem to be risk factors for PD [38]. One large family with PD caused by Parkin mutations included a large number of members with RLS, both with and without concurrent PD [39]. The RLS inheritance pattern was consistent with an autosomal dominant pattern; however, the authors did not find an association between RLS and Parkin mutations within the family. In a South Tyrolean population Parkin status did not independently predict onset or severity of RLS but did synergistically interact with RLS4 to predict a younger age at RLS onset [40].

In summary, there are no clear pathologic similarities between PD and idiopathic RLS. Brain iron is decreased in RLS but increased in PD. Dopamine and dopamine cells are overtly reduced in PD, but not reduced in RLS, where the dopaminergic dysfunction is not clear. Nevertheless, most studies suggest that RLS is more common in subjects with PD than controls.

12.4 Clinical RLS in Patients with PD

Multiple surveys have queried the prevalence of RLS symptoms in PD populations (Table 12.1). Symptoms of RLS in the PD population can overlap with general akathisia and dystonia, both of which can occur when dopaminergic medications wear off. RLS symptoms can also wax and wane, and of course can be treated with PD medications. Therefore, the diagnosis of clinical RLS in PD can be particularly problematic [53, 54]. Most studies were performed at tertiary centers but there is little reason to suspect intrinsic bias. Some reports seek associations and/or include a control group. In general, most studies suggest a higher rate of RLS in PD than control populations or historic controls.

In a prospective survey of 303 consecutive PD patients, we found that 20.8 % of all patients with PD met the diagnostic criteria for RLS [41]. Despite this high number of cases, there are several caveats that tended to lessen its clinical significance. The RLS symptoms in PD patients are often ephemeral, usually not severe, and might be confused with other PD symptoms such as wearing-off dystonia, akathisia, or internal tremor. We specifically attempted to differentiate among these conditions. Most patients in our group were not previously diagnosed with RLS and few recognized that this was separate from other PD symptoms. Finally, the presence of RLS did not affect Epworth scale scores of daytime sleepiness.

Table 12.1 Summary of RLS in PD studies

Study	Population	RLS in PD	Risk factors	Onset of RLS and PD	Comment
Ondo et al. (2002) [41]	USA	63/303 (20.8 %)	Reduced serum ferritin	PD first in 85 %	Older age of onset and less family history than idiopathic RLS
Driver-Dunckly et al. (2006) [42]	USAUndergoing STN DBS	6/25 (24 %)	NR	NR	Improved with STN DBS
Peralta et al. (2005) [43]	Austria	28/113 (24 %)	Younger age Lower "on" H&Y	PD first in 83 %	RLS symptoms during "wearing-off" episodes
Simuni et al. (2000) [44] Abstract	USA	42/200 (21 %)	Tendency for "fluctuators" ($p=0.14$)	PD first in 93 %	RLS undiagnosed in 59 %
Braga-Neto et al. (2004) [45]	Brazil	45/86 (49.9 %)	Longer duration of PD, but not age	NR	RLS not associated with daytime sleepiness
Chaudhuri et al. (2006) [46]	USA and Europe	46/123[a] (37.4) Controls (28.1)		NR	Part of a non-motor survey
Verbaan et al. (2010) [47]	Holland	269 (11 %)	Female	NR	RLS severity correlated with PD severity
Loo et al. (2008) [48]	Singapore	400 (3.0 % vs 0.5 %)	RLS correlated with H&Y and poor sleep	RLS onset 61.7	
Kumar et al. (2002) [49]	India	21/149 (14.1 %) Controls (0.9 %)	NR	NR	RLS diagnosis based on a single question
Krishman et al. (2003) [50]	India	10/126 (7.9 %) Controls (1.3 %)	Older age Depression	NR	
Nomora et al. (2005) [51]	Japan	20/165 (12 %) Controls (2.3 %)	Younger age	PD first in 95 %	RLS worsened PSQI
Tan et al. (2002) [52]	Singapore	1/135 (0.6 %) Controls (0.1 %)	–	–	Motor restlessness in 15.2 %

PSQI Pittsburg sleep quality index
[a]A single written question, not full RLS criteria

After determining the prevalence of RLS in PD, we next evaluated for factors that could predict RLS in this population, and determined that only lower serum ferritin levels predicted RLS symptoms in the PD population. RLS did not correlate with duration of PD, age, H&Y, gender, dementia, use of levodopa, use of dopamine agonists, history of pallidotomy, or history of deep brain stimulation (DBS). PD symptoms preceded RLS symptoms in 35/41 (85.4 %), $X^2 = 20.5$, $p < 0.0001$, of cases in which patients confidently remembered the initial onset of both symptoms. We next compared the PD/RLS group to patients with RLS not associated with PD (idiopathic RLS). Only 20.2 % of all PD/RLS patients reported a positive family history of RLS, compared to more than 60 % of our non-PD RLS population. The serum ferritin was also lower in the PD/RLS group compared to the idiopathic RLS group. In the cases with PD who did have a family history of RLS, the RLS symptoms usually preceded PD and generally resembled typical RLS. In short, our results do not suggest that RLS is a forme fruste or a risk factor for the subsequent development of PD, but rather that PD is a risk factor for RLS, which probably constitutes a non-motor feature of PD.

Peralta reported that 28/113 (24 %) of Austrian PD patients met criteria for RLS [43]. PD/RLS subjects were younger and had lower (less severe) "on" medicine PD severity. PD preceded RLS in 83 %. Two other US studies reported that 24 and 21 % of PD patients had RLS [42, 44]. A Dutch study reported that only 11 % of PD subjects had RLS [47]. Female sex was the only specific predictor of RLS in this population. PD severity did correlate with RLS severity. They did not report a non-PD control group.

Studies done in Asian populations show lower absolute rates of RLS than Caucasian studies but mostly show a relatively increased frequency of RLS in PD. Krishnan et al. evaluated the prevalence of RLS in patients with PD compared to normal controls in a population from India [50]. They found that 10 of 126 cases of PD (7.9 %) versus only 1 of 128 controls ((0.8 %), $p = 0.01$) reported RLS. PD patients with RLS were older and reported more depression. Another report from India similarly found RLS in 14.1 % of PD patients vs. only 0.9 % in controls [49]. Although both prevalence are lower than U.S. reports, the absolute difference in RLS prevalence between PD and controls is similar. This probably reflects baseline epidemiology that suggests RLS is less common in non-Caucasian populations.

A Japanese survey reported similar results. RLS was seen in 12 % of PD subjects compared to 2.3 % of controls [51]. They associated RLS with a younger age of PD and associated it with poor sleep. PD almost always preceded RLS. The only study that did not find any increased risk of RLS in PD was reported from Singapore. Tan, in a mostly Chinese population, found only a single case of RLS out of 125 patients presenting with PD [52]. The study also reported a very low RLS prevalence in the general population [9].

In summary, studies done since modern RLS criteria were established, aside from one Singapore study, report that the absolute differences in the rates of PD/RLS is about 10 % greater (range: 6.6–14 %) than historic controls or actual controls. All reports that queried symptom onset show that PD preceded RLS in the majority.

12.5 Prevalence of PD in RLS Patients

Evaluating the prevalence of PD in populations presenting with RLS is problematic, since PD symptoms would usually be more overt and precipitate an evaluation. Banno et al., however, reported that "extrapyramidal disease or movement disorders" were previously diagnosed in 17.5 % of male RLS patients vs. 0.2 % of male controls, and in 23.5 % of female patients vs. 0.2 % of female controls ($p < 0.05$). They did not clarify whether they felt that these prior diagnoses were correct or truly represented a different disease [3]. In an abstract, Fazzini et al. reported that 19/29 RLS patients had PD symptoms [55]. In contrast Walters et al. reported no patients presenting with RLS who had PD [56]. As part of the Health Professional Follow-up Study, employing only written questionnaires for RLS in men, Gao et al. reported a slight increased risk for PD in mild (<15 days/months) RLS of 1.1 [95 % C.I.: 0.4, 3.0] and a stronger association with more severe (>15 days/month) RLS of 3.09 [95 % C.I.: 1.5, 6.2]; p trend $= 0.003$ [57].

Over 15 years we collected 36 cases in which subjects developed RLS long before PD, and/or had a family history of RLS in a first-degree relative and had well-documented RLS before the onset of their PD. In this RLS/PD group, 13 were female, 18 had a positive family history of RLS, and 6 had a family history of PD. We compared these to a "control" group of idiopathic PD without RLS: $N = 36$, ten females, one with family history of RLS, nine with family history of PD. The age at motor onset of RLS/PD was older (64.25 ± 6.4 years vs. 56.8 ± 10.7) than for patients with idiopathic PD ($p \geq 0.001$). Patients with idiopathic PD developed dyskinesia more (21/36) than RLS/PD (4/32) at last follow-up ($p = 0.0001$). PD phenotype and L-dopa dose were similar. We concluded that idiopathic RLS may actually delay the onset of PD, reduce dyskinesia occurrence, and possibly reduce progression of PD. This is potentially supported by aforementioned pathological studies that show increase dopamine turnover in RLS, and reduced iron, as opposed to increased iron seen in PD. Assessments of brain iron in this unique group (idiopathic RLS followed by PD) have not been done.

Recently Wong et al., using a written RLS questionnaire without interview, evaluated for incident diagnosis of PD in 22,999 U.S. male health professionals age 40–75 years enrolled in the Health Professionals Follow-up Study [58]. They found a moderate increased rate of PD diagnosis within 4 years of RLS but not after 4 years. Since the pathologic process of PD begins years before the clinical diagnosis, they postulated that RLS may be an early feature of PD, preceding motor signs, similar to REM behavioral disorder.

It is the author's opinion that the RLS phenotype is associated with PD but that it derives from a different pathophysiology than idiopathic RLS, perhaps a consequence of reduced CNS dopamine. There is no clear evidence of reduced dopaminergic tone in RLS, despite its robust response to dopaminergics. Therefore, PD is a risk factor for RLS symptoms, but RLS pathophysiology and idiopathic RLS symptoms are not risk factors for PD.

12.6 Periodic Limb Movements of Sleep in RLS and PD

Periodic limb movements of sleep (PLMS) are defined by the American Academy of Sleep Medicine as "at least four periodic episodes of repetitive and highly stereotyped limb movements that occur during sleep." The incidence in the general population increases with age and is reported to occur in as many as 57 % of elderly people [59, 60]. Renal disease and a number of neurological conditions are associated with higher rates. Typically the movements involve various degrees of flexion of the toes, ankles, knees, and hips (triple flexion response), although other patterns are seen. The anterior tibialis is the most affected muscles and the one usually used to assess electromyographic signals to quantify PLM. The physiology of PLM is only partially understood but thought to result from disinhibition of the spinal cord [61]. Autonomic lability with transient hypertension and tachycardia accompany PLM and could be an argument to more aggressively treat the condition when it is not thought to otherwise cause any clinical disability [62]. An expanding body of research has epidemiologically associated PLM with cardiovascular disease [63, 64]. The term periodic limb movement disorder is appropriate when idiopathic PLMS are thought to independently result in disability.

PLMS are strongly associated with RLS. One large study reported that 81 % of RLS patients showed pathologic PLMS [65]. The prevalence increased to 87 % if two nights were recorded. Although PLMS accompany most cases of RLS, data evaluating RLS prevalence in the setting of polysomnographically documented PLMS found that only 9 of 53 (17.0 %) PLMS patients complained of RLS symptoms [66]. Therefore, most people with RLS have PLMS but many patients with isolated PLMS do not have RLS. Although the exact relationship between the two phenotypes is unclear, genetic research suggests a strong biological association [11].

PD is also associated with higher rates of PLMS in most [1, 67, 68], but not all reports [69, 70]. There is more compelling evidence that when present, PLMS correlate with the severity of PD, both clinically and on imaging studies [68, 71]. The clinical consequences of PLMS in PD are less clear. One study reported that greater PLMS was associated with more subjective sleep disturbance, and decreased Quality of Life Scales, but this was largely explained by an association of PLMS with more advanced disease. The same study found and association of PLM and REM behavioral disorder, which interestingly has also been seen in patients presenting with RBD but without PD. Other objective measures of sleep, including sleep efficiency, have not been associated with PLMS in PD [68]. Several other PSG studies, none of which primarily evaluated PLMS, have not reported an association of PLMS with daytime sleepiness. One study that performed PSG studies in PD subjects with and without RLS did find that PLMS were more common in the PPD/RLS group [48]. In contrast another study segregating PD based on the presence of PLMS did not find higher rates of RLS in the PLMS+ group [68].

The assessment of PLMS in PD is clearly confounded by dopaminergic treatment, which improves PLMS in general, and does improve PLMS specifically in

PD in one prospective trial [72]. Another retrospective report in PD suggests benefit of clonazepam for PLMS [73] but there has never been any controlled treatment trial of PLMS in PD.

12.7 Treatment of RLS in PD

No formal study has ever prospectively assessed the treatment of RLS in the setting of PD. Anti-cholinergic and anti-histaminergic drugs, including amitriptyline, mirtazapine, quetiapine, and many others used in PD, can exacerbate RLS in general and should be discontinued if possible. One may consider checking serum ferritin and supplementing this if low; however, it is not known whether this could affect the PD course. Dopamine agonists and levodopa improve RLS as well as PD, so adjustment of these medications may improve RLS. A PSG study found that PD patients already treated with clonazepam had fewer PLM and less daytime sleepiness than those not treated with clonazepam [73].

Interestingly, several reports suggest that CNS surgeries for PD may affect RLS in the PD/RLS population. Rye first reported a single case of RLS symptoms improving in a PD patient following pallidotomy [74]. Driver-Dunkley et al. found RLS in 6/25 PD subjects prior to undergoing bilateral DBS of the subthalamic nucleus (STN) [42]. All six had some improvement in RLS at 3–24 months after DBS. Three had complete resolution and the mean International RLS rating scale improved by 84 %. PD medications were lowered by 56 % and the UPDRS "off" motor scores improved by 63 %, suggesting an excellent clinical response to the DBS. As part of a larger assessment of STN DBS in sleep, Chahine et al. reported improved IRLS scales in six subjects with PD/RLS [75]. In contrast, Kedia et al. reported the emergence of RLS after STN DBS postoperatively in 11 of 195 patients. The mean reduction in antiparkinsonian medication was 74 %, which they felt may have unmasked the RLS symptoms [76]. Parra et al. also reported a case of RLS emergence after DBS [77]. We recently performed a bilateral GPi DBS in a patient with idiopathic RLS without PD. She demonstrated moderate benefit [78].

Conclusions

The majority of studies suggest that RLS is more common in PD than in the general population. Most studies of predominately Caucasian populations demonstrate a >2× rate of RLS in PD compared to the normal population. PD/RLS rates in Asian surveys are less, as are the baseline rates of RLS but still greater than control populations. Reported risk factors for RLS in the PD population include reduced serum iron stores, older age, younger age, depression, and worse PD. RLS symptoms severity is less than those seeking treatment for idiopathic RLS but may be similar to the idiopathic RLS population in entirety. Although the data is mixed, the overall effect of RLS on daytime sleepiness and quality of life in PD is probably modest. Importantly, there is no good evidence to suggest that RLS is a forme fruste of PD, and in fact the pathophysiologies are markedly different, despite similar responses to dopaminergic medications. Therefore, it appears that RLS is one of many non-motor features intrinsic to PD, presumably secondary to dopaminergic loss, although this is not actually known.

References

1. Wetter TC, et al. Sleep and periodic leg movement patterns in drug-free patients with Parkinson's disease and multiple system atrophy. Sleep. 2000;23(3):361–7.
2. Horiguchi J, et al. [Sleep-wake complaints in Parkinson's disease]. Rinsho Shinkeigaku Clin Neurol. 1990;30(2):214–6.
3. Banno K, et al. Restless legs syndrome in 218 patients: associated disorders. Sleep Med. 2000;1(3):221–9.
4. Lang AE. Restless legs syndrome and Parkinson's disease: insights into pathophysiology. Clin Neuropharmacol. 1987;10(5):476–8.
5. Paulson G. Is restless legs a prodrome to Parkinson's disease. Mov Disord. 1997;12 Suppl 1:68.
6. Allen RP, et al. Restless legs syndrome: diagnostic criteria, special considerations, and epidemiology. A report from the restless legs syndrome diagnosis and epidemiology workshop at the National Institutes of Health. Sleep Med. 2003;4(2):101–19.
7. Ondo W, Jankovic J. Restless legs syndrome: clinicoetiologic correlates. Neurology. 1996;47(6):1435–41.
8. Hening W, et al. Impact, diagnosis and treatment of restless legs syndrome (RLS) in a primary care population: the REST (RLS epidemiology, symptoms, and treatment) primary care study. Sleep Med. 2004;5(3):237–46.
9. Tan EK, et al. Restless legs syndrome in an Asian population: a study in Singapore. Mov Disord. 2001;16(3):577–9.
10. Winkelmann J, et al. Genome-wide association study of restless legs syndrome identifies common variants in three genomic regions. Nat Genet. 2007;39(8):1000–6.
11. Stefansson H, et al. A genetic risk factor for periodic limb movements in sleep. N Engl J Med. 2007;357(7):639–47.
12. Chen S, et al. Genomewide linkage scan identifies a novel susceptibility locus for restless legs syndrome on chromosome 9p. Am J Hum Genet. 2004;74(5):876–85.
13. Desautels A, et al. Identification of a major susceptibility locus for restless legs syndrome on chromosome 12q. [see comment]. Am J Hum Genet. 2001;69(6):1266–70.
14. Bonati MT, et al. Autosomal dominant restless legs syndrome maps on chromosome 14q. Brain. 2003;126(Pt 6):1485–92.
15. Earley CJ, et al. Abnormalities in CSF concentrations of ferritin and transferrin in restless legs syndrome. Neurology. 2000;54(8):1698–700.
16. Schmidauer C, et al. Brain parenchyma sonography differentiates RLS patients from normal controls and patients with Parkinson's disease. Mov Disord. 2005;20 Suppl 10:S43.
17. Allen RP, et al. MRI measurement of brain iron in patients with restless legs syndrome. Neurology. 2001;56(2):263–5.
18. Connor JR, et al. Decreased transferrin receptor expression by neuromelanin cells in restless legs syndrome. Neurology. 2004;62(9):1563–7.
19. Connor JR, et al. Neuropathological examination suggests impaired brain iron acquisition in restless legs syndrome. Neurology. 2003;61(3):304–9.
20. Ryu JH, Lee MS, Baik JS. Sonographic abnormalities in idiopathic restless legs syndrome (RLS) and RLS in Parkinson's disease. Parkinsonism Relat Disord. 2010;17(3):201–3.
21. Kwon DY, et al. Transcranial brain sonography in Parkinson's disease with restless legs syndrome. Mov Disord. 2010;25(10):1373–8.

22. Garcia-Borreguero D, et al. Circadian variation in neuroendocrine response to L-dopa in patients with restless legs syndrome. Sleep. 2004;27(4):669–73.
23. Trenkwalder C, et al. Positron emission tomographic studies in restless legs syndrome. Mov Disord. 1999;14(1):141–5.
24. Ruottinen HM, et al. An FDOPA PET study in patients with periodic limb movement disorder and restless legs syndrome. Neurology. 2000;54(2):502–4.
25. Turjanski N, Lees AJ, Brooks DJ. Striatal dopaminergic function in restless legs syndrome: 18F-dopa and 11C-raclopride PET studies. Neurology. 1999;52(5):932–7.
26. Michaud M, et al. SPECT imaging of striatal pre- and postsynaptic dopaminergic status in restless legs syndrome with periodic leg movements in sleep. J Neurol. 2002;249(2):164–70.
27. Linke R, et al. Presynaptic dopaminergic function in patients with restless legs syndrome: are there common features with early Parkinson's disease? Mov Disord. 2004;19(10):1158–62.
28. Eisensehr I, et al. Normal IPT and IBZM SPECT in drug-naive and levodopa-treated idiopathic restless legs syndrome. Neurology. 2001;57(7):1307–9.
29. Earley CJ, et al. The dopamine transporter is decreased in the striatum of subjects with restless legs syndrome. Sleep. 2011;34(3):341–7.
30. Qu S, et al. Locomotion is increased in a11-lesioned mice with iron deprivation: a possible animal model for restless legs syndrome. J Neuropathol Exp Neurol. 2007;66(5):383–8.
31. Stiasny-Kolster K, et al. Normal dopaminergic and serotonergic metabolites in cerebrospinal fluid and blood of restless legs syndrome patients. Mov Disord. 2004;19(2):192–6.
32. Earley CJ, Hyland K, Allen RP. CSF dopamine, serotonin, and biopterin metabolites in patients with restless legs syndrome. Mov Disord. 2001;16(1):144–9.
33. Earley CJ, Hyland K, Allen RP. Circadian changes in CSF dopaminergic measures in restless legs syndrome. Sleep Med. 2006;7(3):263–8.
34. Pittock SJ, et al. Neuropathology of primary restless leg syndrome: absence of specific tau- and alpha-synuclein pathology. Mov Disord. 2004;19(6):695–9.
35. Ye Z, Connor JR. Identification of iron responsive genes by screening cDNA libraries from suppression subtractive hybridization with antisense probes from three iron conditions. Nucleic Acids Res. 2000;28(8):1802–7.
36. Wang X, et al. Thy1 expression in the brain is affected by iron and is decreased in Restless Legs Syndrome. J Neurol Sci. 2004;220(1–2):59–66.
37. Jeng CJ, et al. Thy-1 is a component common to multiple populations of synaptic vesicles. J Cell Biol. 1998;140(3):685–98.
38. Vilarino-Guell C, et al. Susceptibility genes for restless legs syndrome are not associated with Parkinson disease. Neurology. 2008;71(3):222–3.
39. Adel S, et al. Co-occurrence of restless legs syndrome and Parkin mutations in two families. Mov Disord. 2006;21(2):258–63.
40. Pichler I, et al. Parkin gene modifies the effect of RLS4 on the age at onset of restless legs syndrome (RLS). Am J Med Genet B Neuropsychiatr Genet. 2010;153B(1):350–5.
41. Ondo WG, Vuong KD, Jankovic J. Exploring the relationship between Parkinson disease and restless legs syndrome. Arch Neurol. 2002;59(3):421–4.
42. Driver-Dunckley E, et al. Restless legs syndrome in Parkinson's disease patients may improve with subthalamic stimulation. Mov Disord. 2006;21(8):1287–9.
43. Peralta CM, et al. Restless legs syndrome in Parkinson's disease. Mov Disord. 2009;24:2076–80.
44. Simuni T, Wilson R, Stern MB. Prevalence of restless legs syndrome in Parkinson's disease. Mov Disord. 2000;15(Supple 5):1043.
45. Braga-Neto P, et al. Snoring and excessive daytime sleepiness in Parkinson's disease [erratum appears in J Neurol Sci. 2004;219(1–2):171]. J Neurol Sci. 2004;217(1):41–5.
46. Chaudhuri KR, et al. International multicenter pilot study of the first comprehensive self-completed nonmotor symptoms questionnaire for Parkinson's disease: the NMSQuest study. Mov Disord. 2006;21(7):916–23.
47. Verbaan D, et al. Prevalence and clinical profile of restless legs syndrome in Parkinson's disease. Mov Disord. 2010;25(13):2142–7.

48. Loo HV, Tan EK. Case-control study of restless legs syndrome and quality of sleep in Parkinson's disease. J Neurol Sci. 2008;266(1–2):145–9.

49. Kumar S, Bhatia M, Behari M. Sleep disorders in Parkinson's disease. Mov Disord. 2002;17(4): 775–81.

50. Krishnan PR, Bhatia M, Behari M. Restless legs syndrome in Parkinson's disease: a case-controlled study. Mov Disord. 2003;18(2):181–5.

51. Nomura T, et al. Prevalence and clinical characteristics of restless legs syndrome in Japanese patients with Parkinson's disease. Mov Disord. 2006;21(3):380–4.

52. Tan EK, Lum SY, Wong MC. Restless legs syndrome in Parkinson's disease. J Neurol Sci. 2002;196(1–2):33–6.

53. Rijsman RM, et al. Restless legs syndrome in Parkinson's disease. Parkinsonism Relat Disord. 2014;20 Suppl 1:S5–9.

54. Gjerstad MD, Tysnes OB, Larsen JP. Increased risk of leg motor restlessness but not RLS in early Parkinson disease. Neurology. 2011;77(22):1941–6.

55. Fazzini E, Diaz R, Fahn S. Restless legs in Parkinson's disease-clinical evidence for underactivity of catecholamine neurotransmission. [abstract]. Ann Neurol. 1989;26:142.

56. Walters AS, et al. A preliminary look at the percentage of patients with Restless Legs Syndrome who also have Parkinson Disease, Essential Tremor or Tourette Syndrome in a single practice. J Sleep Res. 2003;12(4):343–5.

57. Gao X, et al. Restless legs syndrome and Parkinson's disease in men. Mov Disord. 2010;25(15): 2654–7.

58. Wong JC, et al. Restless legs syndrome: an early clinical feature of Parkinson disease in men. Sleep. 2014;37(2):369–72.

59. Ancoli-Israel S, et al. Periodic limb movements in sleep in community-dwelling elderly. Sleep. 1991;14(6):496–500.

60. Mosko SS, et al. Sleep apnea and sleep-related periodic leg movements in community resident seniors. J Am Geriatr Soc. 1988;36(6):502–8.

61. Bara-Jimenez W, et al. Periodic limb movements in sleep: state-dependent excitability of the spinal flexor reflex. [comment]. Neurology. 2000;54(8):1609–16.

62. Pennestri MH, et al. Nocturnal blood pressure changes in patients with restless legs syndrome. Neurology. 2007;68(15):1213–8.

63. Walters AS, Rye DB. Evidence continues to mount on the relationship of restless legs syndrome/periodic limb movements in sleep to hypertension, cardiovascular disease, and stroke. Sleep. 2010;33(3):287.

64. Winkelman JW, et al. Association of restless legs syndrome and cardiovascular disease in the Sleep Heart Health Study. Neurology. 2008;70(1):35–42.

65. Montplaisir J, et al. Clinical, polysomnographic, and genetic characteristics of restless legs syndrome: a study of 133 patients diagnosed with new standard criteria. Mov Disord. 1997;12(1):61–5.

66. Coleman RM, et al. Sleep-wake disorders in the elderly: polysomnographic analysis. J Am Geriatr Soc. 1981;29(7):289–96.

67. Trenkwalder C. Sleep dysfunction in Parkinson's disease. Clin Neurosci. 1998;5(2):107–14.

68. Covassin N, et al. Clinical correlates of periodic limb movements in sleep in Parkinson's disease. J Neurol Sci. 2012;316(1–2):131–6.

69. Wetter TC, et al. Polysomnographic measures in Parkinson's disease: a comparison between patients with and without REM sleep disturbances. Wien Klin Wochenschr. 2001;113(7–8): 249–53.

70. Ma JF, et al. Efficacy and safety of pramipexole in chinese patients with restless legs syndrome: results from a multi-center, randomized, double-blind, placebo-controlled trial. Sleep Med. 2012;13(1):58–63.

71. Happe S, et al. Periodic leg movements in patients with Parkinson's disease are associated with reduced striatal dopamine transporter binding. J Neurol. 2003;250(1):83–6.

72. Hogl B, et al. The effect of cabergoline on sleep, periodic leg movements in sleep, and early morning motor function in patients with Parkinson's disease. Neuropsychopharmacology. 2003;28(10):1866–70.
73. Shpirer I, et al. Excessive daytime sleepiness in patients with Parkinson's disease: a polysomnography study. Mov Disord. 2006;21(9):1432–8.
74. Rye DB, DeLong MR. Amelioration of sensory limb discomfort of restless legs syndrome by pallidotomy. Ann Neurol. 1999;46(5):800–1.
75. Chahine LM, Ahmed A, Sun Z. Effects of STN DBS for Parkinson's disease on restless legs syndrome and other sleep-related measures. Parkinsonism Relat Disord. 2011;17(3):208–11.
76. Kedia S, et al. Emergence of restless legs syndrome during subthalamic stimulation for Parkinson disease. Neurology. 2004;63(12):2410–2.
77. Parra J, et al. [Severe restless legs syndrome following bilateral subthalamic stimulation to treat a patient with Parkinson's disease]. Rev Neurol. 2006;42(12):766–7.
78. Ondo WG, et al. Globus pallidus deep brain stimulation for refractory idiopathic restless legs syndrome. Sleep Med. 2012;13(9):1202–4.

Fatigue and Sleepiness in Parkinson's Disease Patients

13

Elisabeth Svensson

Contents

Abstract

The main focus of this chapter is fatigue in Parkinson's disease (PD) patients, with particular emphasis on defining and measuring fatigue, describing the epidemiology of fatigue and associated factors, including a brief discussion of the interface between fatigue and sleepiness. Fatigue is a common non-motor symptom in PD patients, but is also a common complaint in the general population. To facilitate research of fatigue in PD it is important to clearly define the concept of fatigue and to use fatigue scales with good psychometric properties. Additionally, it is important to disentangle the effects of fatigue from the effects of other comorbid symptoms in the PD patients, such as depression and sleep problems. Fatigue and sleepiness are two distinct entities; thus, it is important to separate

E. Svensson, PhD
Department of Clinical Epidemiology, Aarhus University, Aarhus, Denmark
e-mail: elisabeth.svensson@clin.au.dk

© Springer-Verlag Wien 2015

A. Videnovic, B. Högl (eds.), *Disorders of Sleep and Circadian Rhythms in Parkinson's Disease*, DOI 10.1007/978-3-7091-1631-9_13

excessive daytime sleepiness from fatigue. Because of scant knowledge on pathophysiology and treatment, these sections are discussed briefly.

13.1　Introduction

Fatigue and sleepiness are commonly seen both in the general and clinical populations, such as Parkinson's disease (PD) patients. Such non-motor symptoms are often under-recognized clinically [1], despite being of uttermost importance for the patients and significantly associated with worse quality of life [2–4]. For many patients and clinicians, the distinction between fatigue and sleepiness is unclear, as there is no clear definition of these concepts, and no consensus on what is normal or pathological. Terms such as fatigued, tired, and sleepy are used interchangeably; while fatigue can be described as an individual's feeling of abnormal tiredness, sleepiness is defined as a tendency to fall asleep. Sleepiness and fatigue frequently co-occur in PD patients; however, it is suggested that they should be regarded as distinct symptoms that must be understood and managed separately [5]. The main focus of this chapter is fatigue, with particular emphasis on defining and measuring fatigue, describing the epidemiology of fatigue and associated factors, including a brief discussion of the interface between fatigue and sleepiness. Finally, the pathophysiology and treatment of fatigue in PD patients are briefly discussed.

13.2　Defining Fatigue

There are two types of fatigue, peripheral fatigue (fatigability) and central fatigue. Fatigability is objectively measured and involves lack of energy associated with repetitive muscular movements. The main focus of this chapter will be on central fatigue, which is a subjective feeling, and thus, objectively immeasurable. There is no universally accepted definition of this type of fatigue, and the division between pathological and normal fatigue is unclear [6]. Focus groups of PD patients operationalized fatigue as abnormal tiredness [7], interfering with normal function. The fatigue experienced by the PD patient is different from the fatigue experienced before developing the disease [7].

Fatigue can be described as physical or mental fatigue [6]. Physical fatigue is the subjective feeling of being exhausted and lacking energy, including muscle weakness, despite being able to perform the tasks. Mental fatigue is the subjective feeling of being mentally exhausted, including difficulty concentrating and lack of mental clarity during and after periods of cognitive strain. It is suggested that mental and physical fatigue are independent of each other [8], as they are not correlated. If the fatigue is persistent over 6 months, it can be defined as chronic fatigue [9]. In patient populations with stable diseases, the concept of chronic fatigue is useful, as it helps to separate acute and transient fatigue from fatigue that is stable over time.

Fatigue can be categorized as primary or secondary fatigue. Primary fatigue is related to the neurologic disease itself, while secondary fatigue is caused by other factors such as infections, anemia, endocrine dysfunction, depression, sleep disturbance, or side effects of the medications. It may be difficult to disentangle these two issues; during a clinical investigation, it is important to rule out fatigue from secondary causes. In research, it is important to define what type of fatigue one seeks to measure.

13.3 Measuring Fatigue

A variety of questionnaires have been developed to measure fatigue and assess its severity, both for clinical and research purposes [10]. These questionnaires encompass different properties, such as being one- or multidimensional, and generic versus disease-specific. A one-dimensional fatigue scale condenses a range of symptoms into a single score. A multidimensional scale incorporates several aspects of fatigue [11]; for example, being able to distinguish between mental and physical fatigue [12]. A generic scale can be used to assess fatigue within the general population, while the use of a disease-specific instrument may better reflect the consequences of disease, such as PD.

As the questionnaires have varying properties, it may be that measurements from different questionnaires yield prevalence estimates that vary. In fact, a comparison between the Fatigue Severity Scale (FSS) and the Functional Assessment of Chronic Illness Therapy—Fatigue scale (FACIT-F)—concludes that they do not appear to measure identical aspects of fatigue [13].

The International Movement Disorder Society has rated all instruments used to measure fatigue in PD [14]. For screening purposes, recommended scales include the FSS, FACIT-F, and the Parkinson Fatigue Scale (PFS) [14]. The Committee suggested further examinations of psychometric properties of the scales, including sensitivity and specificity.

An example of a generic unidimensional scale is the FSS [15], which is probably the most widely used fatigue instrument. The FSS does not distinguish between different aspects of fatigue; and what aspect of fatigue measured is not defined. The FSS is a nine-item instrument; each statement is rated on a scale of 1–7. The individual score is the mean of the numerical responses. A cutoff of four is used to distinguish between fatigued and non-fatigued, but other cutoffs have also been suggested. The psychometric properties of the FSS in PD are good [14].

The Parkinson Fatigue Scale is a PD-specific scale, developed to assess fatigue in PD patients [7]. The scale is unidimensional, encompassing physical fatigue. The focus of the instrument is to distinguish between PD patients who report having fatigue versus not, and between problematic and non-problematic levels of fatigue [7]. Its psychometric properties, including reliability, are good [14].

The FACIT-F scale is another widely used instrument, available in many languages and freely available (http://www.facit.org). While it does not define the type of fatigue it aims to assess, it covers both the experience and impact of fatigue. It consists of 13 items, with 5 response categories, yielding a sum between 0 and 52. The FACIT-F is reported to have good psychometric properties, including data quality, validity, and reliability [14].

One questionnaire not included in the rating by the International Movement Disorder Society is the Fatigue Questionnaire (FQ). The FQ is widely used in cancer research [7], and is an example of a multidimensional fatigue questionnaire that distinguishes between mental and physical fatigue [12]. The FQ also contains two additional items about the duration and extent/impact of disease, enabling the identification of cases with chronic fatigue. The FQ was originally validated in primary care, and has demonstrated good face-and discriminate validity, as well as stable psychometric properties across populations [12].

13.4 The Epidemiology of Fatigue in PD Patients

The prevalence of fatigue in PD patients is found to range between 32 and 70 %, depending on the population examined, the definition of fatigue and the instrument used to measure fatigue (reviewed in [16]). Most of these studies involved small clinical cohorts. Using a population-based cohort approach, two studies have estimated the prevalence of fatigue of 28 % (chronic fatigue, FQ) [17] and 44 % (measured by Nottingham health profile) [18]. This prevalence is likely an underestimation, since studies have not included PD patients who are unable to utilize self-report instruments.

Many of the studies mentioned above have examined whether PD patients experience higher levels of fatigue than those without PD, often using clinical populations. Comparison between PD patients and patients without PD is important as fatigue is common in the general population; one estimation is that 18 % of general population over the age of 65 years experience fatigue (measured as chronic fatigue) [19]. However, clinical populations may have even higher levels of fatigue than the general population, resulting in an underestimation of the importance of fatigue in PD compared with disease-free individuals. Available population-based studies that compared fatigue in the PD population with the general population found significantly higher prevalence of fatigue among PD patients [17, 18].

Women usually report higher levels of fatigue than men in the general population [19]. Examining gender-specific differences, therefore, may be of importance. Few studies have investigated gender differences in PD [16], and results have been inconsistent. One recent study found no evidence of gender differences in fatigue [20], while two earlier studies found a trend towards significantly higher levels of fatigue in women [21] and a significantly higher prevalence of fatigue in women [17].

Most cross-sectional studies reported an association between PD severity and progression and fatigue [17, 20, 22], while others did not confirm these associations [8, 18]. Data from a longitudinal study of a community-based PD cohort reported an increasing lifetime prevalence of fatigue over time [23], and fatigue being related to disease severity. Persistence of fatigue has also been shown to vary, with half of all PD patients experiencing persistent fatigue.

13.5 Factors Associated with Fatigue in PD Patients

Some PD patients have fatigue only, with the absence of other non-motor symptoms [23]. Among patients without sleep problems, depression, and dementia, 43.5 % reported fatigue. Comorbid non-motor symptoms are, however, very common. Among 100 patients who reported the presence of sleep disturbance, depression, anxiety, fatigue or sensory symptoms, 59 % had two or more symptoms, 23 % had four or more, and 11 % had all five symptoms [22]. Thus, it is important to disentangle the effects of the different non-motor symptoms in PD patients, as they are associated and may contribute to secondary fatigue. Here, we focus on sleepiness and depression.

13.5.1 Fatigue and Sleepiness

There has been some focus on the overlap of fatigue and sleep problems, such as sleepiness (or daytime somnolence) in PD patients. Interestingly, while sleep problems overall, as measured by the unidimensional disease-specific Parkinson's Disease Sleep Scale, are significantly associated with fatigue [24, 25], studies assessing daytime sleepiness (using Epworth Sleepiness Scale) generally have not found an association with fatigue [20, 21, 26]. This suggests that fatigue is a distinct entity from sleepiness, as measured by the ESS. Additionally, there are differences in the way fatigue and sleepiness are correlated with other factors such as dopaminergic treatment and depression [27]. This is further underlined by the finding that modaphenil has an effect in treating sleepiness (reviewed in [28]), but not fatigue (reviewed in [29]). Thus, it is important to separate excessive daytime sleepiness from fatigue.

13.5.2 Fatigue and Depression

The presence of fatigue is one of the criteria for diagnosing depression. Thus, in any study of fatigue in PD patients, depression must be taken into account [11]. Accordingly, there are several reports of the association between fatigue and depression. However, nondepressed patients are also fatigued [23], and patients successfully treated for depressive mood may still continue to have fatigue.

13.6 Pathophysiology

The physiological causes of fatigue in PD patients are largely unknown. Evidence is emerging that fatigue is present in early stages of disease, rather than as the result of PD progression. Fatigue is present in 40 % of recently diagnosed PD patients in a representative cohort of patients with incident PD [21]. In a study of levodopa-naïve PD patients, fatigued and nonfatigued PD patients have similar dopamine transporter uptake, while the fatigued patients had more severe Parkinsonism [30]. Although an association between dopamine drugs and fatigue has been observed, there is no evidence of a dose response [20]. Thus, it seems unlikely that the nigrostriatal dopaminergic pathology plays a role for fatigue in PD patients [20].

Fatigue is common not only in other neurologic diseases such as multiple sclerosis but also other somatic diseases such as cancer and rheumatologic conditions, as well as psychiatric disorders such as major depression and chronic fatigue syndrome. The pathophysiology of fatigue in all these states is also largely unknown. It is possible that there are common underlying factors for all of these disease states. While there are several hypotheses implicating immune, metabolic, and endocrine processes, there is little evidence to support them [16].

Further research is necessary to clarify the pathophysiology of fatigue in PD. Investigations must disentangle the effects of the different non-motor symptoms in order to elucidate the effects of primary versus secondary fatigue.

13.7 Treatment

The treatment of subjective fatigue in PD is a challenge, as there is scant knowledge of the pathophysiology. However, treatment of secondary fatigue, such as fatigue due to depression, may lead to improvement in mental and physical dimensions of central fatigue [31]. If pathophysiological studies find a common underlying factor for fatigue across disorders [20], this may result in the development of therapies beneficial for fatigue in PD patients as well.

Treatment of fatigue can broadly be divided into pharmacologic and non-pharmacologic interventions.

13.7.1 Pharmacologic Interventions

There are few studies investigating the efficacy of pharmacological treatments of fatigue in PD patients. A 6-week randomized controlled trial of 36 patients showed methylphenidate (compared to placebo) to significantly reduce FSS and FSI scores [32]. These results have not been replicated. As previously mentioned, modafinil has been reported not to reduce fatigue, but these studies were small (reviewed in [29]). The Movement Disorder Society's evidence-based medicine review update on treatments for non-motor symptoms of PD concluded that there is insufficient evidence of methylphenidate and modafinil for the treatment of fatigue [33].

13.7.2 Non-pharmacologic Interventions

Non-pharmacologic interventions include patient and caregiver education, psychological approaches and physical exercise [34]. This section will focus on exercise.

To date, there has been no randomized controlled trial of exercise for fatigue in PD. However, higher levels of exercise may be associated with lower levels of fatigue in observational studies [35, 36]; in addition to improving fatigue in PD patients, depression may also decrease. The potential effects of exercise in PD patients have been reviewed by Speelman and colleagues [37].

The benefits of exercise as a treatment for fatigue for patients with several medical conditions such as depression, cancer, and multiple sclerosis may extend to PD as well [5]. The difficulties of getting patients, especially those with severe motor dysfunction, to exercise at appropriate levels may be a challenge. However, as there are several benefits of physical activity, exercise programs for patients with PD are warranted [38].

Conclusion

Fatigue is a common non-motor symptom in PD patients as well as a common complaint in the general population. Further research on pathophysiology and treatment is warranted: Improving our knowledge is important to develop effective prevention strategies and treatment for this non-motor symptom of PD. To facilitate further research of fatigue in PD patients, it is of importance to clearly define the concept of fatigue under investigation. Additionally, it is important to disentangle the effects of fatigue from the effects of other comorbid symptoms of PD, such as depression and sleep problems, as these represent distinct entities.

References

1. Shulman LM, Taback RL, Rabinstein AA, Weiner WJ. Non-recognition of depression and other non-motor symptoms in Parkinson's disease. Parkinsonism Relat Disord. 2002;8:193–7.
2. Havlikova E, Rosenberger J, Nagyova I, Middel B, Dubayova T, Gdovinova Z, van Dijk JP, Groothoff JW. Impact of fatigue on quality of life in patients with Parkinson's disease. Eur J Neurol. 2008;15:475–80.
3. Herlofson K, Larsen JP. The influence of fatigue on health-related quality of life in patients with Parkinson's disease. Acta Neurol Scand. 2003;107:1–6.
4. Martinez-Martin P. The importance of non-motor disturbances to quality of life in Parkinson's disease. J Neurol Sci. 2011;310:12–6.
5. Friedman JH, Chou KL. Sleep and fatigue in Parkinson's disease. Parkinsonism Relat Disord. 2004;10 Suppl 1:S27–35.
6. Lou JS. Physical and mental fatigue in Parkinson's disease: epidemiology, pathophysiology and treatment. Drugs Aging. 2009;26:195–208.
7. Brown RG, Dittner A, Findley L, Wessely SC. The Parkinson fatigue scale. Parkinsonism Relat Disord. 2005;11:49–55.
8. Lou JS, Kearns G, Oken B, Sexton G, Nutt J. Exacerbated physical fatigue and mental fatigue in Parkinson's disease. Mov Disord. 2001;16:190–6.
9. Fukuda K, Straus SE, Hickie I, Sharpe MC, Dobbins JG, Komaroff A. The chronic fatigue syndrome: a comprehensive approach to its definition and study. International Chronic Fatigue Syndrome Study Group. Ann Intern Med. 1994;121:953–9.
10. Dittner AJ, Wessely SC, Brown RG. The assessment of fatigue: a practical guide for clinicians and researchers. J Psychosom Res. 2004;56:157–70.

11. Aarsland D, Marsh L, Schrag A. Neuropsychiatric symptoms in Parkinson's disease. Mov Disord. 2009;24:2175–86.
12. Chalder T, Berelowitz G, Pawlikowska T, Watts L, Wessely S, Wright D, Wallace EP. Development of a fatigue scale. J Psychosom Res. 1993;37:147–53.
13. Hagell P, Hoglund A, Reimer J, Eriksson B, Knutsson I, Widner H, Cella D. Measuring fatigue in Parkinson's disease: a psychometric study of two brief generic fatigue questionnaires. J Pain Symptom Manage. 2006;32:420–32.
14. Friedman JH, Alves G, Hagell P, Marinus J, Marsh L, Martinez-Martin P, Goetz CG, Poewe W, Rascol O, Sampaio C, Stebbins G, Schrag A. Fatigue rating scales critique and recommendations by the Movement Disorders Society task force on rating scales for Parkinson's disease. Mov Disord. 2010;25:805–22.
15. Krupp LB, LaRocca NG, Muir-Nash J, Steinberg AD. The fatigue severity scale. Application to patients with multiple sclerosis and systemic lupus erythematosus. Arch Neurol. 1989;46:1121–3.
16. Friedman JH, Brown RG, Comella C, Garber CE, Krupp LB, Lou JS, Marsh L, Nail L, Shulman L, Taylor CB. Fatigue in Parkinson's disease: a review. Mov Disord. 2007;22:297–308.
17. Beiske AG, Loge JH, Hjermstad MJ, Svensson E. Fatigue in Parkinson's disease: prevalence and associated factors. Mov Disord. 2010;25:2456–60.
18. Karlsen K, Larsen JP, Tandberg E, Jorgensen K. Fatigue in patients with Parkinson's disease. Mov Disord. 1999;14:237–41.
19. Loge JH, Ekeberg O, Kaasa S. Fatigue in the general Norwegian population: normative data and associations. J Psychosom Res. 1998;45:53–65.
20. Hagell P, Brundin L. Towards an understanding of fatigue in Parkinson disease. J Neurol Neurosurg Psychiatry. 2009;80:489–92.
21. Herlofson K, Ongre SO, Enger LK, Tysnes OB, Larsen JP. Fatigue in early Parkinson's disease. Minor inconvenience or major distress? Eur J Neurol. 2012;19:963–8.
22. Shulman LM, Taback RL, Bean J, Weiner WJ. Comorbidity of the nonmotor symptoms of Parkinson's disease. Mov Disord. 2001;16:507–10.
23. Alves G, Wentzel-Larsen T, Larsen JP. Is fatigue an independent and persistent symptom in patients with Parkinson disease? Neurology. 2004;63:1908–11.
24. Okuma Y, Kamei S, Morita A, Yoshii F, Yamamoto T, Hashimoto S, Utsumi H, Hatano T, Hattori N, Matsumura M, Takahashi K, Nogawa S, Watanabe Y, Miyamoto T, Miyamoto M, Hirata K. Fatigue in Japanese patients with Parkinson's disease: a study using Parkinson fatigue scale. Mov Disord. 2009;24:1977–83.
25. Svensson E, Beiske AG, Loge JH, Beiske KK, Sivertsen B. Sleep problems in Parkinson's disease: a community-based study in Norway. BMC Neurol. 2012;12:71.
26. Havlikova E, van Dijk JP, Rosenberger J, Nagyova I, Middel B, Dubayova T, Gdovinova Z, Groothoff JW. Fatigue in Parkinson's disease is not related to excessive sleepiness or quality of sleep. J Neurol Sci. 2008;270:107–13.
27. Valko PO, Waldvogel D, Weller M, Bassetti CL, Held U, Baumann CR. Fatigue and excessive daytime sleepiness in idiopathic Parkinson's disease differently correlate with motor symptoms, depression and dopaminergic treatment. Eur J Neurol. 2010;17:1428–36.
28. Arnulf I. Excessive daytime sleepiness in parkinsonism. Sleep Med Rev. 2005;9:185–200.
29. Friedman JH, Abrantes A, Sweet LH. Fatigue in Parkinson's disease. Expert Opin Pharmacother. 2011;12:1999–2007.
30. Schifitto G, Friedman JH, Oakes D, Shulman L, Comella CL, Marek K, Fahn S. Fatigue in levodopa-naive subjects with Parkinson disease. Neurology. 2008;71:481–5.
31. Havlikova E, Rosenberger J, Nagyova I, Middel B, Dubayova T, Gdovinova Z, Groothoff W, van Dijk P. Clinical and psychosocial factors associated with fatigue in patients with Parkinson's disease. Parkinsonism Relat Disord. 2008;14:187–92.
32. Mendonca DA, Menezes K, Jog MS. Methylphenidate improves fatigue scores in Parkinson disease: a randomized controlled trial. Mov Disord. 2007;22:2070–6.
33. Seppi K, Weintraub D, Coelho M, Perez-Lloret S, Fox SH, Katzenschlager R, Hametner EM, Poewe W, Rascol O, Goetz CG, Sampaio C. The movement disorder society evidence-based

medicine review update: treatments for the non-motor symptoms of Parkinson's disease. Mov Disord. 2011;26 Suppl 3:S42–80. doi:10.1002/mds.23884.:S42-S80.
34. Levine J, Greenwald BD. Fatigue in Parkinson disease, stroke, and traumatic brain injury. Phys Med Rehabil Clin N Am. 2009;20:347–61.
35. Abrantes AM, Friedman JH, Brown RA, Strong DR, Desaulniers J, Ing E, Saritelli J, Riebe D. Physical activity and neuropsychiatric symptoms of Parkinson disease. J Geriatr Psychiatry Neurol. 2012;25:138–45.
36. Garber CE, Friedman JH. Effects of fatigue on physical activity and function in patients with Parkinson's disease. Neurology. 2003;60:1119–24.
37. Speelman AD, van de Warrenburg BP, van Nimwegen M, Petzinger GM, Munneke M, Bloem BR. How might physical activity benefit patients with Parkinson disease? Nat Rev Neurol. 2011;7:528–34.
38. van Nimwegen M, Speelman AD, Hofman-van Rossum EJ, Overeem S, Deeg DJ, Borm GF, van der Horst MH, Bloem BR, Munneke M. Physical inactivity in Parkinson's disease. J Neurol. 2011;258:2214–21.

Cognition and the Sleep–Wake Cycle in Parkinson's Disease

14

Jean-Francois Gagnon, Ronald B. Postuma, and Gabrielle Lyonnais-Lafond

Contents

Abstract

Non-motor symptoms of Parkinson's disease (PD) have received increasing attention in the past decade, particularly cognitive and sleep dysfunctions. Moreover, a growing body of evidence suggests an association between sleep and cognition in aging. This chapter outlines the role of sleep in the maintenance of cognition and learning and the high prevalence of cognitive impairment

J.-F. Gagnon, PhD (✉) • G. Lyonnais-Lafond, BSc candidate
Department of Psychology, Université du Québec à Montréal, Montreal, QC, Canada

Centre d'Études Avancées en Médecine du Sommeil, Hôpital du Sacré-Cœur de Montréal, 5400 boul. Gouin Ouest, Montreal, QC H4J 1C5, Canada
e-mail: gagnon.jean-francois.2@uqam.ca

R.B. Postuma, MD, MSc
Centre d'Études Avancées en Médecine du Sommeil, Hôpital du Sacré-Cœur de Montréal, 5400 boul. Gouin Ouest, Montreal, QC H4J 1C5, Canada

Department of Neurology, McGill University,
Montreal General Hospital, Montreal, QC, Canada

© Springer-Verlag Wien 2015
A. Videnovic, B. Högl (eds.), *Disorders of Sleep and Circadian Rhythms in Parkinson's Disease*, DOI 10.1007/978-3-7091-1631-9_14

in PD. We then summarize the evidence for and against associations between rapid-eye-movement (REM) sleep behavior disorder (RBD), excessive daytime sleepiness (EDS), sleep-disordered breathing (SDB), insomnia, sleep quality, sleep architecture abnormalities, and cognitive impairment in PD. Three major sleep outcomes, RBD, EDS, and reduced sleep spindles, are correlated to cognitive impairment in PD, whereas insomnia, sleep quality, and SDB show modest or no correlation. Further longitudinal studies are needed to determine the role of RBD, EDS, and sleep spindle abnormalities as potential markers of cognitive decline in PD.

14.1   Introduction

The non-motor features of Parkinson's disease (PD) have been well identified by clinicians and researchers in the last decade. Two of the most devastating for patients and their caregivers are sleep disorders and cognitive impairment, which affect nearly all patients with PD over the course of the disease. Indeed, patients with PD frequently develop symptoms such as insomnia, rapid-eye-movement (REM) sleep behavior disorder (RBD), sleep-disordered breathing (SDB), excessive daytime sleepiness (EDS), mild cognitive impairment (MCI), and/or dementia. Moreover, sleep and cognition are strongly related: (1) some memory and learning process appear to be mediated by cerebral plasticity mechanisms that occur in part during the sleep–wake cycle and (2) several sleep disorders are associated with varying degrees of cognitive deficits. Both sleep and cognition present age-related changes, which are amplified in pathological aging, such as neurodegenerative diseases. Recent studies suggest that some of these PD-related sleep disorders are associated with an increased risk for cognitive impairment. This chapter reviews the evidence for an association between sleep and cognition in PD.

14.2   Cognition in Parkinson's Disease

Cognitive impairment is a frequent non-motor symptom of PD, and can occur early in the course of the disease [1, 2]. The cognitive profile of patients with PD is heterogeneous and varies widely with the disease stage [1, 2]. The most consistently reported impaired cognitive domains in PD are attention, executive functions, episodic memory, and visuospatial abilities [1, 2]. The severity of the cognitive impairment also differs widely between patients: some patients remain cognitively intact for a long period of time, whereas others develop MCI or dementia early in the disease course.

MCI is defined as significant cognitive decline compared to age- and education-equivalent individuals, without major impact on activities of daily living. It is now a well-recognized feature of PD [1]. Cross-sectional studies using various definitions of PD-MCI have reported MCI in 19–38 % of patients with PD [1]. New criteria for PD-MCI have been proposed by a Movement Disorder Society Task Force [1].

However, the validity of these criteria remains to be determined. MCI is a risk factor for a more severe cognitive decline in PD [1, 3], which is not surprising, given that MCI is often an intermediate stage between normal aging and dementia in the general population [4].

Dementia is one of the most devastating non-motor features of PD. The point prevalence of dementia in PD has been estimated at from 8 to 48 % in cross-sectional studies [2]. This wide range is mainly due to between-study variability in methodology (i.e., population selection, dementia criteria, and population heterogeneity). A point prevalence of 30 % is suggested [2, 5]. The Movement Disorder Society Task Force has also proposed criteria for dementia in PD [2]. Whereas the cross-sectional prevalence is moderately high, prospective long-term studies have reported that most patients with PD eventually develop dementia [2, 5].

There is considerable variation between the time of dementia onset and the time of PD onset [2]. Some demographic and clinical risk factors for dementia in PD have been identified, namely older age, depression, more severe parkinsonism with rigidity, akinetic-rigid subtype, freezing, postural instability, and gait disturbance [2, 5]. In addition, hallucinations, MCI, and apathy increase the risk for dementia in PD, mainly because they are early symptoms of cognitive impairment [1, 2, 5]. Various candidate biomarkers for cognitive decline in PD are currently being investigated, including waking EEG and structural and functional neuroimaging abnormalities, biomarkers in cerebrospinal fluid, and genetic polymorphisms [5]. This chapter focuses on sleep abnormalities as potential risk factors for and markers of dementia in PD.

14.3   Sleep and Cognition in Aging

Sleep is a complex physiological state characterized by coordinated cyclic changes in the activity of diverse neuronal systems. Thus, major changes in neuronal molecular, electrophysiological, and neurochemical activity occur throughout the sleep–wake cycle [6, 7]. Although the specific roles of these physiological events have not been determined, growing evidence suggests that sleep has a significant impact on cognition, particularly memory consolidation and cerebral plasticity [6–8].

In normal aging, age-related changes in sleep are common, and are characterized by increased wake after sleep onset (WASO), reduced duration of slow-wave sleep (SWS), and increased time spent in stage 1 sleep [9, 10]. Consequently, there are more awakenings and sleep quality is poor. Although stage 2 sleep remains relatively unchanged, the EEG features of stage 2 sleep are less pronounced, with reduced frequency of sleep spindles and lower amplitude of K complexes. The REM sleep percentage remains constant, with only a small decrease in older age. Circadian phase advances, characterized by a shift in the sleep–wake cycle toward morningness, have also been reported. Recent studies suggest that age-related changes in sleep parameters are associated with age-related cognitive decline [11, 12].

In addition to sleep-related architecture changes, aging is associated with increased prevalence of sleep disorders such as SDB, EDS, insomnia, and

RBD. These disorders can also impact cognition. In older adults with SDB, impaired vigilance, attention, executive functions, and learning have been reported [13, 14]. In a prospective study in older women, SDB was identified as a risk factor for developing MCI or dementia [15]. However, the mechanism of this effect is unclear (i.e., hypoxia, disrupted sleep, comorbidities such as cerebrovascular disease). Idiopathic RBD is also associated with cognitive impairment, characterized by reduced performance in attention, executive functions, learning, and visuospatial tasks and increased risk for MCI. This is almost certainly due to the fact that RBD is a well-recognized risk factor for dementia with Lewy bodies and PD [16, 17]. Moreover, alterations in the sleep–wake cycle (insomnia, EDS, WASO, and poor sleep quality and duration) may be associated with altered cognitive performance and cognitive decline in the elderly population, although this relationship remains controversial [18–21].

All of these sleep abnormalities are associated with PD, which is characterized by widespread degeneration of the neurons of the reticular activating system and the diverse brain stem structures involved in sleep regulation [9, 10]. This suggests that in pathological aging such as PD: (1) sleep alterations may impact the cerebral plasticity-related mechanisms underlying certain cognitive functions; and/or (2) sleep alterations may indicate more widespread and severe neurodegeneration, particularly in the brain stem, the thalamus and the cortex (thalamo-cortical loop), which indirectly impacts neurobiological systems related to cognitive functions.

14.4 Sleep and Cognition in Parkinson's Disease

As reported in other chapters of this book, sleep complaints and sleep disorders are major non-motor symptoms in PD [9, 10]. The most frequently reported sleep disorders in PD are RBD, EDS, SDB, and insomnia. What are the relationships between these disorders and cognition in PD?

14.4.1 Rapid-Eye-Movement Sleep Behavior Disorder

In studies using polysomnography (PSG) for diagnosis, RBD affects approximately 30–45 % of patients with PD [22, 23]. RBD has been related to disturbances of the brain stem neural networks underlying REM sleep muscle atonia and motor control [24]. These brain stem regions are known to be disrupted in PD [24]. Given that RBD affects only a subgroup of patients with PD, those with concomitant RBD could have a more severe form of PD characterized by more diffuse neurodegeneration, leading to functional impairments such as cognitive deficits.

From 2006 to 2009, some studies reported decreased cognitive performance in patients with PD with RBD. Sinforiani et al. showed altered executive functions performance in patients with PD with clinical RBD compared to patients with PD without RBD [25]. Compared to normative values, patients with PD without RBD did not present any cognitive deficits. A 2-year follow-up of these cohorts confirmed executive dysfunction in patients with PD with RBD, particularly in older individuals at risk for more rapid progression of motor symptoms and hallucinations [26]. Moreover, patients with PD without RBD remained cognitively intact. In 2007, our group performed complete neuropsychological assessments to compare two groups of patients with PD, with and without RBD, to a group of healthy subjects [27]. We found decreased performance on cognitive tests measuring attention, executive functions, verbal learning and memory, and visuospatial abilities in patients with PD with RBD. patients with PD without RBD showed equivalent performance to healthy subjects on all cognitive measures. These results were confirmed in a larger sample drawn from the same cohort in 2009 [28], showing additionally that the presence of MCI in PD is strongly related to RBD. Thus, MCI was present in 73 % of patients with PD with RBD compared to 11 % of patients with PD without RBD and 8 % of controls [28]. Some subsequent studies have confirmed the association between RBD and cognitive dysfunction in PD [29–32] whereas others have not [33–38]. Two recent studies assessed cognition in treatment-naïve newly diagnosed patients with PD [39, 40]. The first reported equivalent cognitive performance and MCI frequency in patients with PD with and without RBD [39]. The second showed no difference in cognitive profile between patients with PD with and without REM sleep behavior events [40]. These two studies suggest that PD duration and the use of dopaminergic medication may modulate cognitive impairment in patients with PD with RBD. Indeed, higher age and more advanced duration of PD are two well recognized risk factors for cognitive decline in PD [41]. Moreover, although still unclear, dopaminergic medication seems to modulate cognition in patients with PD but the positive or negative impact varies according to the type of treatment and concentration used [5]. Note that most previous studies on the impact of RBD in PD have been cross-sectional with certain methodological limitations. Many used screening cognitive tests only, which have poor sensitivity to detect cognitive impairment in PD [31, 34, 36, 38]. Moreover, RBD diagnostic criteria varied, with some studies using clinical criteria without PSG confirmation or nonstandard PSG criteria, which may affect the accuracy of RBD classification, falsely reducing differences between groups [25, 26, 30–32, 34–38, 40]. Others have not included a healthy control group, which limits the interpretation of the results [25, 26, 30–39]. Furthermore, studies of the highest quality, which used PSG criteria for RBD and standard cognitive batteries, were performed on relatively small samples of patients with PD, reducing the statistical power [27–29, 33, 39]. Hence, further longitudinal studies in larger samples are needed, including PSG to confirm RBD, a healthy control group, and complete neuropsychological assessments, in order to better understand the association between RBD and cognition in PD.

The association between RBD and the development of dementia in PD has also been investigated. Marion et al. reported higher prevalence of clinical RBD in PD with dementia and faster cognitive decline in PD with RBD [42]. In a prospective study over a mean 4-year follow-up, we found that 48 % of patients with PD with RBD at baseline developed dementia, whereas no patients with PD without RBD converted to dementia [43]. This finding was confirmed by Nomura et al., who observed faster occurrence of dementia in PD with RBD compared to PD with normal REM sleep features [44]. Taken together, these studies suggest that RBD in patients with PD may be associated with more rapid cognitive decline, and that RBD could be a clinical risk factor for dementia in PD.

Other studies have found functional and structural impairments specific to RBD in PD, which can explain to some degree the higher risk of cognitive deficits in patients with PD with RBD. A distinct clinical profile, often associated with the presence of cognitive impairment in PD, has been identified in patients with PD with RBD, with autonomic dysfunction, higher incidence of visual hallucinations, more freezing and falls, a non-tremor dominant subtype, and symmetric disease [45–50]. Other studies have demonstrated abnormalities in quantitative waking EEG and event-related potentials, mainly in posterior cortical areas, in patients with PD with RBD [51, 52]. Another study using positron emission tomography ([11C] methylpiperidyl propionate acetylcholinesterase) reported relative neocortical, limbic cortical, and thalamic cholinergic denervation in patients with PD with clinical RBD [53]. A further study using diffusion tensor imaging and voxel-based morphometry (VBM) identified subtle (in uncorrected analyses) reductions in cortical gray matter volume (parietal and temporal lobes) and widespread white matter microstructural abnormalities in patients with PD with clinical RBD [54]. Taken together, these studies provide functional and anatomical support, which could explain the higher prevalence of cognitive impairment in PD associated with RBD.

14.4.2 Sleep-Disordered Breathing and Excessive Daytime Sleepiness

Unlike the relatively clear relationship with RBD, the role of SDB in cognition in PD is much less clear. SDB is commonly present in PD, with prevalence varying from 22 to 66 % depending on the apnea-hypopnea index (AHI) cut-off used [55]. However, studies with control subjects have not found increased SDB prevalence in PD compared to healthy age-matched individuals [55]. Despite the high incidence of SDB in PD and its deleterious effects on health reported in the general population, the impact of SDB on motor and non-motor symptoms in PD appears to be minimal. Only a few studies have investigated the impact of SDB on cognition in PD. Cochen de Cock et al. found no significant effect of sleep apnea on nocturia, sleepiness, depression, cardiovascular events, or cognitive impairment in PD [56]. However, they used the standardized mini-mental state examination to measure cognitive functioning, a screening test that is insensitive to cognitive impairment in PD [57]. Our group recently studied 92 patients with PD who underwent PSG, an extensive neurological exam, including several non-motor measures, and a complete neuropsychological assessment [58]. The prevalence of SDB in our cohort, depending on the AHI cut-off, was 11 % (with AHI >15), 21 % (AHI >10), and 33 % (AHI >5). We found no significant differences in motor and non-motor symptoms between apneic and non-apneic patients with PD, regardless of the AHI cut-off. Of note, the two PD groups did not differ on any cognitive measures (attention, executive functions, learning and memory, or visuospatial abilities) or in the proportion of patients with MCI. These results confirm the absence of a strong relationship between SDB and most major outcomes in PD, including cognitive decline.

EDS is another frequent non-motor symptom in PD. Although EDS has been related to cognitive dysfunction in PD [59, 60], several factors may confound this relationship, and other studies have not confirmed it [61–63]. In fact, only a few studies have formally examined the relationship between EDS and cognition in PD. Gjerstad et al. reported that patients with PD with EDS more often had dementia at baseline and showed faster progression of cognitive impairment and disability after a 4-year follow-up [64]. In a subsequent 4-year follow-up on their cohort, the association between cognitive impairment and EDS was confirmed by univariate analysis, but not by multivariate analysis [65]. In another study, Compta et al. reported no significant difference on the Epworth sleepiness scale (ESS) scores between patients with PD with and without dementia [66]. However, the EDS prevalence (ESS > 10) was higher in patients with PD with dementia. Goldman et al. compared EDS symptoms between cognitively intact patients with PD, patients with PD with MCI, and patients with PD with dementia [37]. They found higher ESS scores and higher EDS prevalence in patients with PD with dementia compared to the two other groups. ESS scores correlated with several cognitive measures. However, patients with PD with and without MCI were equivalent on the ESS. In non-demented patients with PD, a significant correlation between EDS and slowed processing speed has been reported, with no differences in other cognitive measures [30]. We recently compared daytime sleepiness symptom severity in 16 patients with PD with MCI, 20 cognitively intact patients with PD, and 36 healthy subjects [67]. All groups were equivalent on sociodemographic variables, and the two PD groups did not differ on clinical signs of PD, including dopaminergic medication dosage. We found no difference on the ESS scores between patients with PD with MCI (mean = 9.60) and patients with PD with normal cognition (mean = 9.55). However, the two PD groups scored higher on the ESS than healthy subjects (mean = 6.42). Of note, EDS in PD may be heterogeneous: in early stages, medication side effects may play a prominent role, whereas EDS becomes less dependent on medication doses as the disease progresses (i.e., it is mostly a primary disease manifestation). Using structural neuroimaging and VBM, Kato et al. found that patients with PD with EDS had marked gray matter atrophy in several brain regions compared to patients with PD without EDS and healthy subjects, whereas patients with PD without EDS showed no gray matter atrophy compared to controls [68]. Taken together, these results suggest that in PD: (1) EDS is a common feature regardless of the presence of cognitive impairment; (2) the severity of EDS increases with cognitive decline and the symptoms are more manifest in patients with dementia; and (3) EDS is associated with more severe neurodegeneration. This suggests that EDS may be a risk factor for dementia in PD, although this hypothesis needs further validation.

14.4.3 Insomnia, Sleep Quality, and Alterations in Sleep Architecture

Insomnia, characterized by difficulty maintaining sleep, and reduced sleep quality are major complaints in PD, affecting the majority of patients [9, 10]. Here again, the association between these symptoms and cognition in PD remains unclear. Erro et al. compared sleep non-motor symptoms between patients with PD with and without cognitive impairment [32]. They found a relationship between sleep non-motor symptoms and cognitive dysfunctions, where insomnia was associated with lower scores on several cognitive tests. Lee et al. also found sleep complaints on the Neuropsychiatric Inventory in 54 % of patients with PD with dementia [69]. However, no patients with PD without dementia or healthy subjects were included as controls. We recently compared insomnia severity complaints on the Insomnia Severity Index (ISI) between patients with PD with MCI, cognitively intact patients with PD, and healthy subjects [67]. We found no difference on the ISI scores between patients with PD with MCI (mean=9.63) and patients with PD with normal cognition (mean=10.95). However, the two PD groups scored higher on the ISI than healthy subjects (mean=5.15), suggesting that insomnia is a core characteristic of PD, independent of cognitive status. Other groups found no association between either insomnia or sleep quality and cognition in PD [37, 63, 70].

Very few studies have investigated the relationships between sleep architecture parameters and cognition in PD. Stavitsky et al. performed a complete neuropsychological assessment and used actigraphy to record sleep in non-demented patients with PD and controls. They found that poorer attention and executive functioning was correlated to poor sleep quality in both groups. Attention and executive functions performance was predicted by sleep efficiency in patients with PD, whereas memory and psychomotor function were not [71]. Recently, we prospectively followed 68 patients with PD and 47 healthy individuals [72]. All participants underwent a comprehensive neuropsychological assessment and PSG recordings in the laboratory. Slow waves (>75 µV and <4 Hz) and sleep spindles (12–15 Hz) were automatically detected by artifact-free non-REM sleep electroencephalography. At follow-up (mean: 4.5 years later), 18 patients with PD developed dementia and 50 remained dementia-free. At baseline, sleep spindle density and amplitude were reduced in patients with PD who converted to dementia compared to both healthy controls and patients who remained dementia-free, mostly in posterior cortical regions. Dementia-free patients with PD were intermediate between control subjects and patients with dementia, with lower baseline sleep spindle density in all cortical areas compared to healthy subjects. Although slow-wave amplitude was lower in patients with PD compared to controls, no difference was observed between those who developed or did not develop dementia. These results suggest that sleep spindle activity are particularly impaired in patients with PD who developed dementia, with a more posterior topographical pattern. Thus, sleep spindle alterations are associated with later development of dementia in patients with PD, and consequently may serve as an additional marker of cognitive decline in these patients.

Preliminary research also suggests that sleep improves cognitive performance in PD. Scullin et al. found that performance on a simple working memory task (backward digit span) improved following a nocturnal sleep interval in patients with PD on dopaminergic medication, but not in medication-free patients [73]. The amount of that patients with PD on dopaminergic medication obtained between training sessions was correlated with improvement on the working memory task. Although their results suggest that improved sleep quality may enhance working memory capacity in patients with PD, further studies are needed to better understand the underlying mechanisms and to generalize this observation to other cognitive domains that are affected in PD.

14.5 Conclusions and Future Directions

In conclusion, good-quality sleep is key for maintaining neurological health. The degenerative process of PD causes numerous sleep abnormalities. Three major sleep outcomes, RBD, EDS, and sleep spindle alterations, are related to decreased cognition in PD, whereas insomnia and SDB have modest or no association. Although much of this relationship is correlative and related to underlying degeneration of sleep–wake structures, some cognitive deficits could also be caused by sleep disturbances. Further research into the associations between sleep and cognition in PD could provide insight into the mechanisms and heterogeneity of the disease, identify new potential risk factors for or markers of cognitive decline, and ultimately enable improving the cognition of patients affected by PD.

References

1. Litvan I, Goldman JG, Tröster AI, Schmand BA, Weintraub D, Petersen RC, et al. Diagnostic criteria for mild cognitive impairment in Parkinson's disease: Movement Disorder Society Task Force guidelines. Mov Disord. 2012;27:349–56.
2. Dubois B, Burn D, Goetz C, Aarsland D, Brown RG, Broe GA, et al. Diagnostic procedures for Parkinson's disease dementia: recommendations from the movement disorder society task force. Mov Disord. 2007;22:2314–24.
3. Pedersen KF, Larsen JP, Tysnes OB, Alves G. Prognosis of mild cognitive impairment in early Parkinson disease: the Norwegian ParkWest study. JAMA Neurol. 2013;70:580–6.
4. Albert MS, DeKosky ST, Dickson D, Dubois B, Feldman HH, Fox NC, et al. The diagnosis of mild cognitive impairment due to Alzheimer's disease: recommendations from the National Institute on Aging-Alzheimer's Association workgroups on diagnostic guidelines for Alzheimer's disease. Alzheimers Dement. 2011;7:270–9.
5. Svenningsson P, Westman E, Ballard C, Aarsland D. Cognitive impairment in patients with Parkinson's disease: diagnosis, biomarkers, and treatment. Lancet Neurol. 2012;11:697–707.
6. Rasch B, Born J. About sleep's role in memory. Physiol Rev. 2013;93:681–766.
7. Cirelli C. Sleep and synaptic changes. Curr Opin Neurobiol. 2013;23:841–6.
8. Stickgold R, Walker MP. Sleep-dependent memory triage: evolving generalization through selective processing. Nat Neurosci. 2013;16:139–45.
9. Gagnon JF, Petit D, Latreille V, Montplaisir J. Neurobiology of sleep disturbances in neurodegenerative disorders. Curr Pharm Des. 2008;14:3430–45.
10. Naismith SL, Lewis SJ, Rogers NL. Sleep-wake changes and cognition in neurodegenerative disease. Prog Brain Res. 2011;190:21–52.
11. Fogel S, Martin N, Lafortune M, Barakat M, Debas K, Laventure S, et al. NREM sleep oscillations and brain plasticity in aging. Front Neurol. 2012;3:176. doi:10.3389/fneur.2012.00176.
12. Harand C, Bertran F, Doidy F, Guénolé F, Desgranges B, Eustache F, et al. How aging affects sleep-dependent memory consolidation? Front Neurol. 2012;3:8. doi:10.3389/fneur.2012.00008.
13. Zimmerman ME, Aloia MS. Sleep-disordered breathing and cognition in older adults. Curr Neurol Neurosci Rep. 2012;12:537–46.
14. Sforza E, Roche F. Sleep apnea syndrome and cognition. Front Neurol. 2012;3:87. doi:10.3389/fneur.2012.00087.

15. Yaffe K, Laffan AM, Harrison SL, Redline S, Spira AP, Ensrud KE, et al. Sleep- disordered breathing, hypoxia, and risk of mild cognitive impairment and dementia in older women. JAMA. 2011;306:613–9.
16. Gagnon JF, Bertrand JA, Génier MD. Cognition in rapid eye movement sleep behavior disorder. Front Neurol. 2012;3:82. doi:10.3389/fneur.2012.00082.
17. Iranzo A, Tolosa E, Gelpi E, Molinuevo JL, Valldeoriola F, Serradell M, et al. Neurodegenerative disease status and post-mortem pathology in idiopathic rapid- eye-movement sleep behaviour disorder: an observational cohort study. Lancet Neurol. 2013;12:443–53.
18. Blackwell T, Yaffe K, Ancoli-Israel S, Redline S, Ensrud KE, Stefanick ML, et al. Association of sleep characteristics and cognition in older community-dwelling men: the MrOS sleep study. Sleep. 2011;34:1347–56.
19. Jaussent I, Bouyer J, Ancelin ML, Berr C, Foubert-Samier A, Ritchie K, et al. Excessive sleepiness is predictive of cognitive decline in the elderly. Sleep. 2012;35:1201–7.
20. Potvin O, Lorrain D, Forget H, Dubé M, Grenier S, Préville M, et al. Sleep quality and 1-year incident cognitive impairment in community-dwelling older adults. Sleep. 2012;35:491–9.
21. Keage HA, Banks S, Yang KL, Morgan K, Brayne C, Matthews FE. What sleep characteristics predict cognitive decline in the elderly? Sleep Med. 2012;13:886–92.
22. Gagnon JF, Bédard MA, Fantini ML, Petit D, Panisset M, Rompré S, et al. REM sleep behavior disorder and REM sleep without atonia in Parkinson's disease. Neurology. 2002;59:585–9.
23. Sixel-Döring F, Trautmann E, Mollenhauer B, Trenkwalder C. Associated factors for REM sleep behavior disorder in Parkinson disease. Neurology. 2011;77:1048–54.
24. Boeve BF, Silber MH, Saper CB, Ferman TJ, Dickson DW, Parisi JE, et al. Pathophysiology of REM sleep behaviour disorder and relevance to neurodegenerative disease. Brain. 2007;130:2770–88.
25. Sinforiani E, Zangaglia R, Manni R, Cristina S, Marchioni E, Nappi G, et al. REM sleep behavior disorder, hallucinations, and cognitive impairment in Parkinson's disease. Mov Disord. 2006;21:462–6.
26. Sinforiani E, Pacchetti C, Zangaglia R, Pasotti C, Manni R, Nappi G. REM behavior disorder, hallucinations and cognitive impairment in Parkinson's disease: a two-year follow up. Mov Disord. 2008;23:1441–5.
27. Vendette M, Gagnon JF, Décary A, Massicotte-Marquez J, Postuma RB, Doyon J, Panisset M, et al. REM sleep behavior disorder predicts cognitive impairment in Parkinson disease without dementia. Neurology. 2007;69:1843–9.
28. Gagnon JF, Vendette M, Postuma RB, Desjardins C, Massicotte-Marquez J, Panisset M, et al. Mild cognitive impairment in rapid eye movement sleep behavior disorder and Parkinson's disease. Ann Neurol. 2009;66:39–47.
29. Marques A, Dujardin K, Boucart M, Pins D, Delliaux M, Defebvre L, et al. REM sleep behaviour disorder and visuoperceptive dysfunction: a disorder of the ventral visual stream? J Neurol. 2010;257:383–91.
30. Naismith SL, Terpening Z, Shine JM, Lewis SJ. Neuropsychological functioning in Parkinson's disease: differential relationships with self-reported sleep-wake disturbances. Mov Disord. 2011;26:1537–41.
31. Wang G, Wan Y, Wang Y, Xiao Q, Liu J, Ma JF, et al. Visual hallucinations and associated factors in Chinese patients with Parkinson's disease: roles of RBD and visual pathway deficit. Parkinsonism Relat Disord. 2010;16:695–6.
32. Erro R, Santangelo G, Picillo M, Vitale C, Amboni M, Longo K, et al. Link between non-motor symptoms and cognitive dysfunctions in de novo, drug-naive PD patients. J Neurol. 2012;259:1808–13.
33. Benninger D, Waldvogel D, Bassetti CL. REM sleep behavior disorder predicts cognitive impairment in Parkinson disease without dementia. Neurology. 2008;71:955; author reply 955–6.
34. Lavault S, Leu-Semenescu S. Tezenas du Montcel S, Cochen de Cock V, Vidailhet M, Arnulf I. Does clinical rapid eye movement behavior disorder predict worse outcomes in Parkinson's disease? J Neurol. 2010;257:1154–9.

35. Yoritaka A, Ohizumi H, Tanaka S, Hattori N. Parkinson's disease with and without REM sleep behaviour disorder: are there any clinical differences? Eur Neurol. 2009;61:164–70.
36. Lee JE, Kim KS, Shin HW, Sohn YH. Factors related to clinically probable REM sleep behavior disorder in Parkinson disease. Parkinsonism Relat Disord. 2010;16:105–8.
37. Goldman JG, Ghode RA, Ouyang B, Bernard B, Goetz CG, Stebbins GT. Dissociations among daytime sleepiness, nighttime sleep, and cognitive status in Parkinson's disease. Parkinsonism Relat Disord. 2013;19:806–11.
38. Bugalho P, da Silva JA, Neto B. Clinical features associated with REM sleep behavior disorder symptoms in the early stages of Parkinson's disease. J Neurol. 2011;258:50–5.
39. Plomhause L, Dujardin K, Duhamel A, Delliaux M, Derambure P, Defebvre L, et al. Rapid eye movement sleep behavior disorder in treatment-naive Parkinson disease patients. Sleep Med. 2013;14:1035–7.
40. Sixel-Döring F, Ellen Trautmann E, Mollenhauer B, Trenkwalder C. REM sleep behavioral events (RBE): a new marker for neurodegeneration in early Parkinson's disease? Sleep. 2014;37:431–8.
41. Aarsland D, Kurz MW. The epidemiology of dementia associated with Parkinson's disease. Brain Pathol. 2010;20:633–9.
42. Marion MH, Qurashi M, Marshall G, Foster O. Is REM sleep behaviour disorder (RBD) a risk factor of dementia in idiopathic Parkinson's disease? J Neurol. 2008;255:192–6.
43. Postuma RB, Bertrand JA, Montplaisir J, Desjardins C, Vendette M, Rios Romenets S, et al. Rapid eye movement sleep behavior disorder and risk of dementia in Parkinson's disease: a prospective study. Mov Disord. 2012;27:720–6.
44. Nomura T, Inoue Y, Kagimura T, Nakashima K. Clinical significance of REM sleep behavior disorder in Parkinson's disease. Sleep Med. 2013;14:131–5.
45. Videnovic A, Marlin C, Alibiglou L, Planetta PJ, Vaillancourt DE, Mackinnon CD. Increased REM sleep without atonia in Parkinson disease with freezing of gait. Neurology. 2013;81:1030–5.
46. Postuma RB, Gagnon JF, Vendette M, Montplaisir JY. Markers of neurodegeneration in idiopathic rapid eye movement sleep behaviour disorder and Parkinson's disease. Brain. 2009;132:3298–307.
47. Postuma RB, Montplaisir J, Lanfranchi P, Blais H, Rompré S, Colombo R, et al. Cardiac autonomic denervation in Parkinson's disease is linked to REM sleep behavior disorder. Mov Disord. 2011;26:1529–33.
48. Romenets SR, Gagnon JF, Latreille V, Panniset M, Chouinard S, Montplaisir J, et al. Rapid eye movement sleep behavior disorder and subtypes of Parkinson's disease. Mov Disord. 2012;27:996–1003.
49. Bliwise DL, Trotti LM, Greer SA, Juncos JJ, Rye DB. Phasic muscle activity in sleep and clinical features of Parkinson disease. Ann Neurol. 2010;68:353–9.
50. Manni R, Terzaghi M, Ratti PL, Repetto A, Zangaglia R, Pacchetti C. Hallucinations and REM sleep behaviour disorder in Parkinson's disease: dream imagery intrusions and other hypotheses. Conscious Cogn. 2011;20:1021–6.
51. Gagnon JF, Fantini ML, Bédard MA, Petit D, Carrier J, Rompré S, et al. Association between waking EEG slowing and REM sleep behavior disorder in PD without dementia. Neurology. 2004;62:401–6.
52. Gaudreault PO, Gagnon JF, Montplaisir J, Vendette M, Postuma RB, Gagnon K, et al. Abnormal occipital event-related potentials in Parkinson's disease with concomitant REM sleep behavior disorder. Parkinsonism Relat Disord. 2013;19:212–7.
53. Kotagal V, Albin RL, Müller ML, Koeppe RA, Chervin RD, Frey KA, et al. Symptoms of rapid eye movement sleep behavior disorder are associated with cholinergic denervation in Parkinson disease. Ann Neurol. 2012;71:560–8.
54. Ford AH, Duncan GW, Firbank MJ, Yarnall AJ, Khoo TK, Burn DJ, et al. Rapid eye movement sleep behavior disorder in Parkinson's disease: magnetic resonance imaging study. Mov Disord. 2013;28:832–6.
55. da Silva-Júnior FP, do Prado GF, Barbosa ER, Tufik S, Togeiro SM. Sleep disordered breathing in Parkinson's disease: a critical appraisal. Sleep Med Rev. 2014;18:173–8.

56. Cochen De Cock V, Abouda M, Leu S, Oudiette D, Roze E, Vidailhet M, et al. Is obstructive sleep apnea a problem in Parkinson's disease? Sleep Med. 2010;11:247–52.

57. Villeneuve S, Rodrigues-Brazète J, Joncas S, Postuma RB, Latreille V, Gagnon JF. Validity of the Mattis Dementia Rating Scale to detect mild cognitive impairment in Parkinson's disease and REM sleep behavior disorder. Dement Geriatr Cogn Disord. 2011;31:210–7.

58. Béland SG, Postuma RB, Latreille V, Bertrand JA, Desjardins C, Panisset M, Chouinard S, Gagnon JF. What is the clinical significance of apnea in PD? Mov Disord. 2013;28 Suppl 1:S228.

59. Tandberg E, Larsen JP, Karlsen K. Excessive daytime sleepiness and sleep benefit in Parkinson's disease: a community-based study. Mov Disord. 1999;14:922–7.

60. Kurtis MM, Rodriguez-Blazquez C, Martinez-Martin P, ELEP Group. Relationship between sleep disorders and other non-motor symptoms in Parkinson's disease. Parkinsonism Relat Disord. 2013;19:1152–5.

61. Arnulf I, Konofal E, Merino-Andreu M, Houeto JL, Mesnage V, Welter ML, et al. Parkinson's disease and sleepiness: an integral part of PD. Neurology. 2002;58:1019–24.

62. Shpirer I, Miniovitz A, Klein C, Goldstein R, Prokhorov T, Theitler J, et al. Excessive daytime sleepiness in patients with Parkinson's disease: a polysomnography study. Mov Disord. 2006;21:1432–8.

63. Boddy F, Rowan EN, Lett D, O'Brien JT, McKeith IG, Burn DJ. Subjectively reported sleep quality and excessive daytime somnolence in Parkinson's disease with and without dementia, dementia with Lewy bodies and Alzheimer's disease. Int J Geriatr Psychiatry. 2007;22:529–35.

64. Gjerstad MD, Aarsland D, Larsen JP. Development of daytime somnolence over time in Parkinson's disease. Neurology. 2002;58:1544–6.

65. Gjerstad MD, Alves G, Wentzel-Larsen T, Aarsland D, Larsen JP. Excessive daytime sleepiness in Parkinson disease: is it the drugs or the disease? Neurology. 2006;67:853–8.

66. Compta Y, Santamaria J, Ratti L, Tolosa E, Iranzo A, Muñoz E, et al. Cerebrospinal hypocretin, daytime sleepiness and sleep architecture in Parkinson's disease dementia. Brain. 2009;132:3308–17.

67. Diab S, Latreille V, Brayet P, Postuma RB, Bertrand JA, Desjardins C, et al. Nonmotor symptoms in Parkinson's disease with mild cognitive impairment. Mov Disord. 2013;28 Suppl 1:S193.

68. Kato S, Watanabe H, Senda J, Hirayama M, Ito M, Atsuta N, et al. Widespread cortical and subcortical brain atrophy in Parkinson's disease with excessive daytime sleepiness. J Neurol. 2012;259:318–26.

69. Lee WJ, Tsai CF, Gauthier S, Wang SJ, Fuh JL. The association between cognitive impairment and neuropsychiatric symptoms in patients with Parkinson's disease dementia. Int Psychogeriatr. 2012;24:1980–7.

70. Gjerstad MD, Wentzel-Larsen T, Aarsland D, Larsen JP. Insomnia in Parkinson's disease: frequency and progression over time. J Neurol Neurosurg Psychiatry. 2007;78:476–9.

71. Stavitsky K, Neargarder S, Bogdanova Y, McNamara P, Cronin-Golomb A. The impact of sleep quality on cognitive functioning in Parkinson's disease. J Int Neuropsychol Soc. 2012;18:108–17.

72. Latreille V, Carrier J, Lafortune M, Postuma RB, Bertrand JA, Panisset M, Chouinard S, Gagnon JF. Sleep spindles in Parkinson's disease may predict the development of dementia. Neurobiol Aging. 2015;36:1083–90.

73. Scullin MK, Trotti LM, Wilson AG, Greer SA, Bliwise DL. Nocturnal sleep enhances working memory training in Parkinson's disease but not Lewy body dementia. Brain. 2012;135:2789–97.

Impact of Surgical Therapies on Sleep and Alertness in Parkinson's Disease

15

Amy W. Amara and Harrison C. Walker

Contents

Abstract

Surgical therapies for Parkinson's disease (PD) play an increasingly important role in the treatment of motor symptoms that are refractory to medical management. These therapies include deep brain stimulation, lesional/ablation surgery of brain structures, and placement of an intrajejunal tube to administer continuous drug delivery of levodopa/carbidopa intestinal gel (LCIG). Sleep dysfunction and excessive daytime sleepiness are very common among patients with Parkinson's disease and negatively impact quality of life. For this reason,

A.W. Amara (✉)
Division of Movement Disorders, Department of Neurology,
UAB Sleep/Wake Disorders Center,
University of Alabama at Birmingham, Birmingham, AL, USA
e-mail: amyamara@uab.edu

H.C. Walker
Division of Movement Disorders, Department of Neurology,
University of Alabama at Birmingham, Birmingham, AL, USA
e-mail: hcwalker@uab.edu

© Springer-Verlag Wien 2015
A. Videnovic, B. Högl (eds.), *Disorders of Sleep and Circadian Rhythms
in Parkinson's Disease*, DOI 10.1007/978-3-7091-1631-9_15

understanding the impact of surgical therapies on these symptoms can provide additional insights into strategies for optimizing outcomes and provide a better understanding of the pathophysiology of sleep disorders in PD patients. In this chapter, we review the available data on the effects of surgical therapies on sleep architecture, sleep quality, and daytime vigilance and discuss the need for further study to fully understand the mechanisms underlying changes in sleep following surgical intervention.

15.1 Historical Overview of Surgical Therapies for Parkinson's Disease

Surgical therapy for movement disorders was introduced as early as 1912 with bilateral cervical rhizotomy for treatment of a patient with Parkinson's disease (PD) in France. Later, other groups performed surgical lesioning of the motor, premotor, and supplementary motor cortices or the corticospinal tract (for an excellent review, see [1]). Lesions of the basal ganglia for Parkinsonism and tremor were explored by Dr. Russell Myers (University of Iowa) and others in the 1940s and 1950s through open surgical approaches excising the head of the caudate, anterior limb of internal capsule, pallidofugal fibers, or globus pallidus interna/ansa lenticularis. Other interventions included ligation of the anterior choroidal artery by Dr. Irving S. Cooper in 1953. These procedures resulted in some relief of Parkinsonian symptoms, but at high risk of mortality and morbidity. As stereotactic techniques advanced, pallidotomy and thalamotomy were introduced and were used frequently prior to the advent of levodopa. The Austrian Ernest Spiegel and his student Henry Wycis at Temple University pioneered many of these techniques, as did Drs. Cooper in Spain and Rolf Hassler in Germany. These ablative surgeries gained favor again as some of the long-term side effects of levodopa were recognized in the 1970s [1].

Stimulation of subcortical brain structures occurred as early as 1947 at Temple University and in these early days stimulation was used for a range of psychiatric and neurological disorders (reviewed in [2]). Most often, electrical stimulation was used to optimize targeting for ultimate ablation surgery. In France, Dr. Alim-Louis Benabid and colleagues introduced modern deep brain stimulation in 1987, with stimulation of the ventral intermediate nucleus (VIM) of the thalamus (contralateral to thalamotomy) for tremor. In 1990, Dr. Hagai Bergman and colleagues demonstrated that pharmacologic lesioning of the subthalamic nucleus (STN) in MPTP-treated monkeys improved Parkinsonian symptoms [3], leading to interest in the STN as a stimulation target. In humans, Dr. Pierre Pollak and colleagues in France first reported the use of high frequency STN DBS for Parkinson's disease in 1993 [4]. Since that time, the body of literature on the effects of deep brain stimulation (DBS) on motor and non-motor symptoms of Parkinson's disease has grown exponentially. While VIM DBS is very effective for tremor, stimulation of the STN and globus pallidus internal segment (GPi) have become the preferred surgical therapeutic targets due to their beneficial effects on bradykinesia, rigidity, and motor

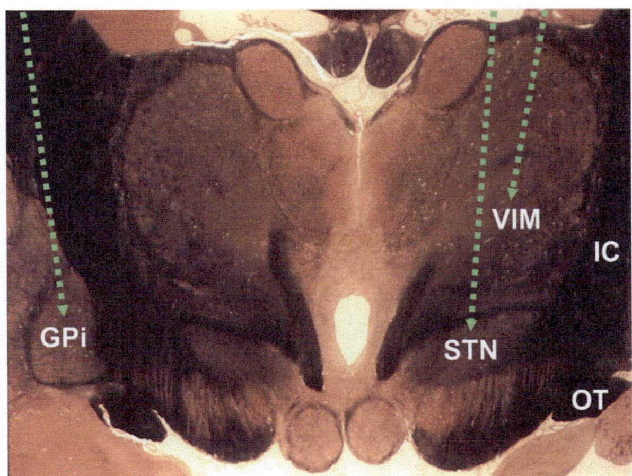

Fig. 15.1 Coronal human Weigert stain (myelin stains black) brain slice with schematic depiction of common anatomic structures targeted for movement disorders surgical therapy, including the subthalamic nucleus (*STN*), globus pallidus interna (*GPi*), and ventral intermediate thalamus (*VIM*). Also depicted are neighboring structures such as the posterior limb of the internal capsule (*IC*) and optic tract (*OT*)

fluctuations in addition to tremor (Fig. 15.1). Potential adverse events of DBS for treatment of PD include mood changes, cognitive dysfunction, speech changes, intracranial hemorrhage, and infection [5]. In this chapter, we summarize the motor effects of surgical therapies for Parkinson's disease and also review the available data on how these therapies impact sleep and vigilance in this patient population.

15.2   Deep Brain Stimulation of the Subthalamic Nucleus

Deep brain stimulation of the bilateral STN provides greater improvement in motor symptoms, motor fluctuations, and quality of life than best medical therapy in patients with PD. However, the surgical therapy does have an increased risk of adverse events [6–8]. Unilateral STN DBS also improves motor symptoms and quality of life in these patients [9–11]. Because of the growing recognition of the prevalence and severity of non-motor symptoms of Parkinson's disease, investigators have increasingly evaluated the effects of STN DBS on sleep and other non-motor symptoms.

Several studies report changes in sleep quality and sleep architecture following bilateral STN DBS. Arnulf and colleagues evaluated 10 subjects 3–6 months after STN DBS with 2 nights of polysomnography (PSG): 1 night with the stimulator on and 1 night with the stimulator off [12]. Compared to the night with DBS off, subjects had a 47 % increase in total sleep time and a 36 % increase in sleep efficiency when DBS was on. In this study, periods of prolonged wakefulness on the DBS-off night coincided with akinesia and dystonia, which were not present during the

DBS-on night. Iranzo and colleagues evaluated 11 subjects pre-surgically and 6 months following bilateral STN DBS and showed post-surgical improvement in subjective sleep quality [13]. Polysomnography showed increased nocturnal mobility, fewer arousals, and an increase in the longest period of uninterrupted sleep. In this study, however, there was no improvement in sleep efficiency and no significant difference in other measures of sleep architecture. Monaca et al. studied 10 subjects with PSG pre-surgically and 3 months after bilateral STN DBS (1 night with DBS on and 1 night with DBS off) [14]. Compared to their pre-surgical evaluation, subjects reported improved sleep quality following STN DBS and post-surgical PSG showed increased sleep duration and sleep efficiency but no change in sleep architecture based on sleep stage percentage. There were no significant differences between the pre-surgical PSG night and the post-surgical DBS off night; therefore, the authors concluded that the lesional/subthalamotomy effect associated with electrode placement was not sufficient to improve sleep in these subjects [14]. However, Merlino and colleagues reported that microsubthalamotomy improved both objective and subjective sleep in 15 subjects who underwent PSG and questionnaire evaluation 1 week before and 1 week after STN DBS before the stimulator was turned on [15]. Cicolin and colleagues investigated polysomnographic changes before and 3 months after bilateral STN DBS in five patients with Parkinson's disease [16]. They found a significant increase in sleep efficiency and a significant reduction in latency to rapid-eye-movement (REM) sleep. They also reported trends toward increased total sleep time and time spent in slow wave sleep and REM sleep, but these did not reach significance. In each of these studies evaluating sleep architecture with PSG, there were no changes in REM Sleep Behavior Disorder or periodic limb movements of sleep before and after STN DBS [12, 16, 13, 14]. However, a recent study by Nishida and colleagues found a reduction in REM sleep without atonia [17]. They evaluated ten subjects (two with unilateral and eight with bilateral STN DBS) 1 week pre-surgically and 1 week after initial DBS programming. In addition to improvement in subjective sleep quality, PSG showed reduced wake after sleep onset, increased time spent in REM, and an increase in normal REM (atonic REM). Of the four subjects who met criteria for REM without atonia pre-surgically, three had restoration of REM atonia following surgery.

Additional studies have evaluated subjective sleep quality before and after STN DBS. Hjort and colleagues evaluated changes in subjective sleep quality using the Parkinson's disease sleep scale (PDSS) in 10 subjects 1 month before and 3 months after bilateral STN DBS compared to changes in sleep quality in 10 control subjects who were on the waiting list for DBS [18]. The subjects who underwent surgery had a significant improvement in sleep quality post-surgically while the control group had no significant change in sleep quality over the 4-month evaluation period, and the STN DBS group had significantly better sleep quality than the control group at the conclusion of the study. Lyons and colleagues evaluated 89 subjects before and 6 months after bilateral STN DBS and followed 83 of these subjects to 12 months and 43 of the subjects to 24 months post-operatively with 2 days of patient diaries at each time point [19]. This analysis showed an improvement in subjective total sleep time following surgery that persisted at 24 months. There was no change in daytime sleepiness post-surgically compared to baseline. Zibetti et al. evaluated 36 subjects with the UPDRS part IV at baseline and 12 and 24 months after bilateral STN DBS and reported an improvement in subjective sleep quality at both time-points based on item 41 of the questionnaire [20].

Unilateral STN DBS also improves subjective sleep quality. Our group evaluated 53 patients with the Pittsburgh Sleep Quality Index at baseline and 6 months after unilateral STN DBS and showed a significant improvement in subjective sleep quality over time [21]. Subjects who underwent right STN DBS had more improvement in sleep quality than subjects who underwent surgery on the left. Chahine and colleagues evaluated 17 subjects (12 with unilateral STN DBS and 5 with bilateral STN DBS) [22]. A combined analysis of all subjects showed improved subjective sleep quality and daytime sleepiness 4 weeks post-operatively that was sustained at 6 months. The 6 subjects in this group who had restless legs syndrome pre-operatively showed subjective improvement in symptoms at 4 weeks and 6 months compared to baseline.

The cause of the improvement in sleep quality and sleep architecture following STN DBS is likely multifactorial, related to improvements in PD motor symptoms, reduction of medications, improved quality of life, and possible stimulation-induced changes in sleep physiology. Further objective study with polysomnography in larger groups of subjects may help to further clarify how STN DBS alters sleep.

Despite the multiple reports of improvement in sleep following STN DBS, a single case report describes onset of severe insomnia following bilateral STN DBS [23]. The patient had continued right-sided motor symptoms and the left STN DBS electrode was determined to be positioned in the extreme external and anterior STN and was therefore repositioned. Following repositioning, the patient's insomnia resolved, with average total sleep time changing from approximately 4 h per night prior to repositioning to 8 h per night afterwards. The authors postulate that the malpositioned electrode disrupted inhibitory connections between the anterior hypothalamus and the upper reticular formation. This report supports the idea that DBS may directly alter sleep architecture in some circumstances.

15.3 Deep Brain Stimulation of the Globus Pallidus Internal Segment

Bilateral DBS of the GPi is also superior to best medical therapy for treatment of Parkinson's disease based on data from a prospective randomized trial [6]. Stimulation at this target is reported to be comparable to STN DBS in terms of motor outcomes up to 36 months post-operatively [24, 25]. Although some studies have shown more motor improvement and more adverse events in subjects undergoing STN versus GPi DBS, as reviewed: [26], a recent randomized study showed greater motor improvement with STN DBS with no difference between the targets in a composite outcome of cognitive and behavioral function [27]. While STN DBS was the preferred target for Parkinson's disease surgical therapy for a number of years, these findings have renewed interest in the use of GPi as a target for treatment of patients with moderate to advanced PD.

Despite the increased interest in GPi DBS for PD, relatively few studies have evaluated the effects of this stimulation site on sleep. One study reported pre- and post-operative quality of life assessments (Parkinson's Disease Questionnaire-39) in 11 subjects who underwent GPi DBS (7 bilateral and 4 unilateral). In this study, 6 of 11 subjects reported an improvement in daytime sleepiness following GPi DBS [28]. Volkmann and colleagues evaluated 20 subjects before surgery and at 6 and 36 months following bilateral GPi DBS with the Sickness Impact Profile as a measure of health related quality of life [29]. They reported a significant improvement in the Sleep and Rest subdomain of the scale at 6 months post-operatively that was not sustained at 36 months. To our knowledge, there are no published reports of polysomnographic outcomes in PD patients with GPi DBS. Future studies evaluating PSG and subjective sleep quality in these patients is important, particularly considering the increasing use of this therapy in PD patients.

15.4 Deep Brain Stimulation of the Ventral Intermediate Nucleus of the Thalamus (VIM)

DBS of the VIM was explored as an alternative to thalamotomy for the treatment of tremor in patients with Parkinson's disease. While it is effective for tremor control in patients with PD and essential tremor, VIM DBS does not provide marked improvement in bradykinesia, rigidity, or dyskinesias in Parkinson's disease [30]. Therefore, with the exception of select patients with tremor predominant Parkinson's disease, thalamic stimulation has largely been abandoned in favor of use of STN or GPi DBS. The proximity of the VIM to the reticular nucleus of the thalamus, where sleep spindles are generated, prompted Arnulf and colleagues to investigate for changes in sleep architecture following VIM DBS in six subjects (four with Parkinson's disease and two with essential tremor) [31]. They evaluated subjects 3–6 months post-operatively with 2 nights of PSG, 1 night with the stimulator at therapeutic settings and 1 night with the stimulator off. At high frequency stimulation (135–185 Hz), there were no changes in sleep architecture or sleep spindles compared to DBS off. In an unsuccessful attempt to induce sleep, the authors also evaluated subjects while awake during low frequency VIM stimulation (1 s bursts of 15 Hz or 30 s trains of 5 Hz) [31].

15.5 Deep Brain Stimulation of the Pedunculopontine Nucleus (PPN)

Due to its role in locomotion, the PPN has been explored as a DBS target in patients with Parkinson's disease who have significant gait disorder refractory to other therapies. Initial studies demonstrated that stereotactic placement of PPN electrodes is safe and that there may be some improvement in gait with bilateral PPN stimulation [32, 33]. Subsequent studies have shown mixed results and have not definitively demonstrated improvement in motor outcomes from stimulation of this novel target. Stefani and colleagues reported motor outcomes in six subjects with bilateral STN and PPN DBS [34], and simultaneous stimulation of PPN and STN produced some degree of additive motor improvement, but was not significantly better than STN DBS alone. Because PPN stimulation was not superior to STN DBS in this group of patients, the authors recommend PPN DBS only as a supplemental therapy to STN DBS [34]. In contrast, Moro and colleagues evaluated six subjects with unilateral PPN DBS and found no significant change in the UPDRS part III. Subjects did report a subjective improvement in falls in the open label phase of the study [35]. Ferraye and colleagues studied six subjects who had previously undergone bilateral STN DBS and evaluated the effects of bilateral PPN DBS. They reported a reduction in falls related to freezing in the off-medication state without significant changes in other gait measures [36]. Khan and colleagues studied seven subjects who underwent bilateral caudal zona incerta (cZI) and PPN DBS with evaluations prior to surgery and 1 year post-operatively [37]. In the on medication state, PPN DBS alone, cZI stimulation alone, or simultaneous stimulation of both targets resulted in statistically significant improvement in motor outcomes compared to baseline, and the combination stimulation was significantly more effective than either target alone [37]. In summary, published reports suggest that PPN DBS may improve balance when used in combination with STN stimulation in the on medication state. However, PPN studies to date have evaluated small numbers of subjects with different surgical approaches (unilateral versus bilateral) and in the context of parallel stimulation at other targets. Further study is needed to determine the benefit of this therapy for gait dysfunction in PD.

In addition to its function in locomotion, the PPN plays a critical role in regulation of behavioral state and sleep. For this reason, several groups have investigated the impact of PPN DBS on sleep in patients with PD. Romigi and colleagues reported polysomnography in one subject before surgery and after bilateral STN and PPN DBS [38]. PSG was performed post-operatively with STN DBS alone and PPN DBS alone. STN stimulation improved sleep efficiency compared to the pre-surgical PSG, but did not alter REM sleep. In contrast, PPN DBS increased the percentage of REM sleep and reduced REM latency. Sleep questionnaires from this patient and four others with bilateral PPN and STN DBS [39] in multiple conditions (PPN and STN on; PPN off and STN on; and PPN-cyclic on (on at night) and STN on) were evaluated at 3 months and 1 year post-operatively. At 3 months, the subjects had improvement in sleep quality based on the Parkinson's disease sleep scale (PDSS) in all three stimulation conditions. Evaluation of individual items from the PDSS suggested more improvement in insomnia when PPN stimulation (either continuous or cyclic) compared to STN stimulation alone. PPN cyclic on also caused further improvement in nocturnal restlessness and daytime dozing compared to the other two stimulation conditions. At 1-year follow-up, the improvement in sleep quality was maintained and subjects also had improvement in daytime sleepiness as measured by the Epworth sleepiness scale [39]. The authors also reported PSG recordings in two of these five subjects (one previously reported [38]) and found reduced REM latency and increase REM sleep [39].

Lim and colleagues investigated the effect of unilateral PPN DBS on sleep in five subjects (three with Parkinson's disease and two with progressive supranuclear palsy) [40]. Polysomnography was performed with PPN DBS on during the first night and with DBS off during the second night. PPN DBS resulted in higher percentage of REM sleep (14 %) compared to DBS off (8 %). REM time was also higher during the PPN DBS on night. PPN DBS did not induce any significant change in total sleep time, non-REM sleep, or wake after sleep onset. Interestingly, two of the five subjects had REM Sleep Behavior Disorder, and REM without atonia was unchanged with PPN DBS on versus off in these subjects [40].

In addition to these reports on the nocturnal effects of PPN DBS on sleep, another group has observed profound effects of PPN DBS on wake-time vigilance. Arnulf and colleagues initiated an investigation using a cross-over, double-blind design after observing that two patients with STN and PPN DBS fell asleep during routine programming of the PPN stimulator when high-frequency stimulation was applied [41]. During the daytime, the two subjects were evaluated with polysomnography for at least 5 min at each parameter: stimulation off, right, left, or bilateral at high frequency or low frequency with 3-min washout between each setting. At low frequency stimulation bilaterally or on either side, both subjects remained alert, but at high frequency stimulation, both subjects reported drowsiness and entered non-REM sleep, predominantly stage N1 and rarely stage N2. Interestingly, in one of the two subjects, abrupt cessation of low frequency PPN stimulation induced REM sleep on five different occasions [41].

In summary, DBS of the PPN likely alters arousal and sleep in complex ways and thus provides a unique opportunity to investigate the effects of stimulation at this site on sleep architecture. The distinct outcomes from high and low frequency PPN stimulation observed in these case reports suggests that altering the stimulation pattern in the PPN region can yield markedly different behavioral states. Further investigation may provide additional clues to the role of the PPN and its connections in both normal sleep architecture and sleep dysfunction in patients with Parkinson's disease.

15.6   Lesional Therapies for Parkinson's Disease

Deep brain stimulation became preferred over lesional therapies for Parkinson's disease because it is reversible, adjustable, and less likely to be associated with speech and bulbar dysfunction when performed bilaterally [42]. Despite this, lesion therapy is still performed commonly worldwide, and there is new interest in focused ultrasound for movement disorders [43]. In this context, review of the available literature on the effects of lesion therapies on sleep and vigilance may provide insights into sleep dysfunction in this patient population. An early case report documented induction of profound insomnia following bilateral thalamotomy for Parkinson's disease. The subject had baseline insomnia that was relieved by initial left thalamotomy. However, 2 years later following subsequent right thalamotomy, he developed severe insomnia and was observed in the hospital with no sleep for more than 96 h. Although he eventually was able to sleep again, he continued to have difficulty with insomnia after discharge [44]. A more recent case report documented a similar outcome following simultaneous left

VIM DBS and right VIM radiofrequency ablation. The patient developed severe insomnia following surgery that was not relieved by turning DBS off or by adjusting DBS parameters. The sleep changes were therefore attributed to lesion effects. The patient reported improvement in insomnia over time, but PSG recording 16 months post-operatively showed continued poor sleep efficiency, prolonged sleep latency, reduced sleep time, and abnormal sleep architecture [45]. Interestingly, the report by Bricolo also mentions anecdotal experience by the author that other patients undergoing bilateral thalamotomy often experience sleep disruption in the immediate post-operative period, but that these symptoms usually resolve quickly [44].

Roth and colleagues investigated the effects of bilateral stereotactic pallido-thalamic tractotomy in three subjects with Parkinson's disease with PSG before and after the surgery. The patients had a significant increase in total sleep time and sleep efficiency and a reduction in latency to REM sleep [46]. The authors propose that the alterations in sleep could be related to improved motor symptoms or post-surgical reduction of medications. Favre and colleagues reported subjective changes in motor and non-motor symptoms based on questionnaires before and after unilateral or simultaneous bilateral pallidotomy in 44 patients [47]. One of the parameters evaluated was sleep, with 59 % of patients reporting improvement in sleep following unilateral pallidotomy and 47 % of patients reporting improvement in sleep following simultaneous bilateral pallidotomy. It is unclear if these changes were related to improvement in motor symptoms, altered medications, or lesional effects on sleep architecture.

15.7 Other Surgical Therapies for Parkinson's Disease

In addition to DBS and lesional therapies for Parkinson's disease, another surgical therapy includes placement of an intrajejunal tube to administer continuous drug delivery with levodopa/carbidopa intestinal gel (LCIG) [48]. In addition to its influence on motor symptoms, the effects of this therapy on sleep quality and other non-motor symptoms have also been investigated. In an open label assessment, 22 subjects who received levodopa/carbidopa intrajejunal infusion were evaluated at baseline and after 6 months with the non-motor symptoms scale (NMSS) as the primary outcome measure. Additionally, 13 subjects were evaluated with the Parkinson's disease sleep scale (PDSS). The results showed a significant improvement in several domains of NMSS, including the sleep/fatigue domain and a significant improvement in the PDSS [49]. In another open label evaluation, 14 subjects were evaluated with the NMSS and the PDSS at baseline and at an average of 24 months after beginning therapy with LCIG. This study also showed a significant improvement in PDSS and a trend toward improvement in the sleep/fatigue domain of the NMSS [50]. Zibetti and colleagues report an additional open label evaluation of 12 subjects at baseline and 2–4 months after initiation of LCIG [51]. They report a 30 % improvement in subjective sleep symptoms and a 31 % improvement in subjective daytime sleepiness. The improvement in subjective sleep quality in these three studies is likely multifactorial, related to improved motor symptoms, altered dopaminergic medications, placebo effect, or other causes. As more patients undergo this therapy, controlled trials with more subjects and with objective PSG evaluation of sleep architecture should help to further elucidate these changes.

Conclusion

Surgical therapies play a key role in the treatment of motor symptoms of Parkinson's disease and provide a unique opportunity to investigate the impact of these therapies on sleep dysfunction in PD patients. To date, most studies have been case reports and small case series. Further objective study in larger patient samples with controls and blinding are required to gain a better understanding of the impact of these therapies on sleep [52]. Additionally, more mechanistic studies are needed to determine the etiology of sleep improvement. The change in sleep is likely multifactorial, related to increased nocturnal mobility due to motor improvement, medication adjustment, changes in mood, placebo effect, or direct effects of the surgical therapy on sleep architecture. Many questions remain to be answered [52]: Is there an influence of laterality of DBS or lesional therapy on sleep outcomes? Are there effects from stimulation of other structures in anatomical proximity to the DBS target? Are there other stimulation settings that are more beneficial for sleep than the conventional settings? Surgical therapies are an important treatment option for PD, and more knowledge about how these therapies alter wakefulness and sleep will provide information to tailor therapies that optimize outcomes for individual patients.

Acknowledgments   This work was supported in part by the Francis and Ingeborg Heide Schumann Fellowship in Parkinson's Disease Research (AA) and the Sartain Lanier Family Foundation (HW), and grant funding from the NIH NINDS K23NS080912 (AW) and NIH NINDS K23NS067053 (HW), and the American Sleep Medicine Foundation (AW). We would also like to sincerely thank Anthony Nicholas for contributing the content of Fig. 15.1.

References

1. Speelman JD, Bosch DA. Resurgence of functional neurosurgery for Parkinson's disease: a historical perspective. Mov Disord. 1998;13(3):582–8. doi:10.1002/mds.870130336.
2. Hariz MI, Blomstedt P, Zrinzo L. Deep brain stimulation between 1947 and 1987: the untold story. Neurosurg Focus. 2010;29(2):E1. doi:10.3171/2010.4.FOCUS10106.
3. Bergman H, Wichmann T, DeLong MR. Reversal of experimental Parkinsonism by lesions of the subthalamic nucleus. Science. 1990;249(4975):1436–8.
4. Pollak P, Benabid AL, Gross C, Gao DM, Laurent A, Benazzouz A, Hoffmann D, Gentil M, Perret J. Effects of the stimulation of the subthalamic nucleus in Parkinson disease. Rev Neurol (Paris). 1993;149(3):175–6.
5. Sako W, Miyazaki Y, Izumi Y, Kaji R. Which target is best for patients with Parkinson's disease? A meta-analysis of pallidal and subthalamic stimulation. J Neurol Neurosurg Psychiatry. 2014;85(9):982–6. doi:10.1136/jnnp-2013-306090.
6. Weaver FM, Follett K, Stern M, Hur K, Harris C, Marks Jr WJ, Rothlind J, Sagher O, Reda D, Moy CS, Pahwa R, Burchiel K, Hogarth P, Lai EC, Duda JE, Holloway K, Samii A, Horn S, Bronstein J, Stoner G, Heemskerk J, Huang GD. Bilateral deep brain stimulation versus best medical therapy for patients with advanced Parkinson's disease: a randomized controlled trial. JAMA. 2009;301(1):63–73. doi:10.1001/jama.2008.929. 301/1/63 [pii].

7. Deuschl G, Schade-Brittinger C, Krack P, Volkmann J, Schafer H, Botzel K, Daniels C, Deutschlander A, Dillmann U, Eisner W, Gruber D, Hamel W, Herzog J, Hilker R, Klebe S, Kloss M, Koy J, Krause M, Kupsch A, Lorenz D, Lorenzl S, Mehdorn HM, Moringlane JR, Oertel W, Pinsker MO, Reichmann H, Reuss A, Schneider GH, Schnitzler A, Steude U, Sturm V, Timmermann L, Tronnier V, Trottenberg T, Wojtecki L, Wolf E, Poewe W, Voges J. A randomized trial of deep brain stimulation for Parkinson's disease. N Engl J Med. 2006;355(9):896–908. doi:10.1056/NEJMoa060281. 355/9/896 [pii].

8. Williams A, Gill S, Varma T, Jenkinson C, Quinn N, Mitchell R, Scott R, Ives N, Rick C, Daniels J, Patel S, Wheatley K. Deep brain stimulation plus best medical therapy versus best medical therapy alone for advanced Parkinson's disease (PD SURG trial): a randomised, open-label trial. Lancet Neurol. 2010;9(6):581–91. doi:10.1016/S1474-4422(10)70093-4. S1474-4422(10)70093-4 [pii].

9. Walker HC, Watts RL, Guthrie S, Wang D, Guthrie BL. Bilateral effects of unilateral subthalamic deep brain stimulation on Parkinson's disease at 1 year. Neurosurgery. 2009;65(2):302–9; discussion 309–10. doi:10.1227/01.NEU.0000349764.34211.74. 00006123-200908000-00011 [pii].

10. Tabbal SD, Ushe M, Mink JW, Revilla FJ, Wernle AR, Hong M, Karimi M, Perlmutter JS. Unilateral subthalamic nucleus stimulation has a measurable ipsilateral effect on rigidity and bradykinesia in Parkinson disease. Exp Neurol. 2008;211(1):234–42. doi:10.1016/j.expneurol.2008.01.024. S0014-4886(08)00057-5 [pii].

11. Slowinski JL, Putzke JD, Uitti RJ, Lucas JA, Turk MF, Kall BA, Wharen RE. Unilateral deep brain stimulation of the subthalamic nucleus for Parkinson's disease. J Neurosurg. 2007;106(4):626–32. doi:10.3171/jns.2007.106.4.626.

12. Arnulf I, Bejjani BP, Garma L, Bonnet AM, Houeto JL, Damier P, Derenne JP, Agid Y. Improvement of sleep architecture in Parkinson's disease with subthalamic nucleus stimulation. Neurology. 2000;55(11):1732–4.

13. Iranzo A, Valldeoriola F, Santamaria J, Tolosa E, Rumia J. Sleep symptoms and polysomnographic architecture in advanced Parkinson's disease after chronic bilateral subthalamic stimulation. J Neurol Neurosurg Psychiatry. 2002;72(5):661–4.

14. Monaca C, Ozsancak C, Jacquesson JM, Poirot I, Blond S, Destee A, Guieu JD, Derambure P. Effects of bilateral subthalamic stimulation on sleep in Parkinson's disease. J Neurol. 2004;251(2):214–8.

15. Merlino G, Lettieri C, Mondani M, Belgrado E, Devigili G, Mucchiut M, Rinaldo S, Craighero C, D'Auria S, Skrap M, Eleopra R. Microsubthalamotomy improves sleep in patients affected by advanced Parkinson's disease. Sleep Med. 2014;15(6):637–41. doi:10.1016/j.sleep.2013.12.016.

16. Cicolin A, Lopiano L, Zibetti M, Torre E, Tavella A, Guastamacchia G, Terreni A, Makrydakis G, Fattori E, Lanotte MM, Bergamasco B, Mutani R. Effects of deep brain stimulation of the subthalamic nucleus on sleep architecture in parkinsonian patients. Sleep Med. 2004;5(2):207–10. doi:10.1016/j.sleep.2003.10.010. S1389945704000061 [pii].

17. Nishida N, Murakami T, Kadoh K, Tohge R, Yamanegi M, Saiki H, Ueda K, Matsumoto S, Ishikawa M, Takahashi JA, Toda H. Subthalamic nucleus deep brain stimulation restores normal rapid eye movement sleep in Parkinson's disease. Mov Disord. 2011;26(13):2418–22. doi:10.1002/mds.23862.

18. Hjort N, Ostergaard K, Dupont E. Improvement of sleep quality in patients with advanced Parkinson's disease treated with deep brain stimulation of the subthalamic nucleus. Mov Disord. 2004;19(2):196–9.

19. Lyons KE, Pahwa R. Effects of bilateral subthalamic nucleus stimulation on sleep, daytime sleepiness, and early morning dystonia in patients with Parkinson disease. J Neurosurg. 2006;104(4):502–5.

20. Zibetti M, Torre E, Cinquepalmi A, Rosso M, Ducati A, Bergamasco B, Lanotte M, Lopiano L. Motor and non-motor symptom follow-up in parkinsonian patients after deep brain stimulation of the subthalamic nucleus. Eur Neurol. 2007;58(4):218–23.

21. Amara AW, Standaert DG, Guthrie S, Cutter G, Watts RL, Walker H. Unilateral subthalamic nucleus deep brain stimulation improves sleep quality in Parkinson's disease. Parkinsonism Relat Disord. 2012;18(1):63–8. doi:10.1016/j.parkreldis.2011.09.001. S1353-8020(11)00298-7 [pii].

22. Chahine LM, Ahmed A, Sun Z. Effects of STN DBS for Parkinson's disease on restless legs syndrome and other sleep-related measures. Parkinsonism Relat Disord. 2011;17(3):208–11. doi:10.1016/j.parkreldis.2010.11.017. S1353-8020(10)00297-X [pii].

23. Monaca C, Ozsancak C, Defebvre L, Blond S, Destee A, Guieu JD, Derambure P. Transient insomnia induced by high-frequency deep brain stimulation in Parkinson's disease. Neurology. 2004;62(7):1232–3.

24. Follett KA, Weaver FM, Stern M, Hur K, Harris CL, Luo P, Marks Jr WJ, Rothlind J, Sagher O, Moy C, Pahwa R, Burchiel K, Hogarth P, Lai EC, Duda JE, Holloway K, Samii A, Horn S, Bronstein JM, Stoner G, Starr PA, Simpson R, Baltuch G, De Salles A, Huang GD, Reda DJ. Pallidal versus subthalamic deep brain stimulation for Parkinson's disease. N Engl J Med. 2010;362(22):2077–91. doi:10.1056/NEJMoa0907083. 362/22/2077 [pii].

25. Weaver FM, Follett KA, Stern M, Luo P, Harris CL, Hur K, Marks Jr WJ, Rothlind J, Sagher O, Moy C, Pahwa R, Burchiel K, Hogarth P, Lai EC, Duda JE, Holloway K, Samii A, Horn S, Bronstein JM, Stoner G, Starr PA, Simpson R, Baltuch G, De Salles A, Huang GD, Reda DJ. Randomized trial of deep brain stimulation for Parkinson's disease: thirty-six-month outcomes. Neurology. 2012;79(1):55–65. doi:10.1212/WNL.0b013e31825dcdc1. WNL.0b013e31825dcdc1 [pii].

26. Follett KA, Torres-Russotto D. Deep brain stimulation of globus pallidus interna, subthalamic nucleus, and pedunculopontine nucleus for PD: which target? Parkinsonism Relat Disord. 2012;18 Suppl 1:S165–7. doi:10.1016/S1353-8020(11)70051-7. S1353-8020(11)70051-7 [pii].

27. Odekerken VJ, van Laar T, Staal MJ, Mosch A, Hoffmann CF, Nijssen PC, Beute GN, van Vugt JP, Lenders MW, Contarino MF, Mink MS, Bour LJ, van den Munckhof P, Schmand BA, de Haan RJ, Schuurman PR, de Bie RM. Subthalamic nucleus versus globus pallidus bilateral deep brain stimulation for advanced Parkinson's disease (NSTAPS study): a randomised controlled trial. Lancet Neurol. 2013;12(1):37–44. doi:10.1016/S1474-4422(12)70264-8. S1474-4422(12)70264-8 [pii].

28. Rodrigues JP, Walters SE, Watson P, Stell R, Mastaglia FL. Globus pallidus stimulation improves both motor and non-motor aspects of quality of life in advanced Parkinson's disease. Mov Disord. 2007;22(13):1866–70. doi:10.1002/mds.21427.

29. Volkmann J, Albanese A, Kulisevsky J, Tornqvist AL, Houeto JL, Pidoux B, Bonnet AM, Mendes A, Benabid AL, Fraix V, Van Blercom N, Xie J, Obeso J, Rodriguez-Oroz MC, Guridi J, Schnitzler A, Timmermann L, Gironell AA, Molet J, Pascual-Sedano B, Rehncrona S, Moro E, Lang AC, Lozano AM, Bentivoglio AR, Scerrati M, Contarino MF, Romito L, Janssens M, Agid Y. Long-term effects of pallidal or subthalamic deep brain stimulation on quality of life in Parkinson's disease. Mov Disord. 2009;24(8):1154–61.

30. Hariz MI, Krack P, Alesch F, Augustinsson LE, Bosch A, Ekberg R, Johansson F, Johnels B, Meyerson BA, N'Guyen JP, Pinter M, Pollak P, von Raison F, Rehncrona S, Speelman JD, Sydow O, Benabid AL. Multicentre European study of thalamic stimulation for parkinsonian tremor: a 6 year follow-up. J Neurol Neurosurg Psychiatry. 2008;79(6):694–9. doi:10.1136/jnnp.2007.118653. jnnp.2007.118653 [pii].

31. Arnulf I, Bejjani BP, Garma L, Bonnet AM, Damier P, Pidoux B, Dormont D, Cornu P, Derenne JP, Agid Y. Effect of low and high frequency thalamic stimulation on sleep in patients with Parkinson's disease and essential tremor. J Sleep Res. 2000;9(1):55–62. jsr171 [pii].

32. Mazzone P, Lozano A, Stanzione P, Galati S, Scarnati E, Peppe A, Stefani A. Implantation of human pedunculopontine nucleus: a safe and clinically relevant target in Parkinson's disease. Neuroreport. 2005;16(17):1877–81. 00001756-200511280-00002 [pii].

33. Plaha P, Gill SS. Bilateral deep brain stimulation of the pedunculopontine nucleus for Parkinson's disease. Neuroreport. 2005;16(17):1883–7. 00001756-200511280-00003 [pii].

34. Stefani A, Lozano AM, Peppe A, Stanzione P, Galati S, Tropepi D, Pierantozzi M, Brusa L, Scarnati E, Mazzone P. Bilateral deep brain stimulation of the pedunculopontine and subthalamic nuclei in severe Parkinson's disease. Brain. 2007;130(Pt 6):1596–607. doi:10.1093/brain/awl346. awl346 [pii].

35. Moro E, Hamani C, Poon YY, Al-Khairallah T, Dostrovsky JO, Hutchison WD, Lozano AM. Unilateral pedunculopontine stimulation improves falls in Parkinson's disease. Brain. 2010;133(Pt 1):215–24. doi:10.1093/brain/awp261. awp261 [pii].
36. Ferraye MU, Debu B, Fraix V, Goetz L, Ardouin C, Yelnik J, Henry-Lagrange C, Seigneuret E, Piallat B, Krack P, Le Bas JF, Benabid AL, Chabardes S, Pollak P. Effects of pedunculopontine nucleus area stimulation on gait disorders in Parkinson's disease. Brain. 2010;133(Pt 1):205–14. doi:10.1093/brain/awp229. awp229 [pii].
37. Khan S, Mooney L, Plaha P, Javed S, White P, Whone AL, Gill SS. Outcomes from stimulation of the caudal zona incerta and pedunculopontine nucleus in patients with Parkinson's disease. Br J Neurosurg. 2011;25(2):273–80. doi:10.3109/02688697.2010.544790.
38. Romigi A, Placidi F, Peppe A, Pierantozzi M, Izzi F, Brusa L, Galati S, Moschella V, Marciani MG, Mazzone P, Stanzione P, Stefani A. Pedunculopontine nucleus stimulation influences rapid eye movement sleep in Parkinson's disease. Eur J Neurol. 2008;15(7):e64–5. doi:10.1111/j.1468-1331.2008.02167.x. ENE2167 [pii].
39. Peppe A, Pierantozzi M, Baiamonte V, Moschella V, Caltagirone C, Stanzione P, Stefani A. Deep brain stimulation of pedunculopontine tegmental nucleus: role in sleep modulation in advanced Parkinson's disease patients: one-year follow-up. Sleep. 2012;35(12):1637–42. doi:10.5665/sleep.2234.
40. Lim AS, Moro E, Lozano AM, Hamani C, Dostrovsky JO, Hutchison WD, Lang AE, Wennberg RA, Murray BJ. Selective enhancement of rapid eye movement sleep by deep brain stimulation of the human pons. Ann Neurol. 2009;66(1):110–4.
41. Arnulf I, Ferraye M, Fraix V, Benabid AL, Chabardes S, Goetz L, Pollak P, Debu B. Sleep induced by stimulation in the human pedunculopontine nucleus area. Ann Neurol. 2010;67(4):546–9. doi:10.1002/ana.21912.
42. Hariz M. Twenty-five years of deep brain stimulation: celebrations and apprehensions. Mov Disord. 2012;27(7):930–3. doi:10.1002/mds.25007.
43. Elias WJ, Huss D, Voss T, Loomba J, Khaled M, Zadicario E, Frysinger RC, Sperling SA, Wylie S, Monteith SJ, Druzgal J, Shah BB, Harrison M, Wintermark M. A pilot study of focused ultrasound thalamotomy for essential tremor. N Engl J Med. 2013;369(7):640–8. doi:10.1056/NEJMoa1300962.
44. Bricolo A. Insomnia after bilateral stereotactic thalamotomy in man. J Neurol Neurosurg Psychiatry. 1967;30(2):154–8.
45. Quigg M, Frysinger RC, Harrison M, Elias WJ. Acute insomnia following surgery of the ventralis intermedius nucleus of the thalamus for tremor. J Clin Sleep Med. 2007;3(1):58–9.
46. Roth C, Jeanmonod D, Magnin M, Morel A, Achermann P. Effects of medial thalamotomy and pallido-thalamic tractotomy on sleep and waking EEG in pain and Parkinsonian patients. Clin Neurophysiol. 2000;111(7):1266–75. S1388-2457(00)00295-9 [pii].
47. Favre J, Burchiel KJ, Taha JM, Hammerstad J. Outcome of unilateral and bilateral pallidotomy for Parkinson's disease: patient assessment. Neurosurgery. 2000;46(2):344–53; discussion 353–5.
48. Nyholm D, Askmark H, Gomes-Trolin C, Knutson T, Lennernas H, Nystrom C, Aquilonius SM. Optimizing levodopa pharmacokinetics: intestinal infusion versus oral sustained-release tablets. Clin Neuropharmacol. 2003;26(3):156–63.
49. Honig H, Antonini A, Martinez-Martin P, Forgacs I, Faye GC, Fox T, Fox K, Mancini F, Canesi M, Odin P, Chaudhuri KR. Intrajejunal levodopa infusion in Parkinson's disease: a pilot multicenter study of effects on non-motor symptoms and quality of life. Mov Disord. 2009;24(10):1468–74. doi:10.1002/mds.22596.
50. Fasano A, Ricciardi L, Lena F, Bentivoglio AR, Modugno N. Intrajejunal levodopa infusion in advanced Parkinson's disease: long-term effects on motor and non-motor symptoms and impact on patient's and caregiver's quality of life. Eur Rev Med Pharmacol Sci. 2012;16(1):79–89.
51. Zibetti M, Rizzone M, Merola A, Angrisano S, Rizzi L, Montanaro E, Cicolin A, Lopiano L. Sleep improvement with levodopa/carbidopa intestinal gel infusion in Parkinson's disease. Acta Neurol Scand. 2013;127(5):e28–32. doi:10.1111/ane.12075.
52. Amara AW, Watts RL, Walker HC. The effects of deep brain stimulation on sleep in Parkinson's disease. Ther Adv Neurol Disord. 2011;4(1):15–24. doi:10.1177/1756285610392446.

Sleep Disorders in Atypical Parkinsonisms

16

Alex Iranzo

Contents

Abstract

Atypical parkinsonism includes dementia with Lewy bodies (DLB), multiple system atrophy (MSA), and progressive supranuclear palsy (PSP). In DLB, insomnia, circadian rhythm changes, frequent daytime napping, confusional awakenings, and REM sleep behavior disorder (RBD) are frequent. Severity of dementia is linked to abnormal sleep architecture even in the forms of ambiguous sleep and status dissociatus. In DLB, RBD may be the presenting symptom and is considered a red flag of the disease. About 70 % of the MSA patients report sleep problems such as insufficient and fragmented sleep, hypersomnia, RBD, and stridor. RBD

A. Iranzo, MD, PhD
Neurology Service, Hospital Clínic de Barcelona
and Institut d'Investigació Biomèdiques August Pi i Sunyer (IDIBAPS),
C/Villarroel 170, Barcelona 08036, Spain
e-mail: airanzo@clinic.ub.es

© Springer-Verlag Wien 2015
A. Videnovic, B. Högl (eds.), *Disorders of Sleep and Circadian Rhythms in Parkinson's Disease*, DOI 10.1007/978-3-7091-1631-9_16

and stridor are considered red flags of MSA and may be their initial manifestation. Death during sleep is not infrequent in MSA subjects with untreated stridor. Nasal continuous positive airway pressure and tracheostomy abolish stridor in MSA. PSP patients complain of insomnia and have reduced and abnormal sleep architecture on polysomnography. RBD occurs in PSP but is much less frequent than in DLB and MSA. The cause of sleep disorders in atypical parkinsonisms are multifactorial and they include the degenerative process itself; parkinsonism leading to immobility; coexistent disturbances such as depression, dementia, and anxiety; and the effect of some medications. Treatment should be individualized.

Atypical parkinsonisms are neurological conditions where parkinsonism (defined as the combination of bradykinesia, rigidity, and tremor) is present with the exception of idiopathic Parkinson's disease (PD). These conditions include DLB, MSA, PSP, corticobasal degeneration, and others. Besides parkinsonism, other symptoms occur such as ataxia, oculomotor abnormalities, dysautonomic features, dementia, and sleep problems. Disorders of sleep in atypical parkinsonisms include insomnia, excessive daytime sleepiness (EDS), RBD, restless legs syndrome (RLS), and sleep-disordered breathing (SDB). This chapter reviews the sleep disorders occurring in DLB, MSA, and PSP, as three most common of neurodegenerative atypical parkinsonian disorders (Tables 16.1 and 16.2).

Table 16.1 Main sleep disturbances in the atypical parkinsonisms dementia with Lewy bodies, multiple system atrophy, and progressive supranuclear palsy

1. Dementia with Lewy bodies
1.1. Insomnia
1.2. Circadian rhythmic dysregulation
1.3. Excessive daytime sleepiness
1.4. Confusional awakenings
1.5. Nocturnal wandering
1.6. Ambiguous sleep and status dissociatus
1.7. Periodic leg movements in sleep
1.8. REM sleep behavior disorder
2. Multiple system atrophy
2.1. Insomnia
2.2. Excessive daytime sleepiness
2.3. Periodic and aperiodic limb movements in non-REM sleep
2.4. REM sleep behavior disorder
2.5. Central hypoventilation
2.6. Central sleep apnea
2.7. Obstructive sleep apnea
2.8. Stridor due to vocal cord obstruction at the larynx
3. Progressive supranuclear palsy
3.1. Insomnia
3.2. Subclinical REM sleep without atonia
3.3. Mild form of REM sleep behavior disorder

Table 16.2 Main sleep disturbances in other atypical parkinsonisms

1. Corticobasal degeneration
1.1. Insomnia
1.2. Anecdotal descriptions of REM sleep behavior disorder
2. Autosomal dominant spinocerebellar ataxias
2.1. Restless legs syndrome (SCA 3 and less frequently in SCA 1, SCA 2, and SCA 6)
2.2. Periodic leg movements in sleep (SCA 1,2,3, and 6)
2.3. Subclinical REM sleep without atonia (SCA 2)
2.4. REM sleep behavior disorder (SCA 3 and not in SCA 1 and in SCA 2)
2.5. Anecdotal descriptions of stridor due to vocal cord abductor paralysis in SCA 3
3. Huntington disease
3.1. Insomnia
3.2. Circadian rhythmic dysregulation
3.3. Excessive daytime sleepiness
3.4. Mild form of restless legs syndrome
3.5. Subclinical periodic leg movements in sleep
3.6. Mild form of REM sleep behavior disorder

16.1 Dementia with Lewy Bodies (DLB)

DLB is the second most common cause of neurodegenerative dementia after Alzheimer's disease (AD). It is characterized by parkinsonism, recurrent visual hallucinations, and fluctuations in cognition and alertness. DLB is diagnosed if dementia precedes or appears within 1 year before onset of parkinsonism. Neuronal loss and Lewy bodies are found in the brainstem, limbic system, and neocortex [1].

16.1.1 Studies Evaluating Sleep Disorders

Overall, insomnia, circadian rhythm disorder with early awakening, EDS due to frequent napping, nocturnal hallucinations, and confusional nocturnal wandering are frequent. In contrast, SDB and RLS seem to be no more common than in the general population of similar age. RBD is very common and may antedate the onset of dementia by several years. Detection of RBD in a patient with dementia point toward DLB because this parasomnia is rare in other forms of dementia including AD, frontotemporal dementia, and PSP.

In a large multicenter study, Bliwise et al. [2] compared nocturnal sleep disturbance between 339 patients with DLB and 4,192 with AD. Sleep problems were estimated by the informant report through the Neuropsychiatric Inventory Questionnaire (NPI-Q) item "Does the patient awaken you at night, rise too early in the morning, or takes excessive naps during the day?" Nocturnal sleep disturbance was more frequent in DLB (63 %) than in AD (27 %) and was not linked to more advanced disease, depressive symptoms, apathy, hallucinations, delusions, or agitation.

In a retrospective study, Pao et al. [3] reviewed the polysomnographic (PSG) findings of 78 DLB patients (71 male, mean age 71 years) with sleep-related complaints. Seventy-five (96 %) patients had histories of dream-enactment behaviors with 65 (83 %) showing confirmation of RBD during PSG. The remaining 13 subjects did not attain any REM sleep, and hence RBD could not be confirmed by PSG. Mean respiratory disturbance index (RDI, number of apneas and hypopneas per hour of sleep) was 12, and this was greater than 5 in 60 % and greater than 10 in 36 %. The mean periodic leg movements in sleep (PLMS) index (number of PLMS per hour of sleep) associated with arousals was 6. Sleep efficiency was less than 80 % in 72 % of the subjects, and about 75 % of the sample had isolated arousals. Among the six patients who underwent multiple sleep latency test (MSLT) two showed a sleep latency onset of less than 5 min and none showed REM sleep.

Terzaghi et al. [4] evaluated the clinical and video-PSG findings of 29 consecutive DLB patients. Patients were taking levodopa but no dopamine agonists, benzodiazepines, cholinergics, neuroleptics, or antidepressants. Patients were 21 males, their mean age was 75 years and mean disease duration was 3 years. Eleven (38 %) patients reported insomnia, 17 (59 %) EDS, 1 (3 %) had RLS, 3 (10 %) nightmares, 23 (79 %) hallucinations at night, 19 (65 %) episodes suggestive of confusional arousals, and 18 (62 %) episodes suggestive of RBD. Video-PSG showed a mean sleep efficiency of 55 %, mean RDI of 6, and mean PLMS index of 50. REM sleep without atonia was found in 46 %, RDI greater than 5 in 35 % and PLMS index greater than 15 in 61 %. Dissociated or ambiguous sleep was found in six patients who had severe dementia. Disruptive motor behaviors during sleep were found in 70 % and consisted in RBD in 11 subjects, confusional episodes from NREM sleep in 7 cases, and arousal-related episodes from REM or NREM sleep mimicking RBD in 2. Of note, these REM and NREM sleep enactment behaviors have also been described to occur in PD associated with dementia [5].

16.1.2 REM Sleep Behavior Disorder (RBD)

The most studied sleep disturbance in DLB is RBD. Available data indicate that in subjects with DLB, RBD is common, may be the first symptom of the disease, is associated with less AD pathology in the brain, and can be considered a red flag of the disease. RBD is very rare in AD and other forms of dementia with the exception of PD associated with dementia. Current diagnostic criteria of DLB consider RBD as a *suggestive* feature of the disease because "it has been demonstrated to be more frequent than in other dementing disorders" [1]. This statement was initially based on a single retrospective study involving 37 consecutive patients with dementia plus RBD [6]. Thirty-four of these patients (92 %) were male. In 35 (96 %) RBD symptoms preceded or occurred simultaneously with the cognitive complaints. Of the 37 patients, 23 fulfilled the 1996-consensus criteria for probable DLB (dementia plus at least two of the following: parkinsonism, visual hallucinations, and fluctuations), and all fulfilled criteria for possible DLB (dementia plus one of the following:

parkinsonism, visual hallucinations, and fluctuations) [7]. The diagnosis of DLB was confirmed in the three patients that underwent autopsy and supported the notion that the combination of dementia and RBD most often reflects DLB. This is in agreement with neuropathological studies in patients with antemortem diagnosis of DLB plus RBD showing cell loss and Lewy bodies in the brainstem, limbic system, and neocortex [8, 9]. In a cohort of 234 autopsy-confirmed dementia patients followed longitudinally, a history of definite or probable RBD was present in 76 % of 98 with autopsy confirmed DLB, indicating that RBD is a common feature of DLB. In contrast, only 6 of the 136 patients without autopsy-confirmed DLB exhibited RBD [9]. Thus, inclusion of RBD improves the diagnostic accuracy of DLB [9]. Dugger et al. [10] compared the clinical characteristics of 71 DLB patients with RBD and 19 without RBD. Those with RBD were predominantly male, had shorter duration of dementia, earlier onset of parkinsonism and visual hallucinations, and less AD-related pathology on autopsy. In 54 of the 71 (76 %) RBD patients this parasomnia coincided or developed before dementia onset. This group of patients in whom RBD developed before cognitive impairment were characterized by earlier onset of visual hallucinations and parkinsonism, more severe baseline parkinsonism and shorter duration of dementia.

On the other hand, patients initially diagnosed with idiopathic RBD frequently are diagnosed with DLB and other synucleinopathies (mainly PD and less frequently MSA) with time. We reported that in a cohort of 44 IRBD subjects, 36 (82 %) were eventually diagnosed with a defined neurodegenerative syndrome: 14 with DLB, 16 with PD, 1 with MSA and 5 with mild cognitive impairment [11]. All 14 subjects diagnosed with DLB were men. In these subjects with DLB, recurrent visual hallucinations occurred in 13 (93 %), parkinsonism in 11 (79 %), and fluctuating cognition in 9 (65 %). Dementia was preceded by a recognized period of mild cognitive impairment characterized by executive, visuospatial and memory dysfunction. The median interval between the diagnosis of mild cognitive impairment and the diagnosis of DLB was 2 years. Median age at DLB diagnosis was 76 years, median RBD duration at the time of the diagnosis of DLB was 12 years, and the median interval between diagnosis of RBD with PSG and clinical diagnosis of DLB was 7 years.

16.2 Multiple System Atrophy (MSA)

MSA is a progressive neurodegenerative disorder characterized by a combination of parkinsonism, cerebellar syndrome, and autonomic failure [12]. Neuropathology shows neuronal loss and alpha-synuclein positive glial cytoplasmic inclusions in many brain structures. About 70 % of the MSA patients, regardless of the parkinsonian or cerebellar clinical subtype, report sleep problems. Insufficient and fragmented sleep, EDS, RBD, nocturnal stridor, and SDB are common in MSA. RBD and stridor are considered red flags of the disease and may be initial manifestation. Death during sleep is not infrequent and may be related to laryngeal narrowing.

16.2.1 Sleep Fragmentation

Sleep onset insomnia and interrupted sleep are common complains. PSG studies have consistently found low sleep efficiency between 40 and 60 %, increased sleep latency and excessive sleep fragmentation, with relatively long periods of wakefulness throughout the night, sometimes without a clear cause [13–22]. However, there is a small subgroup of patients that report no sleep problems despite PSG shows dramatic fragmented sleep, severe PLMS and intense RBD. In MSA, many causes may contribute to sleep fragmentation and these include urinary incontinence, anxiety, depression, PLMS, inability to change body position in the bed because of parkinsonism, and the use of several medications. Abnormal nighttime sleep increases with progression of the disease. It is unclear, though, if interrupted sleep contributes to EDS in MSA.

16.2.2 Excessive Daytime Sleepiness (EDS)

EDS is frequent but in most of the cases is not a major complaint. Many variables may induce EDS in MSA but studies have not found consistent clues of which are the most relevant. Moreno-López et al. [21] evaluated EDS in 86 European MSA subjects (73 with the parkinsonian and 13 with the cerebellar subtypes) with the Epworth sleepiness scale (ESS). Mean EES score was higher (more indicative of hypersomnia) in MSA than in healthy subjects (7.72 versus 4.5). EDS (defined as an ESS greater than 10) was present in 28 % of the patients and in 2 % of the healthy subjects. EDS was associated with SDB and low sleep efficiency, and not with disease duration and dopaminergic therapy. Shimohata et al. [22] evaluated EDS in 25 Japanese patients (21 with the cerebellar and 4 with the parkinsonian subtypes) and found that the mean ESS was 6.2 and that the score was greater than 10 in 24 %. PSG detected SDB in 96 % and PLMS in 44 % but these variables were not linked to ESS score. Guo et al. [19] found a mean EES score of 8.2 in a sample of 37 subjects from China. In one small study [23] in which MSLT was performed in five MSA patients, the sleep latency was normal in four, despite poor nocturnal sleep quality. Hypocretin neurons have been found to be moderately decreased in the brain of patients with MSA [24] but hypocretin-1 levels in the cerebrospinal fluid were normal [23]. Sleep attacks induced by the introduction of levodopa have been reported in a few MSA patients with the parkinsonian subtype.

16.2.3 Restless Legs Syndrome (RLS)

There are only a few studies addressing whether RLS is common in the backdrop of MSA and they have shown different results. An optimal strategy would be to study untreated MSA patients and to exclude other conditions with symptoms that may resemble RLS. None of the published studies, however, have excluded other forms of sensory and motor problems that are common in MSA and that may mimic the symptoms of RLS (e.g., rigidity, stiffness, central pain, dystonia, etc.). Most of these studies evaluated the presence of RLS in subjects already treated for parkinsonism with dopaminergic agents, a therapy that may mask the symptoms of true RLS. Thus, the prevalence of RLS given in these studies may have been either underestimated or overestimated. Moreno et al. [21] found RLS in 24 (28 %) of 86 subjects, 23 with the parkinsonian subtype and 1 with the cerebellar subtype, and RLS was unrelated to the amount of dopaminergic therapy. Other studies reported RLS in 3 % [20] and 12 % [16, 22] of the patients.

16.2.4 Periodic Leg Movements in Sleep (PLMS)

It is not clear whether PLMS are more frequent in MSA than in the general population of similar age. One small study comparing PLMS in untreated ten MSA patients, ten PD patients, and ten matched controls found an increase in PLMS in PD only [25]. Compared to controls, MSA patients had more PLMS (mean PLMS index of 34 versus 14), but the difference did not reach the level of significance. Overall, PSG studies commonly disclose PLMS in untreated and dopaminergic-treated patients with MSA, both with the predominantly parkinsonian and cerebellar presentations [15, 19, 20, 22]. Most patients with MSA who experience PLMS are unaware of these leg movements probably because they are generally not associated with arousals. Therefore, PLMS in MSA do not appear to be a main contributing factor for developing sleep fragmentation and EDS. In MSA, it is common to find aperiodic leg and upper limb movements in non-REM sleep which in some cases resemble visually those typical jerky and brisk movements seen in RBD during REM sleep.

16.2.5 REM Sleep Behavior Disorder (RBD)

A majority of patients with MSA have RBD with a prevalence of 70–100 % [13, 15, 20, 26–28]. The finding that in MSA brainstem cell loss is consistently widespread and severe may explain the high prevalence of RBD in this disease. In one study, 21 consecutive MSA patients without sleep behavioral complaints underwent video-PSG that demonstrated RBD in 19 (90.5 %) [27]. In another study, video-PSG showed RBD in 35 out of 37 (95 %) consecutive patients [13]. In our experience, all 78 MSA patients who were referred to our sleep center from April 1997 to October 2013 for different reasons (suspected RBD, stridor, or sleep fragmentation) had RBD on video-PSG. Taken together, we think that in a patient with suspected MSA, the absence of RBD (particularly if it is formally excluded by video-PSG) should seriously question the diagnosis of this disease. RBD is currently considered a red flag for the diagnosis of MSA [12].

Self-awareness of abnormal sleep behaviors and unpleasant dream recall is variable among MSA subjects with RBD. In one study, 27 of 39 (69 %) consecutive MSA patients with RBD or their relatives reported dream-enacting behaviors.

Interestingly, most of the 12 patients that did not report dream-enacting behaviors were sleeping alone at their home [13]. In another study, only 7 of 21 (33 %) MSA patients with RBD recalled vivid dreams [27]. In our first published case series comprising 26 consecutive MSA cases with RBD free of psychoactive drugs, 77 % of the patients were unaware of their abnormal behaviors, which were only noticed by bed partners. Recall of unpleasant dreams was absent in 35 % of the patients [26]. Bed partners report that RBD-related movements are faster, stronger, and smother than during wakefulness [28].

The strong male predominance seen in idiopathic RBD, and in those RBD forms associated with PD and DLB is much less evident in MSA, where 33–61 % of the patients are men [13, 26–28]. This may be explained by the simple fact that most, if not all, patients with MSA have RBD. The male/female ratio of RBD in MSA reflects the roughly 1:1 male/female ratio of the disease. RBD in MSA is unrelated to age, disease severity, disease duration, clinical subtype (parkinsonian or cerebellar), or to any other demographic or clinical feature [26].

RBD may be the first symptom of MSA. In one study of 27 RBD patients aware of their dream-enacting behaviors, RBD preceded the waking motor symptoms in 12 (44 %) [26]. In another study with 19 patients, RBD features were reported by the patients or their relatives as the first manifestation of the disease in 3, concomitant with other symptoms in 9, and developed after the onset of waking symptoms in the remaining 7 [15]. In our series, RBD onset antedated parkinsonian, cerebellar and dysautonomic onset in 35 of 67 (52 %) patients by a mean of 7 years (range, 1–38 years). MSA is eventually diagnosed in only a few subjects with the initial diagnosis of idiopathic RBD (most of them are diagnosed with PD and DLB), probably because in the general population MSA is much more rare than PD and DLB [11]. We reported a patient presenting with dysautonomia, stridor during sleep and RBD without parkinsonism or cerebellar syndrome in whom brain pathology disclosed MSA after sudden death during wakefulness [29].

16.2.6 Sleep Disordered Breathing and Stridor

Breathing problems in MSA may be of central and peripheral (obstructive) origin. During wakefulness intermittent involuntary gasping, abnormal hypoxic ventilatory responses, cluster breathing, irregular breathing, abnormal hypoxic and hypercapnic respiratory responses, periodic breathing in the erect posture, respiratory failure and laryngeal stridor have been described. These disturbances during wakefulness have mainly a central origin due to neurodegeneration of the respiratory center in the lower brainstem. Breathing problems during sleep include central apneas, obstructive apneas/hypopneas, Cheyne-Stokes breathing pattern, apneustic breathing, snoring and stridor, either alone or combined with other sleep breathing abnormalities. These abnormalities occurring during sleep may be of either central or peripheral (upper airway, particularly in the larynx involving the vocal cords) origin.

One of the most relevant sleep related symptoms of MSA is nocturnal stridor. In clinical series, stridor is considered a relatively common finding in MSA occurring in about 19 % of the patients [16]. Its frequency increases when patients are formally studied with video-PSG where stridor of variable intensity is found in 30–42 % [14–18]. Stridor is considered one of the red flags that should raise suspicion of MSA in a patient with parkinsonism [12]. Stridor may occur in all stages of the disease, it may rarely be the first symptom of the disease [30], and is not related to MSA clinical subtype. The presence of stridor indicates obstruction of the airway at the level of the larynx. As the disease advances, nocturnal stridor progresses into wakefulness due to an increasing reduction in the glottic aperture. Stridor (as a sign of obstruction in the larynx) and snoring (as a sign of obstruction in the oropharynx) may coexist in the same MSA patient.

MSA patients, particularly those with stridor, may have typical obstructive sleep apnea episodes with oxyhemoglobin desaturations [15, 17, 18]. Stridor during wakefulness indicates severe obstruction of the glottic aperture and this may lead in some cases to subacute episodes of respiratory failure and death [30]. In the majority of patients with nocturnal stridor the clinical exam of the vocal cords during wakefulness with laryngoscopy is very useful showing unilateral or bilateral partial or complete vocal cord abduction restriction, paradoxical vocal cord movements, flickering of the vocal cords, and floppy epiglottis [18, 31]. In almost all MSA patients with stridor during wakefulness, laryngoscopy shows severe laryngeal narrowing.

The presence of stridor in MSA has been linked to decreased survival and sudden death during sleep. MSA patients with stridor treated with tracheostomy and nasal continuous positive airway pressure (CPAP) show similar survival trends than patients without stridor. Sudden death, however, may occur in patients already treated with tracheostomy and CPAP. It has been reported that tracheostomy may increase fatal central sleep apneas [32], emphasizing the idea that respiratory impairment in MSA is complex and occurs at multiple levels. However, the clinical relevance of these central apneas, which are usually not related to severe oxyhemoglobin desaturations, is not clear. Nevertheless it can be speculated that the association of impaired central hypoxic ventilatory response with upper airway obstruction during sleep and with physiological decreased ventilatory response during sleep, particularly during REM sleep, may render MSA patients at risk of sudden death during sleep.

The cause of stridor in MSA is not completely understood. There are currently two opposed views suggesting completely different mechanisms with different treatment implications. One view suggests that stridor occurs as a result of a dystonic contraction of the thyroarytenoid (TA) muscles, in essence, the muscles that adduct the vocal cords [33]. An alternative view suggests that stridor is due to paralysis of the posterior cricoarytenoid (PCA) muscles, the only muscles that abduct the vocal cords, probably as a result of degeneration of the nucleus ambiguus neurons and/or the nerve fibers innervating them [31]. There are findings supporting both views and it cannot be excluded that stridor may be produced by different mechanisms in different patients. An alternative explanation that fits better the available data comes from a study by Isono et al. [34] who performed a very detailed study of MSA patients with stridor during sleep under general anesthesia. They suggested that stridor during sleep is the result of a reflex contraction of the abductors (PCA) combined with a reflex contraction of the adductors (TA). This reflex co-contraction is a normal response of all the muscles of the larynx to an increase in airway resistance in order to protect the patency of the upper airway. In patients with MSA, however, the selective weakness of the abductors makes that the net result of this reflex contraction is the narrowing of the glottic aperture, due to the predominance of the adductors, resulting in stridor. There are many causes of increased upper airway resistance in MSA, particularly the weakness of the vocal cord abductors as well as the presence of decreased oropharyngeal space. This may explain why relatively low pressures of CPAP are able, by decreasing upper airway resistance, to diminish this adductor reflex response of the TA and subsequently to eliminate stridor.

Nocturnal stridor should alert the clinician about the possibility of respiratory complications during sleep including sudden death. It is reasonable to confirm its presence by video-PSG recording, although a simple audio home recording may be useful. In cases where stridor occurs only during sleep, treatment with CPAP should be first offered, given that in most cases stridor and obstructive sleep apneic events can be completely eliminated, the reasonable tolerance, improved nocturnal sleep of the patient and their family as well as the reported increase in survival [18]. Laryngoscopy during spontaneous sleep (sleep not induced by drugs) in a MSA subject with stridor documented inspiratory adduction of the vocal cords with downward displacement of the larynx. Application of CPAP resulted in improvement of stridor, distension of the hypopharynx, separation of the vocal cords and reduction of the downward displacement of the larynx [35]. During CPAP titration central sleep apneic event may appear, but its clinical relevance is not known. When CPAP does not fully eliminate stridor, cannot be tolerated and especially as soon as stridor appears during wakefulness, thracheostomy needs to be considered. Botulinum toxin has been reported to relieve stridor in three patients with diurnal stridor [33] but there is not enough information available to recommend it in patients with stridor. Unilateral cordectomy and laser arytenoidectony have also been proposed, but again there are not enough studies to determine when and how it should be used. It is important to realize that the vocal cord weakness induced by botulinum toxin or the persistent glottic aperture produced by surgery may render MSA patients more prone to bronchial aspiration, a frequent cause of death in MSA.

16.3 Progressive Supranuclear Palsy (PSP)

PSP is a neurodegenerative disease clinically characterized by dementia, parkinsonism, falls, and vertical gaze palsy. PSP is a tauopathy involving the brainstem, basal ganglia, frontal lobe and several other brain areas [36]. PSG studies show decreased

REM sleep percentage and features also seen in other neurodegenerative diseases such as decreased total sleep time and reduction in sleep spindles and K complexes. These abnormalities are mainly due to neurodegeneration of the sleep structures that regulate and modulate the sleep-wake cycle. Sleep complains include insomnia and sometimes symptoms suggestive of RBD. In some patients, RBD-like symptoms may reflect true nocturnal wandering and confusional awakenings which are frequent in patients with any type of dementia. Sleep disorder breathing, EDS, PLMS, and RLS are not major concerns in PSP.

RBD in PSP occurs but is less frequent than in the synucleinopathies PD, DLB, and MSA. In PSP, the subclinical form of RBD (asymptomatic REM sleep without atonia) is more frequent than full-blown RBD with dream-enacting behaviors and nightmares. There are no reported cases from sleep centers of patients with idiopathic RBD who were later diagnosed with PSP. The first reported case of RBD linked to PSP was a 70-year-old woman presenting with inhibition of speech during wakefulness and intelligible somniloquy at night due to RBD. In this patient, parkinsonism developed 1 year before the onset of RBD [37]. In a series of 15 PSP patients who underwent PSG, 2 had clinical RBD and 4 exhibited asymptomatic REM sleep without atonia. Clinical manifestations of RBD were severe in one patient, but none of the patients were aware of their abnormal sleep behaviors [38]. Nomura et al. [39] evaluated PSG in 20 PSP patients and 93 subjects with PD. When compared with PD, PSP group had lower sleep efficiency, lower total sleep time and a small number of subjects showing subclinical REM sleep without atonia (20 % in PSP versus 60 % in PD). None of the PSP patients experienced RBD symptoms in contrast to 32 % with PD. In another study, Sixel-Döring et al. [40] evaluated sleep in 20 PSP and 20 PD subjects. On PSG, PSP patients had significantly lower sleep efficiency (43 %) compared to PD patients (62 %). Seventeen PSP patients and 19 PD patients had asymptomatic REM sleep without atonia. Seven PSP patients and 13 PD patients had clinical RBD. The finding that RBD may be found in a tauopathy such as PSP argues against RBD as an exclusive feature of the synucleinopathies (PD, DLB, and MSA), and implies that RBD may be explained by dysfunction of the brainstem structures that regulate REM sleep.

Conclusion

Sleep disorders are common in the atypical parkinsonisms DLB, MSA, and PSP. They mainly include insomnia, hypersomnia, sleep disordered breathing of either central or peripheral origin, and RBD. In DLB and MSA, RBD may be the initial symptom of the disease and it is considered a red flag. Stridor during sleep in MSA is linked to sudden death and may be eliminated with CPAP and tracheostomy. Origins of sleep disorders in the atypical parkinsonism are multifactorial and associated with degeneration of the brain structures that regulate sleep and coexistent clinical features such as immobility, dementia, nocturia, depression, and anxiety.

References

1. McKeith IG, Dickson DW, Lowe J, et al. Diagnosis and management of dementia with Lewy bodies. Third report of the DLB consortium. Neurology. 2005;65:1863–72.
2. Bliwise DL, Mercaldo ND, Avidan AY, Boeve BF, Greer SA, Kukull WA. Sleep disturbance in dementia with Lewy bodies and Alzheimer's disease: a multicenter analysis. Dement Geriatr Cogn Disord. 2011;31:239–46.
3. Pao WC, Boeve BF, Ferman TJ, et al. Polysomnographc findings in dementia with Lewy bodies. Neurologist. 2013;19:1–6.
4. Terzaghi M, Arnaldi D, Rizzetti MC, et al. Analysis of video-polysomnographic sleep findings in dementia with Lewy bodies. Mov Disord. 2013;28:1416–23.
5. Ratti PL, Terzaghi M, Minafra A, et al. REM and NREM sleep enactment behaviors in Parkinson's disease, Parkinson's disease dementia and dementia with Lewy bodies. Sleep Med. 2012;13:926–32.
6. Boeve BF, Silber MH, Ferman TJ, et al. REM sleep behavior disorder and degenerative dementia. An association likely reflecting Lewy body disease. Neurology. 1998;51:363–70.
7. McKeith IG, Galasko D, Kosaka K, et al. Consensus guidelines for the clinical and pathological diagnosis of dementia with Lewy bodies (DLB): Report of the consortium on DLB international workshop. Neurology. 1996;47:113–1124.
8. Boeve BF, Silber MH, Parisi JE. Synucleinopathy pathology and REM sleep behavior disorder plus dementia or parkinsonism. Neurology. 2003;61:40–5.
9. Ferman TJ, Boeve BF, Smith GE, et al. Inclusion of RBD improves the diagnostic classification of dementia with Lewy bodies. Neurology. 2011;77:875–82.
10. Dugger BN, Boeve BF, Murray ME, et al. Rapid eye movement sleep behavior disorder and subtypes in autopsy-confirmed dementia with Lewy bodies. Mov Disord. 2012;27:72–8.
11. Iranzo A, Tolosa E, Gelpi E, et al. Neurodegenerative disease status and post-mortem pathology in idiopathic rapid-eye-movement sleep behaviour disorder. Lancet Neurol. 2013;12:443–53.
12. Wenning GK, Colosimo C, Geser F, et al. Multiple system atrophy. Lancet Neurol. 2004;3:93–103.
13. Plazzi G, Corsini R, Provini F, et al. REM sleep behavior disorders in multiple system atrophy. Neurology. 1997;48:1094–7.
14. Iranzo A, Santamaria J, Tolosa E, et al. Continuous positive air pressure eliminates nocturnal stridor in multiple system atrophy. Lancet. 2000;356:1329–30.
15. Vetrugno R, Provini F, Cortelli P, et al. Sleep disorders in multiple system atrophy: a correlative video-polysomnographic study. Sleep Med. 2004;5:21–30.
16. Ghorayeb I, Yekhlef F, Chrysostome Y, et al. Sleep disorders and their determinants in multiple system atrophy. J Neurol Neurosurg Psychiatry. 2002;72:798–800.
17. Manni R, Morini R, Martignoni E, et al. A nocturnal sleep in multisystem atrophy with autonomic failure: polygraphic findings in ten patients. J Neurol. 1993;240:247–50.
18. Iranzo A, Santamaria J, Tolosa E, et al. Long-term effect of CPAP in the treatment of nocturnal stridor in multiple system atrophy. Neurology. 2004;63:930–2.
19. Guo XY, Cao F, Lei F, et al. Clinical and polysomnographic features of patients with multiple system atrophy in Southwest China. Sleep Breath. 2013;17(4):1301–7.
20. Muntenan ML, Sixel-Döring F, Trenkwalder C. No difference in sleep and RBD between different types of patients with multiple system atrophy: a pilot video-polysomnographic study. Sleep Disorders. 2013;2013:258390.
21. Moreno-López C, Santamaria J, Salamero M, et al. Excessive daytime sleepiness in multiple system atrophy (SLEEMSA study). Arch Neurol. 2011;68:223–30.
22. Shimohata T, Nakayama H, Tomita M, Ozawa T, Nishizawa M. daytime sleepiness in Japanese patients with multiple system atrophy. BMC Neurol. 2012;12:1–6.
23. Martinez-Rodriguez JE, Seppi K, Cardozo A, et al. Cerebrospinal fluid hypocretin-1 levels in multiple system atrophy. Mov Disord. 2007;22:1822–4.

24. Benarroch EE, Schmeichel AM, Sandroni P, et al. Involvement of hypocretin neurons in multiple system atrophy. Acta Neuropahtol. 2007;113(1):75–80.
25. Wetter TC, Collado-Seidel V, Pöllmacher T, et al. Sleep and periodic leg movement patterns in drug-free patients with Parkinson's disease and multiple system atrophy. Sleep. 2000;23:1–7.
26. Iranzo A, Rye DB, Santamaria J, et al. Characteristics of idiopathic REM sleep behavior disorder and that associated with MSA and PD. Neurology. 2005;65:247–52.
27. Tachibana N, Kimura K, Kitajama K, Shinde A, Kimura J, Shibasaki H. REM sleep motor dysfunction in multiple system atrophy: with special emphasis on sleep talk as its early clinical manifestation. J Neurol Neurosurg Psychiatry. 1997;63:678–81.
28. De Cock V, Debs R, Oudiette D, et al. The improvement of movement of speech during rapid eye movement sleep behavior disorder in multiple system atrophy. Brain. 2011;134:856–62.
29. Gaig C, Iranzo A, Tolosa E, Vilaseca I, Rey MJ, Santamaria J. Pathological description of a non-motor variant of multiple system atrophy. J Neurol Neurosurg Psychiatry. 2008;79:1399–400.
30. Glass GA, Josephs KA, Ahlskog JE. Respiratory insufficiency as the primary presenting symptom of multiple system atrophy. Arch Neurol. 2006;63:978–81.
31. Isozaki E, Naito A, Horiguchi S, et al. Early diagnosis and stage classification of vocal cord abductor paralysis in patients with multiple system atrophy. J Neurol Neurosurg Psychiatry. 1996;60:399–402.
32. Jin K, Okabe S, Chida K, et al. Tracheostomy can fatally exacerbate sleep-disordered breathing in multiple system atrophy. Neurology. 2007;68:1618–21.
33. Merlo IM, Ochinni A, Pacchetti C, et al. Not paralysis, but dystonia causes stridor in multiple system atrophy. Neurology. 2002;58:649–52.
34. Isono S, Shiba K, Yamaguchi M, et al. Pathogenesis of laryngeal narrowing in patients with multiple system atrophy. J Appl Physiol. 2001;536:237–49.
35. Kuzniar TJ, Morgenthaler TI, Prakash UBS, et al. Effect of continuous positive airway pressure on stridor in multiple system atrophy-sleep laryngoscopy. J Clin Sleep Med. 2009;5:65–7.
36. Williams DR, Lees AJ. Progressive supranuclear palsy: clinicopathological concepts and diagnostic challenges. Lancet Neurol. 2009;8:270–9.
37. Pareja JA, Caminero AB, Masa JF, Dobato JL, Schenck C. A first case of progressive supranuclear palsy and pre-clinical REM sleep behavior disorder presenting as inhibition of speech during wakefulness and somniloquy with phasic muscle twitching during REM sleep. Neurologia. 1996;11:304–6.
38. Arnulf I, Merino-Andreu M, Bloch F, et al. REM sleep behavior disorder and REM sleep without atonia in progressive supranuclear palsy. Sleep. 2005;28:349–54.
39. Nomura T, Inoue Y, Takigawa H, Nakashima K. Comparison of REM sleep behaviour disorder variables between patients with progressive supranuclear palsy and those with Parkinson's disease. Parkinsonism Relat Disord. 2012;18:394–6.
40. Sixel-Döring F, Schweitzer M, Mollenhauer B, Trenkwalder C. Polysomnographic findings, video-based sleep analysis and perception in progressive supranuclear palsy. Sleep Med. 2009;10:407–15.

Future Directions

Aleksandar Videnovic and Birgit Högl

Clinical observations and research performed on sleep and alertness issues in PD have attracted the attention of the medical and scientific PD community. This provides a unique opportunity to further examine interactions between sleep and circadian regulation and PD outcomes. Numerous avenues for future investigations need to be considered. Given the complexities of sleep and circadian research, these efforts will require a collaborative and multidisciplinary approach of clinicians and investigators involved in various aspects of PD.

Better understanding of the natural history of sleep and circadian disorders in the PD population will require multicenter longitudinal studies. Optimization of the existing methods and tools, as well as the development of new instruments for the ascertainment of PD-specific sleep and alertness problems and issues related to the circadian dysregulation, will be critical for further advancements. Further, an educational outreach is needed to implement best practices and appropriate use of methodologies currently available to assess various aspects of sleep-wake cycle in the PD population.

New screening instruments will need to be developed in order to facilitate timely and cost-effective diagnosis of sleep disorders in PD as well as to enable early detection and sharpen the profile of sleep-specific pre-motor forms of PD. The latter is of utmost importance in the field, as it will provide means to identify individuals at risk for development of synuclein-related neurodegeneration, as well as allow for timely testing of therapies that may modify the progression of the disease.

Systematic study of sleep in genetically homogeneous PD cohorts will help overcome obstacles related to sleep research within quite heterogeneous phenotypic expression profiles of PD. This will further facilitate our understanding how

A. Videnovic, MD, MSc (✉)
Department of Neurology, Massachusetts General Hospital
Harvard Medical School, Boston, MA, USA
e-mail: avidenovic@mgh.harvard.edu

B. Högl, MD
Department of Neurology, Medical University of Innsbruck,
Innsbruck, Austria
e-mail: birgit.ho@i-med.ac.at

© Springer-Verlag Wien 2015
A. Videnovic, B. Högl (eds.), *Disorders of Sleep and Circadian Rhythms in Parkinson's Disease*, DOI 10.1007/978-3-7091-1631-9

sleep-wake regulation in this disease affects its motor, cognitive, neuropsychiatric and autonomic features.

Circadian dysregulation has started to emerge as an important component of sleep-wake disruption in neurodegenerative disorders. Further exploration of bidirectional relationship between circadian disruption and sleep problems on one side, and between neurodegenerative disease process and circadian function on the other side, will position circadian system as a potential novel diagnostic and therapeutic target in PD.

Despite the wide range of sleep disturbance in PD and its major clinical impact, almost no systematic treatment studies have been performed. This is a strong impetus to focus efforts on design and execution of clinical treatment studies that will lead to optimized and new treatments for the various aspects of sleep, wakefulness and circadian disturbances in PD.

Index

© Springer-Verlag Wien 2015
A. Videnovic, B. Högl (eds.), *Disorders of Sleep and Circadian Rhythms
in Parkinson's Disease*, DOI 10.1007/978-3-7091-1631-9

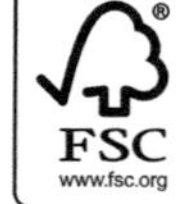

MIX
Papier aus verantwortungsvollen Quellen
Paper from responsible sources
FSC® C105338

If you have any concerns about our products,
you can contact us on
ProductSafety@springernature.com

In case Publisher is established outside the EU,
the EU authorized representative is:
Springer Nature Customer Service Center GmbH
Europaplatz 3, 69115 Heidelberg, Germany

Printed by Libri Plureos GmbH
in Hamburg, Germany